LIBRARY

An Atlas of Investigation and Management

HELICOBACTER PYLORI

An Atlas of Investigation and Management

HELICOBACTER PYLORI

By
John Holton, BSc, MB ChB, PhD, MRCPath
Reader Clinical Microbiology
Centre for Infectious Diseases and International Health
Windeyer Institute of Medical Sciences
Royal Free and University College London Medical School
London, UK

Natale Figura, MD
Associate Professor in Gastroenterology
Department of Internal Medicine, Endocrine-Metabolic Sciences and Biochemistry
University of Siena and Policlinico S. Maria alle Scotte
Siena, Italy

Berardino Vaira, MD
Associate Professor, Department of Internal Medicine and Gastroenterology
University of Bologna
Bologna, Italy

CLINICAL PUBLISHING
OXFORD

Clinical Publishing
an imprint of Atlas Medical Publishing Ltd
Oxford Centre for Innovation
Mill Street, Oxford OX2 0JX, UK

Tel: +44 1865 811116
Fax: +44 1865 251550
E mail: info@clinicalpublishing.co.uk
Web: www.clinicalpublishing.co.uk

Distributed in USA and Canada by:
Clinical Publishing
30 Amberwood Parkway
Ashland OH 44805, USA

Tel: 800-247-6553 (toll free within US and Canada)
Fax: 419-281-6883
Email: order@bookmasters.com

Distributed in UK and Rest of World by:
Marston Book Services Ltd
PO Box 269
Abingdon
Oxon OX14 4YN, UK

Tel: +44 1235 465500
Fax: +44 1235 465555
Email: trade.orders@marston.co.uk

A catalogue record for this book is available from the British Library

ISBN-13   978 1 904392 89 7
ISBN e-book   978 1 84692 630 3

Project manager: Gavin Smith, GPS Publishing Solutions, Herts, UK
Typeset by Phoenix Photosetting, Chatham, Kent, UK
Printed and bound in the United Kingdom by Latimer Trend & Company Ltd, Plymouth.

Contents

Abbreviations

ABC	ATP-binding cassette
ACh	acetylcholine
ADH	alcohol dehydrogenase
AG	atrophic gastritis
Alp	adherence-associated lipoprotein
AMP	adenosine monophosphate
AP-PCR	Arbitrarily primed PCR
AS	aphthous stomatitis
ATP	adenosine triphosphate
BabA2	Lewis blood group antigen-binding protein
BHIA	brain heart infusion agar
BLAST	Basic Local Alignment Search Tool
BMI	body mass index
bp	base pairs
BRENDA	bacteria restriction endonuclease analysis
CAD	coronary artery disease
CagA	cytotoxin-associated gene A protein
cAMP	cyclic-AMP
CARD	caspase recruitment domains
CD	Crohn's disease
cDNA	complementary DNA
Che	chemotaxis protein
CLO	*Campylobacter*-like organism
CM	cytoplasmic membrane
CoA	coenzyme A
COPD	chronic obstructive pulmonary disease
COX	cyclo-oxygenase
ECG	electrocardiogram
EGF	epidermal growth factor
EGFR	EGF receptor
EHSG	European *Helicobacter* Study Group
Erk	extracellular signal regulated kinase
EYA	egg yolk agar
FADH	flavin adenine dinucleotide (reduced)
FD	functional dyspepsia
Fec	ferric citrate transporter
FlaA/-B	flagellin protein subunit A or B
Flg	flagellar basal body rod protein
Fli	flagellar motor switch protein
Frp	NAD(P)H-flavin oxidoreductase
GH	growth hormone
GlcNAc	*N*-acetyl glucosamine
GORD	gastro-oesophageal reflux disease
GroEL	a chaperonin
HLA	human leukocyte antigen
HopZ	*Helicobacter* outer membrane adhesin protein
Hpa	flagellar sheath adhesin
HSP	heat shock protein
IBD	inflammatory bowel disease
ICAM	intracellular adhesion molecule
IceA	restriction endonuclease (induced by contact with epithelium)
Ig	immunoglobulin
IL	interleukin
iNOS	inducible nitric oxide synthase
InvA	invasion protein
ITP	idiopathic thrombocytopenic purpura
ITT	intention to treat
Le	Lewis antigen
LPS	lipopolysaccharide
MALDI-TOF	matrix-assisted laser desorption/ionization time-of-flight
MALT	mucosal-associated lymphoid tissue
Mbp	megabase pairs
MCA	MacConkey agar
MCP	macrophage chemoattractant protein
MLEE	multilocus enzyme electrophoresis
MLST	multilocus sequence typing
MLVA	multiple loci VNTR analysis
Mot	flagellar motor protein
MTM	modified Thayer–Martin agar
MurNAc	*N*-acetyl muramic acid
NAD	nicotinamide adenine dinucleotide
NADH	nicotinamide adenine dinucleotide (reduced)
NADPH	nicotinamide adenine dinucleotide phosphate (reduced)
NFAT	nuclear factor of activated T cell
NixA	nickel-transport protein

NOD1/-2	nucleotide-binding oligomerization domain-containing protein 1 or -2	RuvABC	Holliday junction resolvase
		SabA	sialic acid-binding adhesin protein
NSAID	non-steroidal anti-inflammatory drug	SCC	squamous cell carcinoma
NSF	N-ethylmaleimide-sensitive factor	Sec	preprotein translocase subunit
OipA	outer inflammatory protein A	SHP-2	Src homology-2 domain
PAF	platelet-activating factor	σ	sigma factor (RNA polymerase factor)
PAI	pathogenicity island	SNARE	soluble NSF attachment protein receptor
PAMP	pathogen associated molecular pattern		
Pbp	penicillin-binding protein	spp.	species (note: sp. singular)
PCR	polymerase chain reaction	Src	proto-oncogene tyrosine-protein kinase Src
PG	peptidoglycan		
PGE_2	prostaglandin E_2	SST	somatostatin
PLA	phospholipase A	TNF	tumour necrosis factor
PPIs	proton pump inhibitors	TonB	T-one (bacteriophage T1) ferric hydroxamate transporter B
PSGN	pepsinogen		
PUD	peptic ulcer disease	TSA	trypticase soy agar
RecG	ATP-dependent DNA helicase	TTI	'test and treat' intervention
RecN	DNA repair protein	UKCRC	UK Clinical Research Collaboration
RFLP	restriction fragment length polymorphism	Uvr	excision endonuclease subunit
		VCAM	vascular cell adhesion molecule
RT-PCR	reverse transcription PCR	VNTR	variable-number tandem repeat
RUT	rapid urease test		

Acknowledgement

The authors are grateful to the contribution made to this book by Dr Carla Vindigni, Pathology Unit, Department of Oncology, Policlinico Santa Maria alle Scotte, Siena, Italy

Chapter 1

Discovery, metabolism, genome and taxonomy

Discovery

In 2005, Warren and Marshall were awarded the Nobel Prize for Medicine and Physiology for a discovery made by Warren over 25 years ago. Warren, a histopathologist, noted an association between a helical-shaped organism in the stomach of humans and gastritis. Several investigators had seen similar organisms over the preceding decades in a variety of animals, including humans. However, they were considered to be commensals by most who noticed them and were therefore ignored. However, because of the very close association between presence of the organism and presence of inflammation in the stomach, Warren thought there might be a causal relationship. Warren and Marshall studied 100 patients and found the organism to be present in every patient who had a duodenal ulcer and suggested it might also be related to peptic ulceration as well as gastritis. Warren and Marshall's perseverance paid off and, in 1984, they informed the scientific community. Few people believed them: in order to satisfy Koch's Postulates, Marshall and, at a later date, Morris self-administered a culture of the isolated organism. They developed dyspeptic symptoms and on endoscopy had gastritis. They successfully eradicated the organism by taking bismuth and antibiotics. Slowly, evidence accumulated from a number of sources as to the causal relationship between *Helicobacter pylori* (as it is now called) and serious gastroduodenal and possibly extra-gastrointestinal disease.

Helicobacter pylori was initially called a *Campylobacter*-like organism (CLO), then for a short time *Campylobacter pyloridis* and *Campylobacter pylori*. A new genus, *Helicobacter*, was proposed in 1989 (with *Helicobacter pylori* as the type species) based on a number of differences between the newly isolated bacterium and the genus *Campylobacter* (*Table 1.1*). Major differences in the fatty acid profile also exist between *Campylobacter* and *Helicobacter*. The former is characterized by the presence of 3-hydroxyltetradecanoic acid (14:0), hexadecanoic acid (16:0), octadecanoic acid (18:1) and C19 cyc (cyclopropane); the latter by tetradecanoic acid (14:0), hydroxyhexadecanoic acid (3-OH 16:0), hydroxyoctadecanoic acid (3-OH 18:0) and C19 cyc (cyclopropane). The lipopolysaccharide (LPS) is relatively under-phosphorylated compared with other Gram-negative bacteria and comprises steric, β-hydroxysteric and β-hydroxy palmitic acids. It is much less effective as an endotoxin. The genomes of *Helicobacter* and *Campylobacter* are approximately the same size but the former has a cytotoxin-associated gene A (*cagA*) pathogenicity island (PAI) and codes for a vacuolating cytotoxin. *Helicobacter* has a type IV secretion apparatus while *Campylobacter* uses an ancestral type III secretion apparatus—the flagellum. Both genera are oxidase positive but *Helicobacter pylori* is urease positive while *Campylobacter* spp. are urease negative. Some species of both genera are thermo-tolerant and can grow at 42°C.

Helicobacter structure

Helicobacter pylori (**1.1**) has the typical structure of a Gram-negative bacterium consisting of a cytoplasmic membrane (CM; see **1.2**), a layer of peptidoglycan (PG; see **1.3**) and an outer hydrophobic LPS layer (**1.4**). A

Table 1.1 Main microbiological characteristics of *Helicobacter pylori* compared with *Campylobacter jejuni*

Characteristic	*H. pylori* J99	*C. jejuni* RM1221
Genome size (bp)	1.64 Mbp	1.77 Mbp
GC ratio (%)	38.87	30.30
Open reading frame	1637	1654
Type III or IV secretion	Present IV	Absent system
cagA/vacA homologues	Present	Absent
Flagella	Multiple polar	Single polar
Oxidase	Positive	Positive
Rapid urease	Positive	Negative

typical Gram-negative cell wall consists of the inner layer of phospholipid known as the CM, containing proteins necessary for respiration and permeability and covered by a PG layer. On the external surface of the PG layer is a second hydrophobic phospholipid membrane, the LPS (or endotoxin). On electron microscopy, a Gram-negative cell wall has a tri-laminar appearance with a periplasmic space between the CM-PG and the PG-LPS. This space contains enzymes required for cell wall synthesis—transpeptidases (proteins that bind β-lactam antibiotics called penicillin-binding proteins), which are the target for inhibition by β-lactam antibiotics.

Peptidoglycan is a heteropolymer of *N*-acetyl glucosamine (GlcNAc) and *N*-acetyl muramic acid (MurNAc) in which adjacent glycan chains are cross-linked by peptides. The amino acid composition of these peptides varies between bacteria. The amino acids in *H. pylori* are *meso*-diaminopimelic acid, alanine and glutamic acid. The short peptide chain attached to the glycan units consist of alternating D- and L- amino

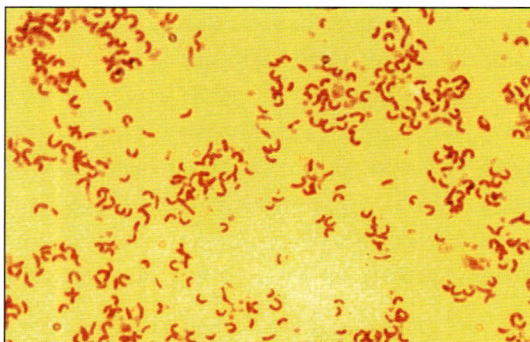

1.1 Gram stain of *H. pylori* showing predominant curved bacilli. *H. pylori* is a non-spore forming, motile Gram-negative bacterium with a helical shape measuring 2.5–4.5×0.5–1.0 μm. It has four to eight unipolar sheathed flagella. In addition to the helical shape, curved forms occur and the bacillus also converts to a coccoid morphology when under environmental stress. The role of this coccoid form in infection or persistence is uncertain.

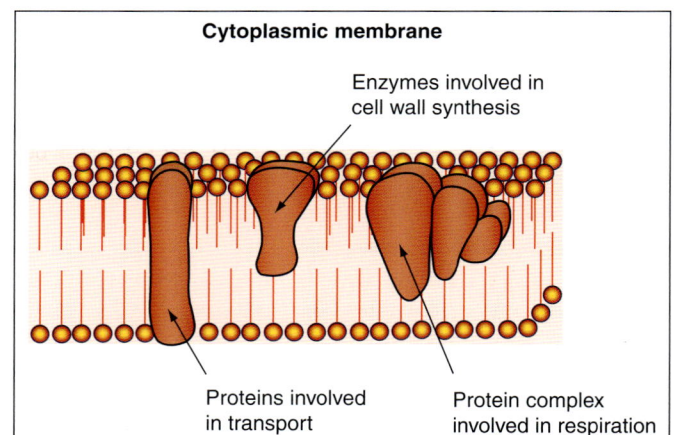

1.2 Diagram of a typical bacterial cytoplasmic membrane (CM). The CM of a bacterium contains all the proteins necessary for respiration, because prokaryotic cells do not have mitochondria. In addition, as the lipid bilayer is hydrophobic, protein channels are required to allow access of water-soluble molecules. Generally, the bacterial CM does not contain sterols.

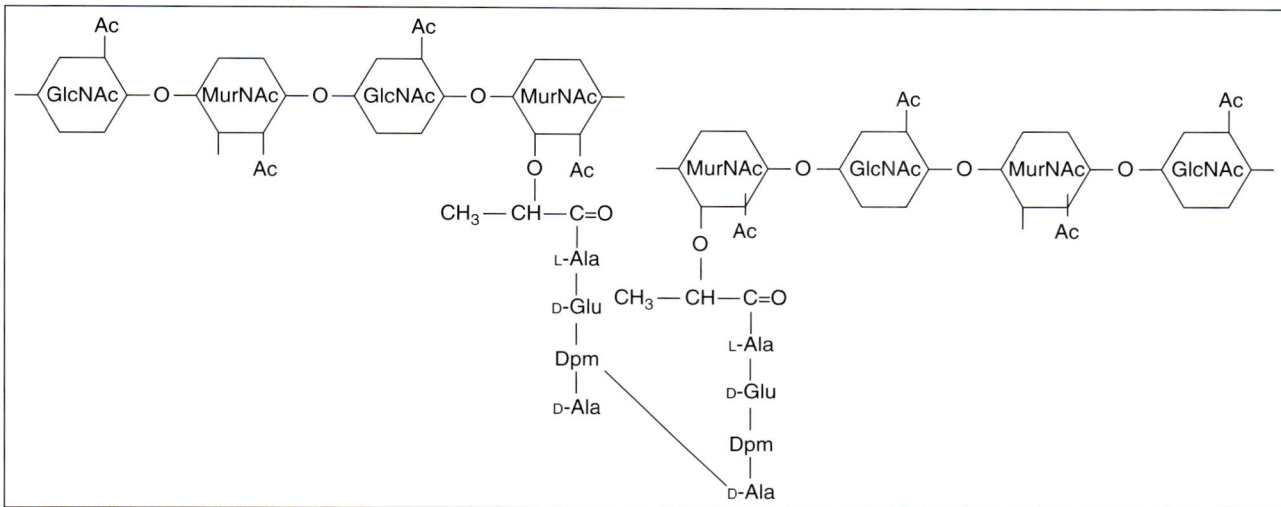

1.3 Diagram showing the structure of peptidoglycan. Ac = acetate; Ala = alanine; Dpm = *meso*-diaminopimelic acid (2,6-diaminoheptanedioic acid); Glu = glutamic acid; GlcNAc = *N*-acetyl glucosamine; MurNAc = *N*-acetyl muramic acid.

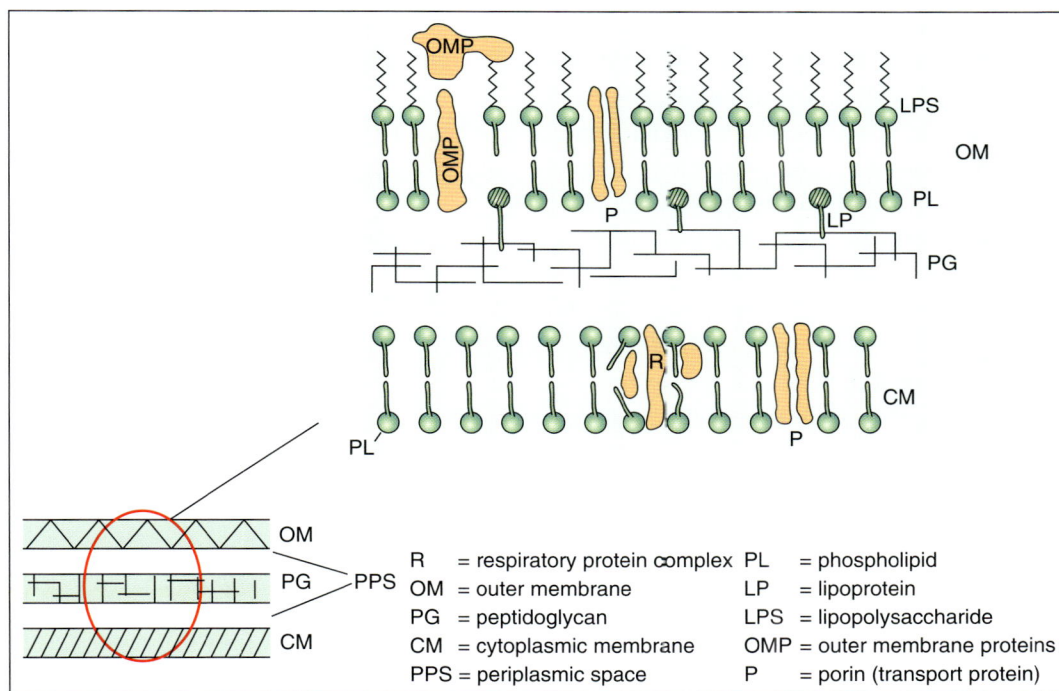

R	= respiratory protein complex	PL	= phospholipid
OM	= outer membrane	LP	= lipoprotein
PG	= peptidoglycan	LPS	= lipopolysaccharide
CM	= cytoplasmic membrane	OMP	= outer membrane proteins
PPS	= periplasmic space	P	= porin (transport protein)

1.4 Structure of a typical Gram-negative cell wall such as *Helicobacter pylori*.

acids, including variously alanine, glutamic acid, diaminopimelic acid, lysine or ornithine. The terminal two amino acids on this peptide are usually alanine. The cross-links can be direct, or with a short peptide chain. The various arrangements of how the cross-links are formed lead to a classification of cell wall peptidoglycans

and *Helicobacter pylori* falls into the A1 subgroup with direct cross-linking from the third position, where meso-diaminopimelic acid is located. The cross-linking of the PG layer provides shape and structure to the micro-organism. PG is a substance not encountered in eukaryotic cells and can be recognized by the host innate immune system as foreign, thus initiating the host response. These and similar microbial molecules are called pathogen-associated molecular patterns. PG is found in nearly all cell walls and is most abundant in Gram-positive cell walls. *Helicobacter pylori* is Gram-negative and thus has an outer hydrophobic membrane containing LPS.

LPS, also known as the 'O' antigen or endotoxin, is composed of three areas: the inner lipid A component; an intermediate, so-called core component; and an outer variable region. Lipid A is a relatively conserved structure between different bacteria but variation occurs in the type and chain length of the fatty acid attached to the carbohydrate moeity and the degree of phosphorylation and acylation. Lipid A is the most active component of the endotoxin but this activity is modified by the type of carbohydrate backbone and degree of substitution. In *Helicobacter pylori*, lipid A is sparsely phosphorylated compared with *Escherichia coli* and has much less endotoxin activity. The core is fairly stable in composition across all Gram-negative bacteria, consisting of a small number of sugars, including 3-deoxy-D-manno-octulosonic acid, galactose and heptose. In *Helicobacter pylori*, an unusual D-glycero-D-manno-heptose is found in the core region compared with the more usual L- and D-heptose.

The outer variable region consists of a larger number of different monosaccharides, with different substituents arranged in various ways, all giving rise to the high degree of antigenic variability in this region. The sugars include hexoses, deoxyhexoses, pentoses and uronic acids. In *Helicobacter pylori*, the variable region contains *N*-acetylglucosamine substituted with fucose residues and carrying Lewis x (Le^x) and Lewis y (Le^y) blood group epitopes. The LPS is phosphorylated to different degrees in different bacteria. LPS is an important pathogen-associated molecular pattern and in some bacteria activates many host functions such as coagulation, complement, cytokine production, etc. leading to endotoxic (septic) shock. In *Helicobacter pylori*, LPS is a poor endotoxin, which may also in part contribute to the chronicity of infection. In addition, strains of *Helicobacter pylori* express an immunodominant epitope and a weakly antigenic epitope in the LPS, which is distinct from the expression of Lewis antigens. Avoidance of binding by surfactant protein D, part of the innate immune system in the stomach, occurs

through phase variation of the LPS. The increased relative amounts of fucose compared with glucose/galactose on the LPS is brought about by slipped-strand mispairing of a fucosyltransferase in wild type bacteria leading to fewer fucose residues, more glucose/galactose residues and greater binding to surfactant protein D. The structure of the LPS is shown in **1.5** and contains Lewis antigens related to human blood group antigens.

Lewis antigens (**1.6**), resembling human blood group antigens, are expressed on the LPS of *Helicobacter pylori*. *In vitro*, they are expressed during logarithmic phase growth and shed into the media during stationary phase growth. Expression is subject to phase variation due to slipped-strand mispairing within a homopolymeric (PolyC) strand in the α-1,3-fucosyltransferase. These

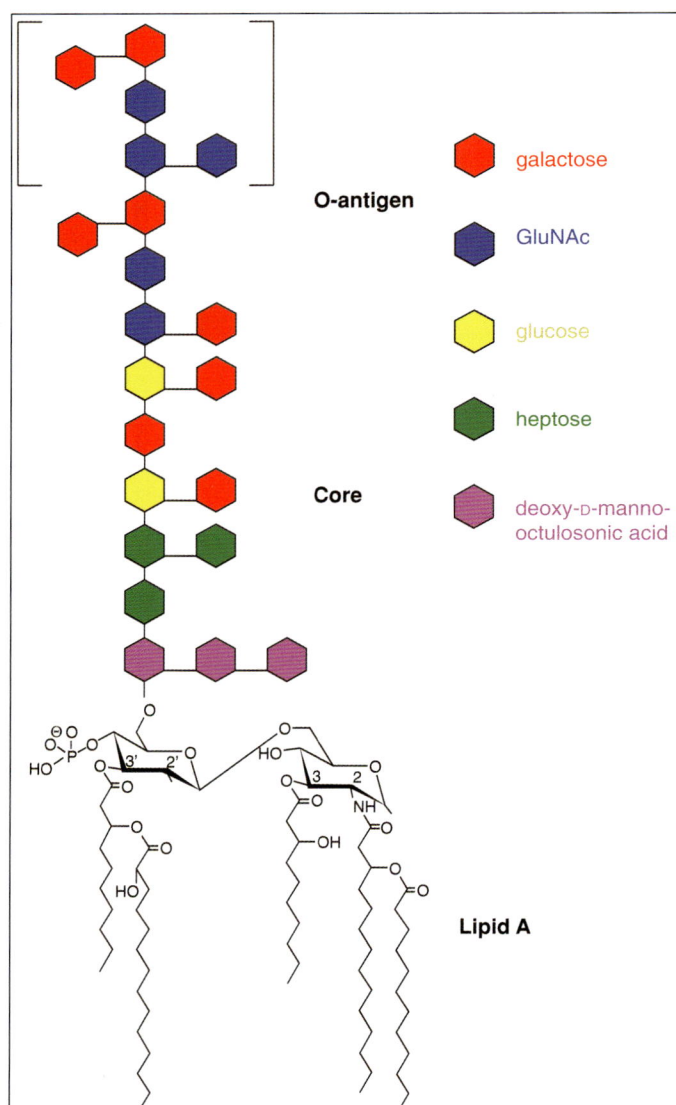

1.5 Typical structure of LPS.

structures mimic host cell structures and this may account in part for the chronicity of infection. Expression of Lewis antigens by *Helicobacter pylori* is not only phase variable and dependent upon growth dynamics but is also strain dependent with some strains expressing Lewis antigen a (Le^a) or Lewis antigen b (Le^b) and many strains expressing Le^x/Le^y. The principal adhesin for *Helicobacter pylori* is Le^b, which is found on the surface of gastric epithelial cells and the cognate ligand is BabA2 expressed on the surface of *Helicobacter pylori*. If the stomach is inflamed then sialyl-Le^x is expressed on gastric cells, to which *Helicobacter pylori* can also bind.

The organism is helical in shape, which is likely to be an adaptation, aiding its penetration through viscid mucus. Under metabolic stress, such as nutrient limitation or in the presence of antibiotics, *Helicobacter pylori* undergoes a morphological change to a coccoid form, passing through a U-shaped form, which appears to be enclosed in a membranous structure. During transition from the helical to the coccoid form, the cell wall undergoes significant changes in composition. There is a reduction in percentage of the classical peptidoglycan unit (*see* **1.3**) and an increase in GlcNAc-MurNAc-L-Ala-D-Glu (GM-dipeptide), with an increase in anhydro-PG dimers (GlcNAc-anhydroMurNAc-L-Ala-D-Glu-Dpm-D-Ala and GlcNAc-MurNAc-L-Ala-D-Glu-Dpm-D-Ala-D-Ala moieties). Mutants of a putative MurNAc-L-Ala-amidase, *amiA*, do not accumulate the GM-dipeptide, suggesting it may have some role in this morphological transformation. Additionally, there is a marked change in the lipid profile of the coccoid form compared with the bacillary form, with levels of cholesteryl-6-*O*-tetradecanoyl-α-D-glucopyranoside, cholesteryl-6-*O*-phosphatidyl-α-D-glucopyranoside and cardiolipin increasing,

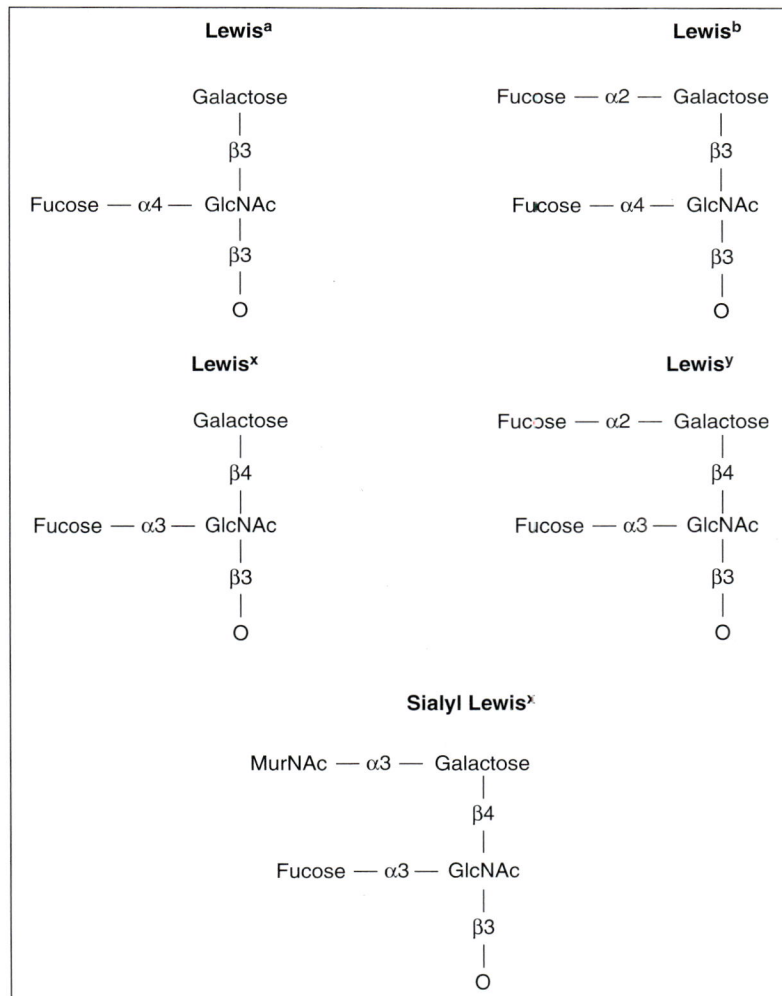

1.6 Structure of the Lewis antigens.

while cholesteryl-α-D-glucopyranoside, phosphatidyl ethanolamine and phosphatidyl glycerol levels decrease. During this transformation (**1.7**), there is also a decrease in the 94 kDa and 30 kDa antigen components present in the bacillary form, as shown by Western blot. There is a progressive reduction in the nucleic acid content, with evidence of DNA cleavage after prolonged incubation (as shown by DNA A and B), and a progressive reduction of DNA, RNA and cellular adenosine triphosphate (ATP) over a period of 7 days. The DNA and RNA decrease from 2.5 genome equivalents/cell (DNA) and $6 \mu g/5 \times 10^8$ cells (RNA) to 0.23 genome equivalents/cell and $1.8 \mu g/ 5 \times 10^8$ cells at day 7. There is also a decrease in the synthesis of new proteins as illustrated by labelling with ^{35}S-methionine. In parallel with these changes, the percentage of coccoid forms increases from 0% to 100% and the total viable count decreases to 0%. Under anaerobic conditions, polyphosphate can still be detected at day 7, as can the global sigma factor RpoD. The coccoid form retains metabolic activity as shown by its ability to reduce tetrazolium salts and is viable as shown by Live/Dead staining. This activity is greatly prolonged at 4°C compared with 37°C. This suggests limited but decreasing viability despite the coccoid form being non-culturable. However, when introduced

in vivo into mice, the coccoid form may revert to the helical form. These coccoid forms have been detected in naturally acquired infection in humans and occur in the majority of infections where they can be detected by staining with anti-*Helicobacter* antibodies. Coccoid forms appear to bind less well to gastric tissue and to induce less interleukin (IL)-8 compared with the bacillary form. Sensing of PG in gastric epithelial cells is dependent on NOD1 (*see* p.79) and the accumulation of GM-dipeptide, which is detected by NOD2, explains the lack of NFκB activation and subsequent IL-8 production. This lack of an inflammatory response may contribute to the chronicity of infection.

The role of this coccoid form in relation to spread of the organism is uncertain. Some bacteria possess flagella (**1.8**) necessary for motility, or pili (fimbriae) important in adhesion or conjugation. The flagella of *Helicobacter pylori* are composed of two flagellin subunits: a minor 57 kDa (FlaB) protein found below the hook assembly, and a major 56 kDa (FlaA) protein, which forms the flagella. Both proteins are post-translationally modified with *N*-acetyl pseudaminic acid. The flagellar assembly resembles a typical Gram-negative flagellum and requires about 20 structural proteins and 30 regulatory proteins. The tip of the flagellum in *Helicobacter pylori* is bulbous

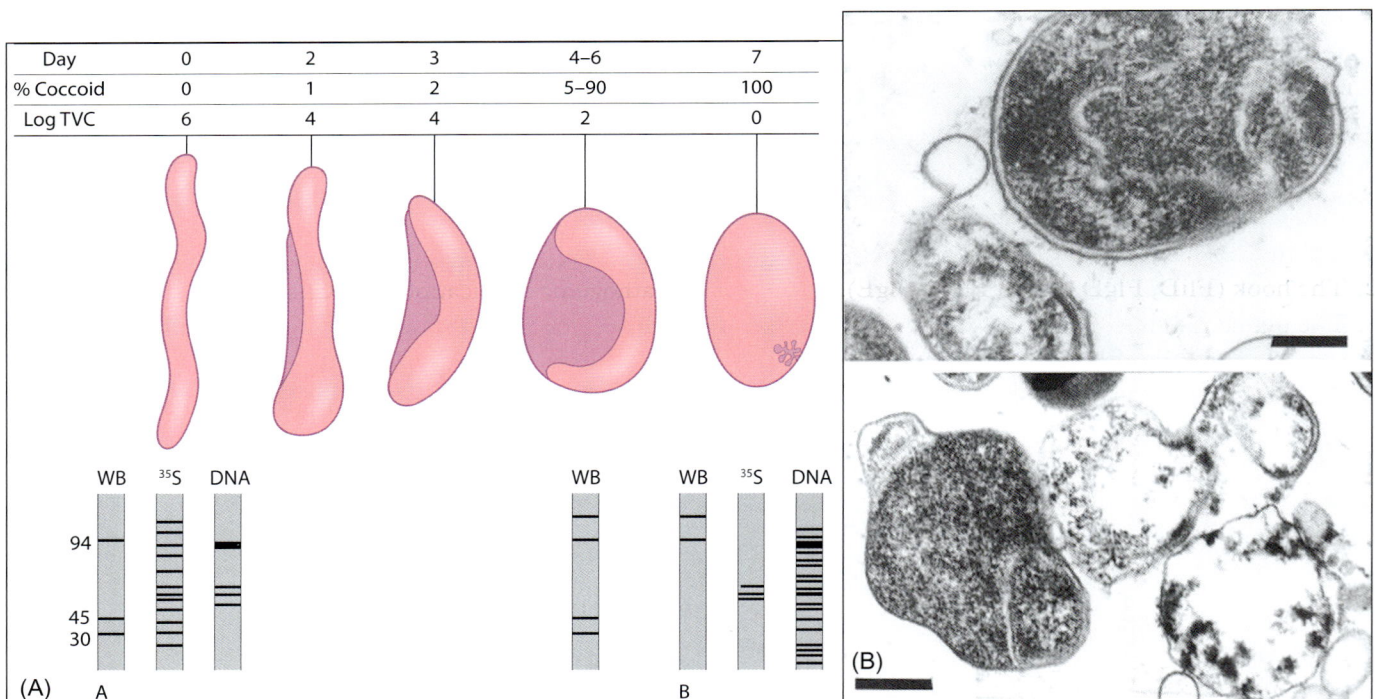

Day	0	2	3	4–6	7
% Coccoid	0	1	2	5–90	100
Log TVC	6	4	4	2	0

1.7 (A) Transformation of the helical to coccoid form of *Helicobacter pylori*. (B) Electron micrograph of the coccoid form of *Helicobacter pylori*. WB = Western blot.

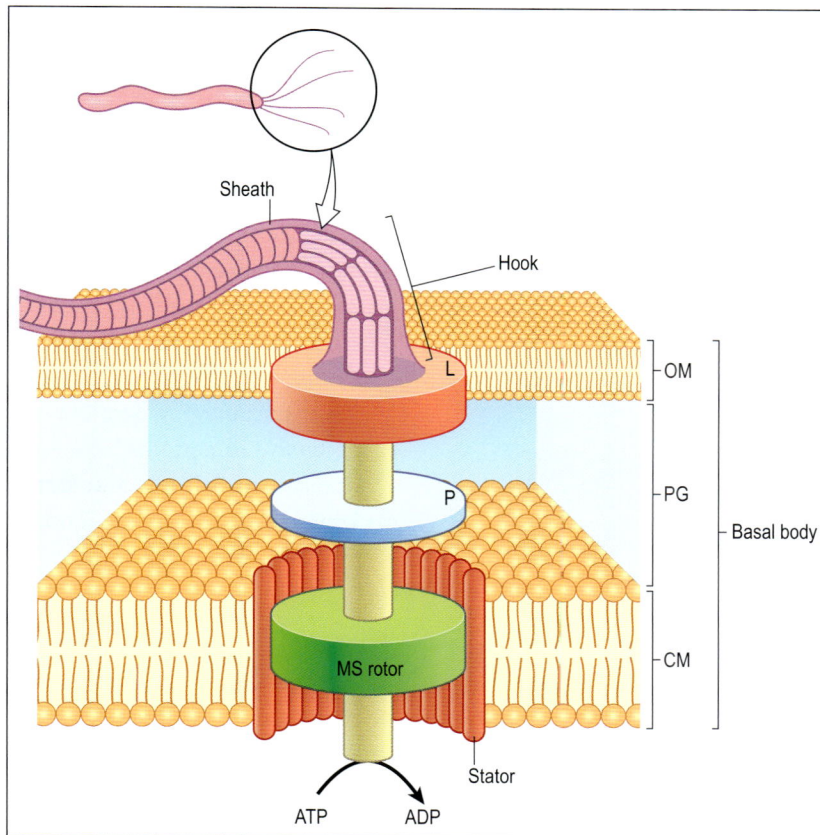

1.8 Structure of a bacterial flagellum.

and the sheath is an extension of the outer membrane. The three components of the flagellum assembly comprise:

1. The basal body consisting of motor rotary proteins (MotA, MotB), motor switch proteins (FliM, FliN, FliG), MS ring (FilF), P ring (FlgI), L ring (FlgH) and rod (FlgB, FlgC, FlgG).
2. The hook (FliD, FlgD, FlgK, FlgL, FlgE).
3. The filament (FlaA, FlaB) and sheath (HpaA).

The initial anchoring proteins of the basal body are secreted by the Sec secretory pathway, whereas the other structural components are secreted by a flagellar type III secretion system, which consists of about eight proteins (e.g. FliL, FliH, FliQ). The remaining proteins involved in flagellar assembly and function are the regulatory proteins for synthesis (FlgR, σ^{28}, σ^{54}, σ^{80}) and chemotaxis (CheA, CheY, CheW, CheZ).

Both fimbriae and flagella can also act as a binding site for bacteriophage. *Helicobacter pylori* has from two to six polar-sheathed flagella. There is a strong evolutionary link between flagella and secretion and adhesion systems in bacteria. *Helicobacter pylori* has a type IV secretion system. This is encoded on a PAI called the *cag*PAI and used to secrete the CagA protein along with cell wall peptidoglycan into the host cell. Like many Gram-negative bacteria, *Helicobacter pylori* releases outer membrane vesicles of cell wall components, which have pathogenic implications (*see* Chapter 4).

Bacteria secrete enzymes and toxins from the cytoplasm to the exterior environment and it is estimated that about 20% of all anabolites are transported to the outside environment. To achieve this, the product must be transported across the cytoplasm from its site of production to and across the (hydrophobic) cytoplasmic membrane into the periplasmic space, from the periplasmic space across the (hydrophilic) PG cell wall and, in Gram-negative bacteria (such as *Helicobacter pylori*), across the (hydrophobic) outer LPS membrane to the exterior. Several types of export mechanisms exist, which are described below, with **1.9** illustrating Types I–IV.

Type I

These systems are part of a large family of proteins called the ATP-binding cassette (ABC) transporters, which are also found in eukaryotic cells and the Archaea. The transport channel crosses the inner and outer membranes of Gram-negative bacteria and consists of the ABC protein (which hydrolyses ATP thus providing energy for the process), a membrane fusion protein and an outer membrane protein. Many toxins are transported by this mechanism, particularly the repeat-in-toxin cytotoxins.

Type II (general secretory pathway)

This pathway is the commonest secretory pathway in bacteria and consists of two branches. The first part of the pathway that secretes proteins across the CM is all that is required in Gram-positive bacteria; however, in Gram-negative bacteria, a terminal branch of the general secretory pathway is an additional requirement. Proteins secreted by this pathway have an N-terminal leader sequence, which is cleaved at the CM by a signal peptidase. The leader sequence is about 20–30 amino acids in length. The export pathway consists of a Sec translocase comprising subunits Y, E and G, which form the pore and two other protein subunits, SecD and SecF. The cytoplasmic chaperone, SecB, keeps the protein in an unfolded exportable state and delivers it to the membrane-linked SecA (an ATPase), whence the protein is transported through the pore into the periplasmic space.

The second part of a type II export pathway is the main terminal branch and consists of a multiprotein complex. Most of these proteins are integral CM proteins that have a strong homology to type IV pili subunits, suggesting an evolutionary relationship. The outer membrane protein of the complex belongs to a protein family called secretins, which form multimers in the outer membrane to act as the pore through which the protein is secreted. Because of the evolutionary link between the main terminal branch of type II secretion and pili synthesis, it is speculated that during protein secretion a temporary trans-periplasmic pseudo-pilus is formed that assists secretion of the protein.

However, once in the periplasmic space, a protein can by transported to the outside environment by pathways other than the main terminal branch of the type II export pathway:

1. The protein may be able to transport itself (autotransporter or type V pathway). Proteins exported by this pathway form a β-barrel at their C-terminus, which inserts into the outer membrane, allowing the rest of the peptide to reach the outside of the cell. The β-barrel domain may be left in the outer membrane, freeing the passenger domain.
2. The chaperone–usher pathway: this pathway is normally involved in transport of type I and P-pili structures that are important in adhesion.
3. The twin-arginine translocation pathway (type VI). This pathway is similar to the general secretory pathway, except that the leader sequence contains a characteristic amino acid motif (Arg-Arg-X-Phe-X-Lys) at the N-terminal end. The proteins are already in a folded configuration.

Type III

The type III export mechanism is analogous to a micro-syringe that delivers bacterial products, usually toxins, directly into a eukaryotic cell cytoplasm. The secretion of the virulence factor by this pathway is Sec-independent but some components of the pathway are secreted into the periplasm by the Sec pathway. The type III export apparatus is composed of many CM proteins. The most likely mode of action is that the pore of the apparatus is blocked by a protein(s), which on some signals is removed, allowing the 'syringe' component to engage with the eukaryotic cell membrane to form a pore and allow ingress of the virulence factors to the eukaryotic cell cytoplasm. In some bacteria with a type III export mechanism, one of the signals that unblocks the 'syringe' barrel is in contact with the eukaryotic cell membrane. The type III export apparatus shows strong homology in many of the proteins in the basal body of the flagella apparatus.

Type IV

This export mechanism is found in *Helicobacter pylori*. It has a strong homology to DNA conjugation systems (e.g. the Vir B system of *Agrobacterium tumefaciens*) and consists of a micro-syringe (similar to the type III export mechanism) that delivers virulence factors into host cell cytoplasm. In *Helicobacter pylori*, it is known that the type IV apparatus delivers the CagA protein and PG into the gastric epithelial cell. Although the exact details of functioning of the type IV export apparatus in *Helicobacter pylori* are still to be worked out, it seems likely that CagL—found on the surface of the growing micro-syringe barrel—binds to host cell $\alpha_5\beta_1$ integrins, which in turn activates Src kinases and modulates the actin cytoskeleton and the host cell membrane, allowing injection of CagA and PG (*see also* Chapter 4). The CagA is phosphorylated on tyrosine residues by the Src kinases, which leads to downstream signalling and, eventually, production of IL-8 from the host cell.

Types V and VI

Type V and type VI secretion apparatuses are structurally similar to type IV. Type V is used for conjugal transfer of plasmids (e.g. *Agrobacterium* spp.), and some type VI proteins are homologous to the basal apparatus of bacteriophage.

Helicobacter metabolism

The tricarboxylic acid (TCA) cycle is central to metabolism: it converts the end products of the catabolic pathways for carbohydrates, proteins and fats into precursors for anabolic pathways; it alo produces energy in the form of ATP, and reducing equivalents in the form of nicotinamide adenosine dinucleotide (NADH in its reduced form), NADH phosphate (NADPH [reduced]) and flavin adenine dinucleotide (FADH [reduced]), which are in turn utilized in the respiratory chain with oxygen as the terminal electron acceptor in oxidative respiration. The metabolism of one molecule of glucose to pyruvate via the Embden–Meyerhof–Parnas pathway yields two molecules of ATP by substrate-level phosphorylation (**1.10**). The TCA cycle starts with conversion of pyruvate to acetyl coenzyme A (acetyl-CoA), which is subsequently incorporated into the TCA cycle by reaction with oxaloacetate to form citrate. This yields one molecule of GTP by substrate-level phosphorylation, three molecules of NADH, one molecule of FADH and two molecules of carbon dioxide. Eleven molecules of ATP are produced by the four electron donors formed in the TCA cycle (three per molecule of NADH and one by FADH).

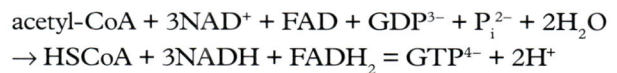

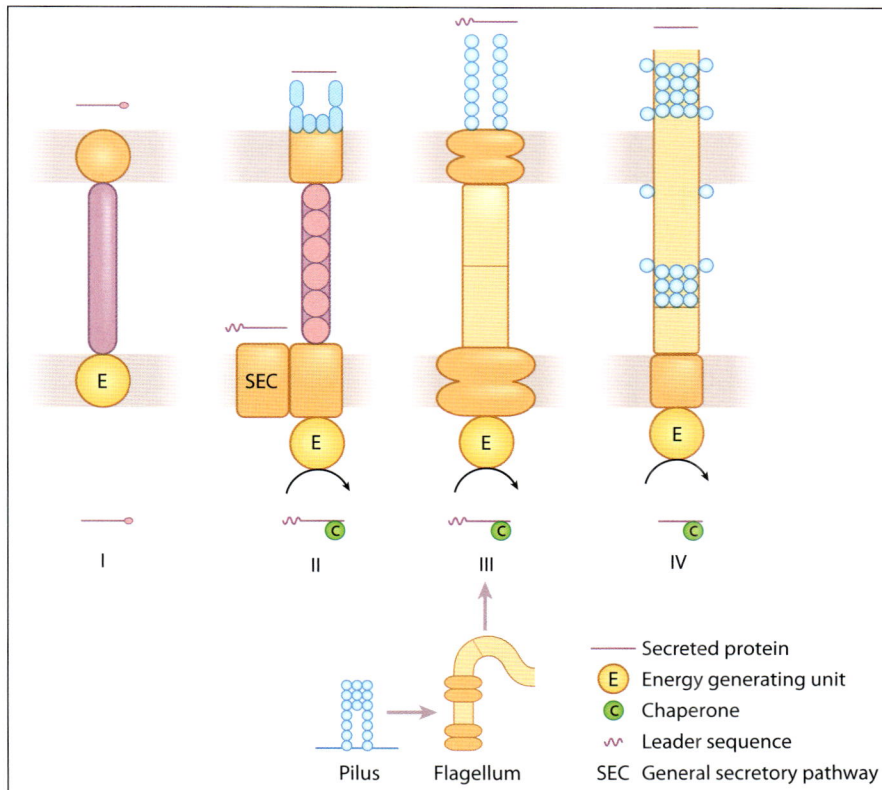

$$\text{acetyl-CoA} + 3NAD^+ + FAD + GDP^{3-} + P_i^{2-} + 2H_2O$$
$$\rightarrow HSCoA + 3NADH + FADH_2 = GTP^{4-} + 2H^+$$

1.9 Structure of a type IV secretion system.

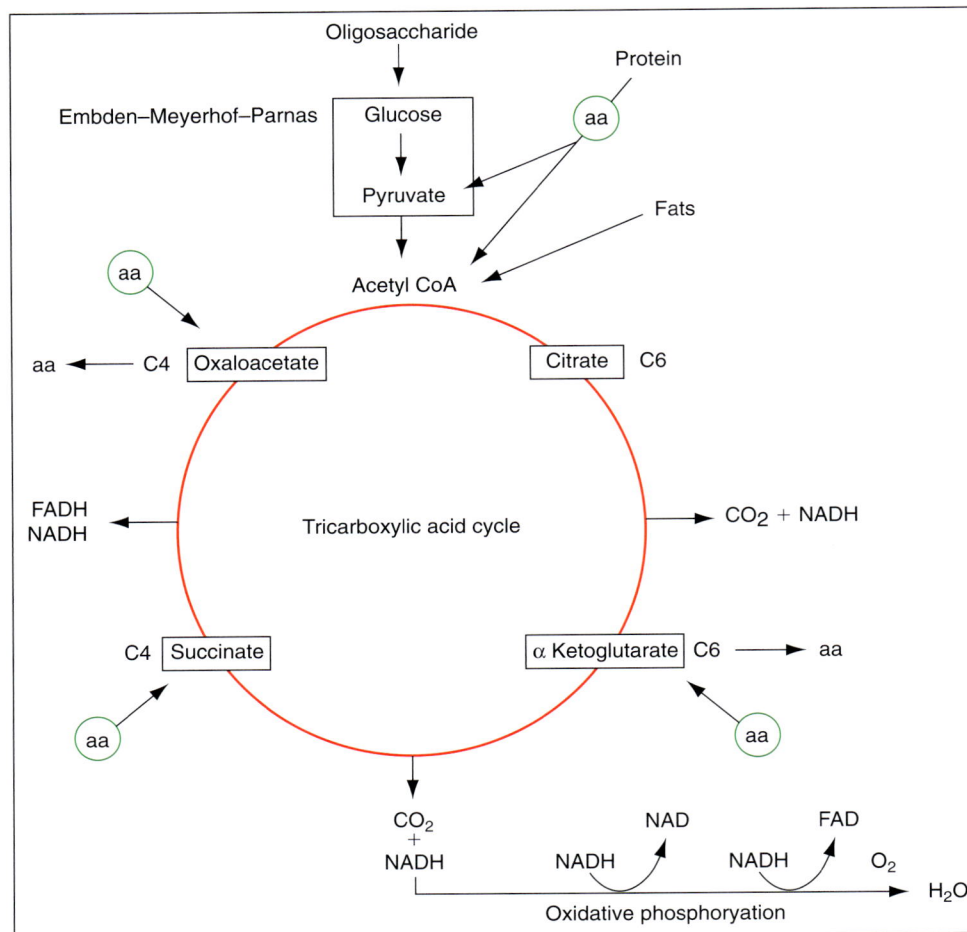

1.10 Embden–Meyerhof–Parnas and TCA biochemical pathways. aa = amino acid.

Bioinformatic studies on the genome of *Helicobacter pylori* combined with investigations using labelled substrates and nuclear magnetic resonance spectroscopy show that, compared with many organisms, *Helicobacter pylori* has a limited set of metabolic pathways, an incomplete TCA cycle and a limited oxygen transport chain. In *Helicobacter pylori*, the TCA cycle is incomplete with the absence of three key enzymes (α-ketoglutarate dehydrogenase, succinyl CoA synthetase and succinate dehydrogenase). The lack of these enzymes converts the TCA cycle into a branched pathway whose end products are succinate and α-ketoglutarate. This is similar to *E. coli* when grown under anaerobic conditions. In *Helicobacter pylori*, the two branches are linked by the presence of α-ketoglutarate oxidase. *Helicobacter pylori* has a hexose monophosphate shunt and, in keeping with some bacteria (e.g. *Pseudomonas* spp.), possesses an

Entner–Doudoroff pathway that also converts glucose to pyruvate (**1.11**).

Helicobacter pylori can phosphorylate glucose via glucokinase rather than hexokinase, which may explain the limited use of carbohydrates as carbon and energy sources. Oxidation of glucose-6-phosphate is via the Entner–Doudoroff pathway rather than the Embden–Meyerhof–Parnas pathway. This suggests that *Helicobacter* can also use aldoses as metabolic sources. The hexose monophosphate shunt provides NADPH for reductive catabolism and a supply of C5 sugars for DNA synthesis. Pyruvate from the Entner–Doudoroff pathway can be converted to acetyl-CoA by pyruvate flavidoxin oxidoreductase.

The principal metabolic source for energy and carbon is catabolism of amino acids rather than carbohydrates, although this is still questionable. *Helicobacter* cannot

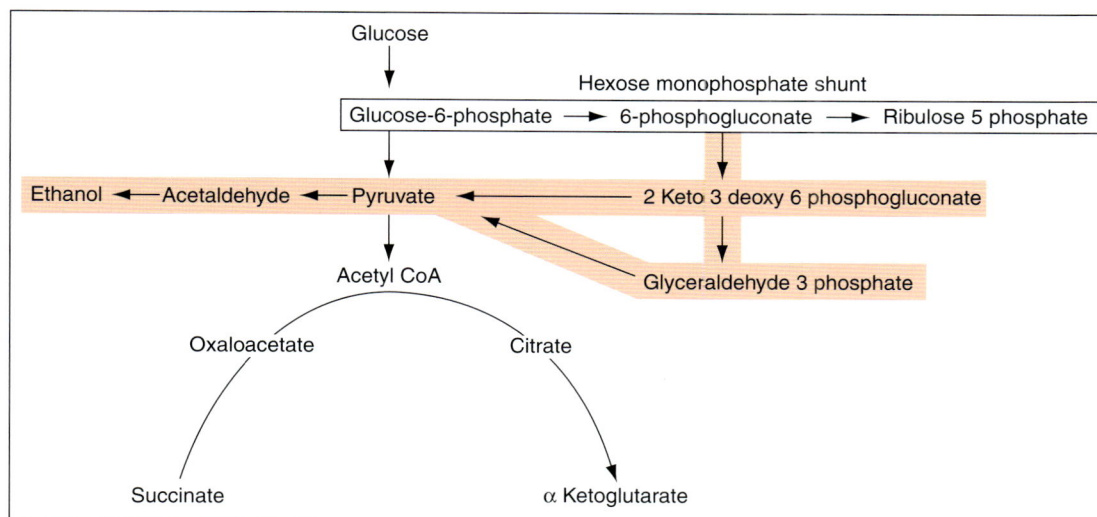

1.11 Biochemical pathways in *Helicobacter pylori*.

synthesize a small number of amino acids (arginine, histidine, leucine, isoleucine, methionine and valine). Amino acids are metabolized by fermentative pathways to acetate, formate and succinate. Lipid metabolism is not well explored. The major fatty acids are tetradecanoic acid (14:0) and methyleneoctadecanoic acid (19:0) with smaller quantities of hexadecanoic acid (16:0) and octadecanoic acid (18:0, 18:1); compare this with other Gram-negative bacteria, which have significant amounts of hexadecanoic (16:0), hexadecenoic (16:1) and octadecanoic acid (18:0). The organism also possesses cholesterol glycosides, which is unusual in bacteria, as they are more commonly found in plants. The overall structure of the LPS is similar to other Gram-negative bacteria with lipid A, a core region and an O (variable) side chain, but the molecule has fewer phosphate groups and consists of 3-hydroxyhexadecanoic acid (16:0) and 3-hydroxy octadecanoic acid (18:0). Le^x and Le^y blood group antigens are found in the O side chains.

Helicobacter has both pyrimidine and purine *de novo* synthesis as well as nucleotide salvage pathways, although for purines the salvage pathway is probably the primary pathway for synthesizing purine nucleotides.

The respiratory chain is relatively simple with a terminal oxidase of the cytochrome cbb3-type, although quinol oxidase and cb-type cytochromes are also present in *Helicobacter*. The organism has several reductive dehydrogenases: NADH quinine oxidoreductase; nickel/iron dehydrogenase; and glyceraldehyde-3-phosphate

dehydrogenase, although there is a preference for NADPH over NADH. Quinones pass on the electrons from the dehydrogenases to the terminal oxidoreductase and in *Helicobacter* the major respiratory quinine is menaquinone 6, which is typical of an anaerobic type of metabolism. *Helicobacter* possesses a fumarate reductase for anaerobic respiration.

In-silico predictions of metabolic pathways have been used to investigate *Helicobacter pylori*. The genome of *Helicobacter pylori* has been incorporated into the BioCyc website (http://BioCyc.org), which has set up a database of predicted biochemical pathways with visualization and query tools. This can be used to identify unique metabolic pathways that may serve as therapeutic targets. The input of the PathoLogic algorithm requires an annotated genome sequence (from *Helicobacter pylori* in this case) and a comparator pathway EcoCyc (based upon *E. coli*) or MetaCys (a database with pathways from over 130 organisms). In a comparison of the *in silico* prediction with manual pathway identification, some 40 pathways were consistent. Further computational investigations using extreme pathway (flux) analysis demonstrated a fairly rigid metabolic network; redundancy in amino acid pathways were twice that of ribonucleotide pathways and importantly a large proportion of the amino acid flux was directed into ammonia production.

A number of different iron uptake mechanisms exist in *Helicobacter pylori* but there is no evidence to suggest under what circumstances they are used or whether expression is related to colonizability or pathogenicity.

The pathways that have been detected are similar to those in *E. coli*: a Fec pathway (a ferrous uptake system); a lactoferritin uptake mechanism; a TonB pathway; a Frp pathway; and a Ceu (*Campylobacter* enterochelin uptake) pathway. *Helicobacter* also contains a bacterioferritin and a non-haem iron containing ferritin, which forms paracrystalline inclusions, as storage forms of iron. An ATPase transition metal uptake mechanism (NixA) also exists, which is involved in the uptake of nickel, copper and cobalt. Nickel is an important metal in the enzyme urease.

Helicobacter synthesizes about 6% of its protein anabolism as a urease, which has high substrate affinity. It is found both in the cytoplasm and on the surface of the organism and is important in maintaining the periplasmic pH of *Helicobacter* at 6. Its presence is important for the ability of *Helicobacter* to colonize the stomach.

Helicobacter pylori is auxotrophic for the following amino acids: arginine, histidine, isoleucine, leucine, methionine, phenylalanine and valine. It acquires these essential amino acids from the digestive milieu of the stomach, which are transported by specific amino acid uptake systems. An alternative nitrogen source is from urea (*see* Chapter 4).

Helicobacter culture

Helicobacter pylori is micro-aerobic, taking up to 5 days to grow on primary isolation media and producing small (1–2 mm diameter) colonies on horse blood agar (5% horse blood in Columbia agar base). The colonies are domed, glistening, entire, grey or water-clear, and are sufficiently characteristic to suggest the presence of the organism. A number of selective media are also available, but *Helicobacter pylori* grows perfectly well on 5% horse blood agar in Columbia agar base (**1.12**). Amphotericin can be added to suppress fungal growth that may mask the small colonies of the bacterium during prolonged growth.

Several different culture media have been proposed, usually with Columbia agar base, but Brucella or brain–heart infusion agar (BHIA) base have also been used. Most media contain either horse or sheep blood, although egg yolk, serum or cyclodextrose are used as substitutes. Selective agents vary but include some

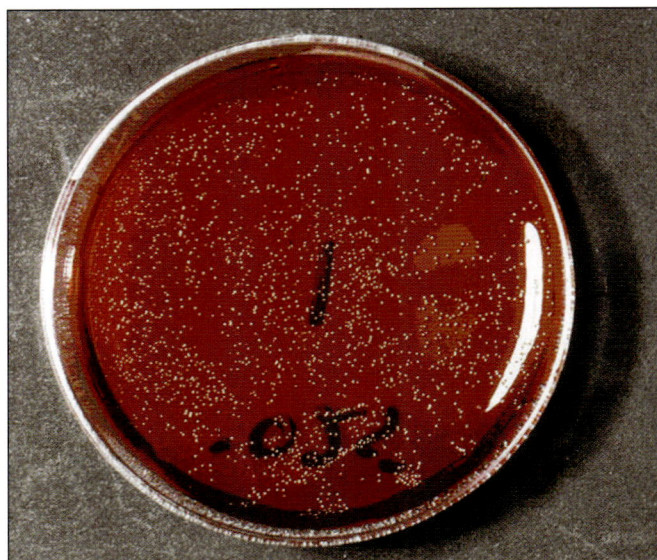

1.12 Photograph of *Helicobacter pylori* colonies on Colombia agar with 5% horse blood. It is recommended that for primary isolation a selective and non-selective medium is used (see also *Table 1.2*).

combination of trimethoprim, vancomycin, polymyxin and amphotericin.

The organism grows in an atmosphere of 5–15% oxygen, 5–12% carbon dioxide and 70–90% nitrogen. A number of selective media have been utilized (*Table 1.2*). *Helicobacter pylori* can also be grown in a chemically defined serum-free medium that is useful for metabolic studies. Growth can be enhanced in this medium (Ham's F12) with the addition of bovine serum albumin, cholesterol or cyclodextrin.

The organism can be cultured from clinical samples such as gastric biopsies, dental plaque or faeces. Although detected by molecular means, *H. pylori* has thus far not been cultured from water samples.

Helicobacter genome

The *Helicobacter pylori* genome is about 1.60 Mbp long, about half the size of that of *E. coli*, and consists of about 1600 predicted genes. The organism has a large number of outer membrane proteins and putative adhesions testifying to the importance of adhesion in its biology. It also codes for about 25 restriction endonucleases and 27 methylases, underpinning the importance of genetic exchange to *Helicobacter pylori*. Additionally, there are

Table 1.2 Composition of media used to isolate *Helicobacter pylori*

Medium	Agar base	Tm (mg/L)	V (mg/L)	Cef (mg/L)	Polyene (mg/L)	Polym (IU)	Additives
Dent	Columbia	5	10	5	A 5		7% sheep blood
Glupczynski	BHIA	5	10	5	A 10		10% FCS; 2 g activated charcoal; 40 mg TPT
Skirrow	Columbia	5	10			2500	7% lysed horse blood
EYA	Columbia	5	6	5	A 6		10% egg yolk; 1% Vitox; 40 mg TPT
MTM	GC	5	3		N 12 500		10% soluble Hb; 10 g YE; 1.5 g dextrose; 15 g NaHCO$_3$; 7.5 mg colistin
Brucella	Brucella						5% sheep blood; 1% Vitox
TSA	Trypticase						5% sheep blood
BHIA	Brain–heart						7% horse blood
MCA	Columbia						5% sheep blood; 1% Vitox
Columbia	Columbia				A 10		5% horse blood

Red = selective media; Black = non-selective media.
A = amphotericin; Cef = cefsulodin; FCS = fetal calf serum; Hb = haemoglobin; N = neomycin; Polyene = polyene antimycotic; Polym = polymyxin; Tm = trimethoprim; TPT = triphenyl tetrazolium; V = vancomycin; YE = yeast extract.

large numbers of homopolymorphic tracts, which is in part the basis for the known genetic diversity of the organism. *Helicobacter pylori* has relatively few regulatory proteins compared with organisms with similar sized genomes.

Three important areas of the *Helicobacter* genome are the locus for the vacuolating cytotoxin A protein (VacA), *cag*PAI and plasticity region. The *vacA* gene is not carried within the PAI but at a separate location on the *Helicobacter* genome. The *vacA* gene is present in nearly all strains of *Helicobacter pylori* but only half of them secrete VacA as a mature protein of 95 kDa. Various polymorphisms are found in the gene as illustrated in **1.13**. Variation occurs in the leader sequence (LS), the mid-region (m) of the gene and in the intermediate region (i) between the leader sequence and m regions. There are two types of leader sequence (s1 and s2), two

of the intermediate (i1 and i2), and two of the m (m1 and m2) regions. The s region affects the vacuolating activity of the toxin, and the m region determines the specificity of toxin binding to host cells. The i region seems to be a marker for clinical outcome.

The *vacA* gene carried by the type strain CCUG 17874, which is cytotoxic, contains a single open reading frame, flanked by consensus promoter sequences, the ribosomal binding site and terminator sequences. Some regions are highly conserved, while other regions are divergent. The divergent regions are constituted by a 50 bp segment included in the signal sequence (s), and a fragment of ca. 700 bp contained in the middle part (m) of the gene. Strains with *vacA* subtype s1/m1 produce increased levels of cytotoxin, while strains with the mosaic structure s2/m2 are completely devoid of toxic activity. The *vacA* signal sequence type s1a

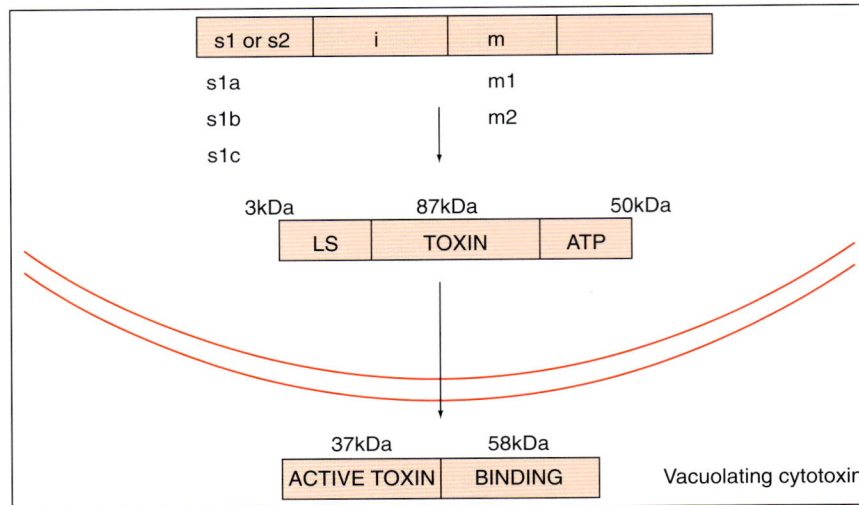

1.13 The vacuolating cytotoxin gene and secretion. LS = leader sequence.

is associated with increased mucosal inflammation, duodenal ulcer, enhanced gastric epithelial damage and gastric cancer.

Some researchers have noticed the existence of geographic differences in the sequence of *Helicobacter pylori* virulence determinants. More precisely, they found a subtle diversity in the *vacA* sequences of strains isolated from Japanese people or from populations living in Western countries. In addition, although almost all Japanese isolates are *vacA* subtype s1/m1, the levels of cytotoxic activity exhibited by these strains are not high and no difference was found in the middle region of cytotoxic and non-cytotoxic strains. The low genetic diversity of strains isolated in Japan may reflect the homogeneity of the Japanese individuals, due to little mixing of this population with other ethnic groups and geographic isolation. Alternatively, we could suppose that the predominance of a certain *vacA* type in Japan might reflect a better adaptation of strains with *vacA* s1a/m1 subtype to the gastric environment. Studies carried out in different Japanese areas with high or low risk of gastric carcinoma showed that, while infection by *Helicobacter pylori* strains with *vacA* subtype s1 was associated with duodenal ulcer, the possession of *vacA* subtype m1 was statistically more frequent in patients with gastric carcinoma.

The s1 LS is found in type I strains and the s2 LS in type II strains, which produce less toxin and are less frequently associated with severe disease.

The vacuolating cytotoxin is translated from the gene as a 140 kDa pro-toxin that has a 33 amino acid leader sequence and thus is excreted by the general secretory (Sec) pathway. The leader sequence is cleaved during transfer across the CM into the periplasmic space. The C-terminus of the pro-toxin has a 50 kDa region that resembles the IgA protease of *Neisseria gonorrhoea* and may act in a similar fashion as an auto-transporter for the VacA toxin. During transfer across the outer membrane C-terminal processing occurs, releasing a 94 kDa toxin into the surrounding medium. This undergoes further cleavage to produce a 37 kDa N-terminal and a 58 kDa C-terminal fragment, which remain associated after cleavage.

Figure **1.14** shows the general structure of the *cag*PAI. Strains with *cag*PAI are called type I strains and those lacking *cag*PAI are type II strains. Type I strains are more likely linked to severe gastroduodenal disease than type II strains. The *cag*PAI comprises 30 genes involved in the synthesis of the type IV secretion apparatus and a gene for the CagA protein. The PAI may be complete and it may be separated into two sections (cag I and cag II) by an insertion element, IS605. This insertion sequence encodes two putative transposons, called TnpA and TnpB. One or other part of the PAI may be missing or the strain may lack a PAI. Of the 31 genes contained in the *cag*PAI, eight encode for the conjugative apparatus through which CagA is injected into the colonized cells. The *cagA* gene is divided into an N-terminal constant region and the C-terminal variable region. The variable region encompasses nucleotide repeats that recur with varying frequency. The importance of repeats is the fact that they encode tyrosine phosphorylation sites. Based on the polymorphisms of the tyrosine phosphorylation sites, CagA can be subclassified into two main types: the Western CagA and the Eastern Asia CagA. The tyrosine motif undergoes phosphorylation at the level of the amino acidic sequence Glu-Pro-Ile-Tyr-Ala, also called EPIYA, which is present in the carboxy-terminal sequence of the protein. The EPIYA motif can be subdivided into four distinct sites from A–D, depending on the amino acid sequence that encircles the motif. The type IV secretion apparatus is a complex structure that acts as a micro-syringe and is used to transfer material such as CagA and part of the peptidoglycan from the cell wall of *Helicobacter pylori* into the host cell.

The first locus codes for a protein which has an important virulence characteristic—a cytotoxin that induces vacuolation in exposed cells. The second locus is a region of DNA that has undergone horizontal transfer from an as yet unknown organism; this region codes for 30 genes, many of which are involved in the synthesis of a type IV secretion apparatus, and also contains the *cagA* coding region. CagA is transferred to the host cell along with peptidoglycan and interferes with host cell signalling, leading to altered cell morphology, cell division or apoptosis. The plasticity region is an area of hypermutation.

Helicobacter pylori can be divided into type I and type II strains based upon the presence of *cagA* and the secretion of VacA. Type I strains are *cagA* positive and secrete VacA, while type II stains are *cagA* negative and do not secrete VacA. However, the totality of *cag*PAI is important, since if the type I secretion system is not functional (due to deletion in *cag*PAI) then CagA will not be injected into the host cell. This feature is important, as the ability to induce IL-8 production in cells is correlated with the presence of the complete *cag*PAI; thus, the presence of an intact *cag*PAI is correlated with the development of more severe pathology.

Even though the sequence of an organism may be available, it is recognized that variation may exist between different strains of the same organism and that these differences may have significance in relation to virulence. Such differences can be identified either by microarray technology, or by the process of subtractive hybridization, a method that amplifies differences between genomes. In the former, only sequences absent from the unsequenced strain can be identified. In subtractive hybridization the genome sequence of one strain (called the 'driver') is known and endonuclease-generated DNA fragments from this strain are mixed with fragments from the related strain (called the 'tester'); the 'tester'-specific sequences, which self-anneal rather than anneal with 'driver' DNA, are amplified by polymerase chain reaction (PCR). Using *Helicobacter pylori*, two separate isolates (strain 26695 and J99) show about 7% unique sequences. The *Helicobacter pylori* 26695 genome

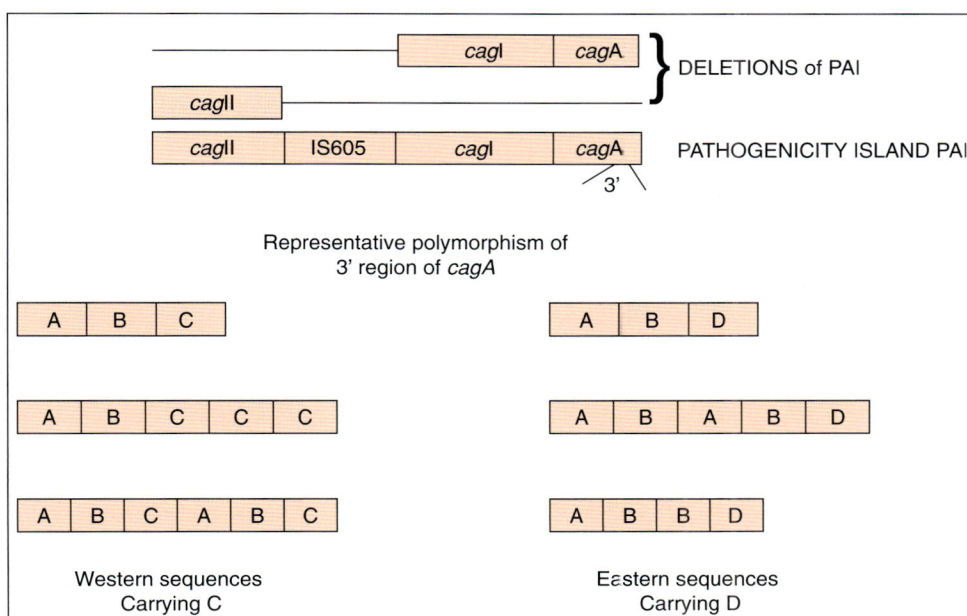

1.14 Arrangement and polymorphisms of the *cag*PAI.

is approximately 1.68 Mbp long and contains about 1590 predicted genes (**1.15**). It has a well-developed system for motility, iron scavenging and for DNA restriction and modification. There are many adhesins, lipoproteins and other outer membrane proteins. Homopolymeric tracts and dinucleotide repeats occur frequently, suggesting the use of recombination and slipped-strand mispairing as a genetic mechanism for variation. There is a relatively limited metabolic ability and few regulatory pathways.

The *Helicobacter pylori* J99 genome is 1.64 Mbp long and contains about 1754 predicted genes (**1.16**). Like *H. pylori* 26695, *H. pylori* J99 has a well-developed system for motility, iron scavenging and for DNA restriction and modification, with many adhesins and other outer membrane proteins. Homopolymeric tracts and

dinucleotide repeats are frequent and there is a relatively limited metabolic ability and few regulatory pathways. Of the 7% of genes specific to J99 and 26695, about 50% are in a single hypervariable region, suggesting acquisition of DNA by horizontal transfer.

The proteome of different organisms can be compared and identical sequences used to annotate proteins for functionality. Algorithms based on a modular approach to homology are thought to provide a more accurate identification of function. Currently, it is recognized that *Helicobacter pylori* has evolved with a large investment in adhesion ligands.

The investigation of whole genome expression of *Helicobacter pylori* under natural conditions may throw light on the host–pathogen interaction and aid

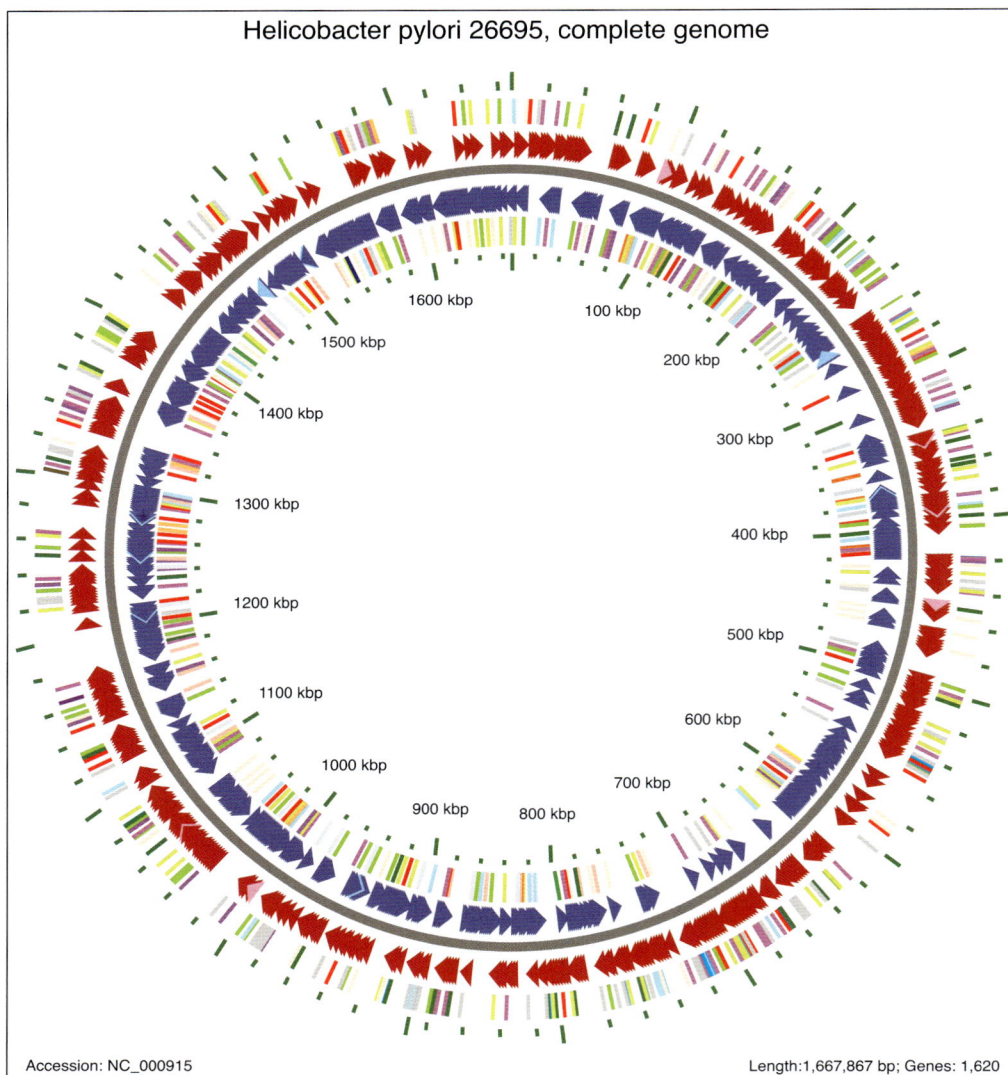

Helicobacter pylori 26695, complete genome

Accession: NC_000915   Length:1,667,867 bp; Genes: 1,620

1.15 Genome map of *Helicobacter pylori* strain 26695.

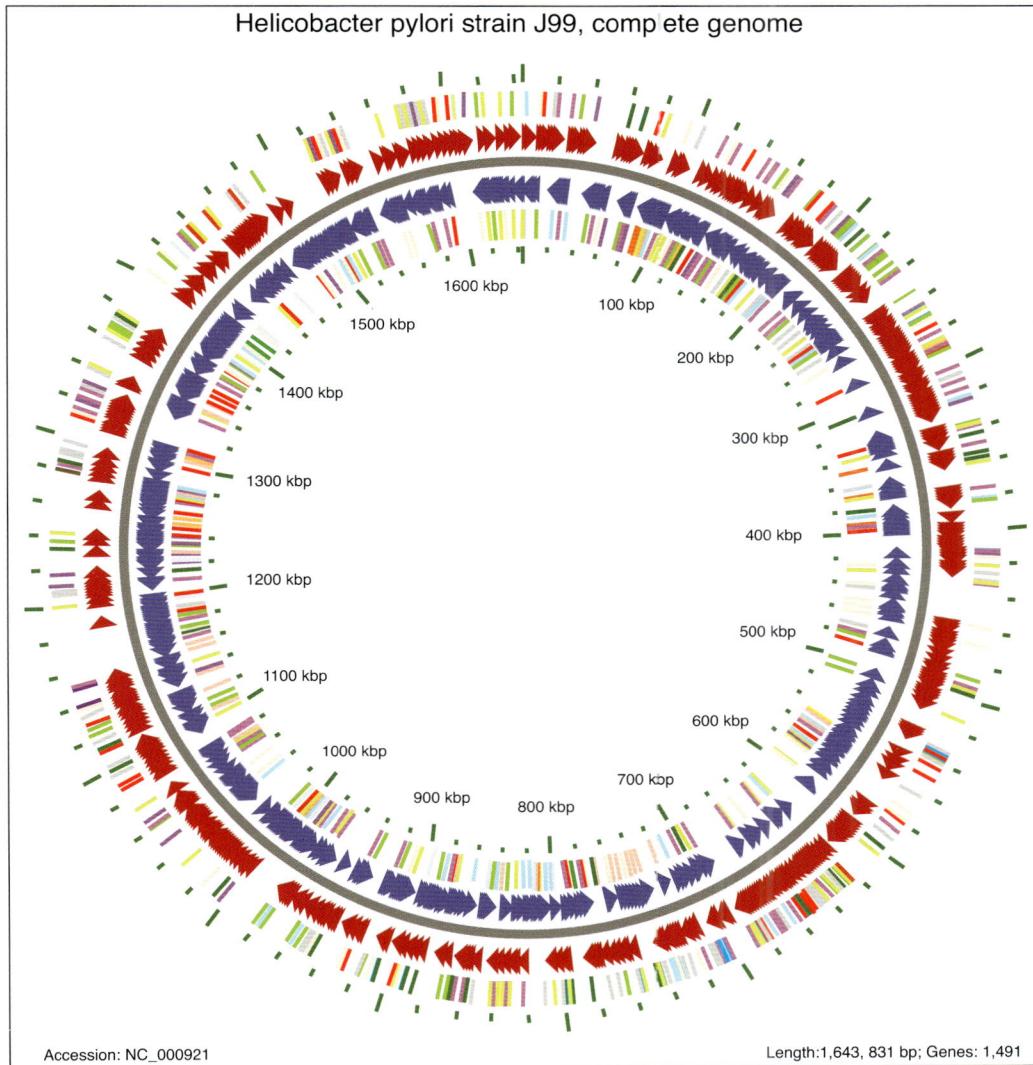

1.16 Genome map of *Helicobacter pylori* strain J99. This figure and the previous one opposite illustrate BacMap, an interactive visual data base of over 2000 bacterial genomes. Each map can be expanded and rotated, with gene labels linked to a textual description. The site allows a Text or BLAST search of the genome and a brief description of the species is available. Both the proteomic and genomic characteristics are available online or as file downloads. BacMap can be accessed at http://wishart. biology.ualberta.ca/BacMap/ and the full description of this bioinfomatic tool is found in Stothard *et al*. (2005).

understanding of *Helicobacter pylori* pathogenesis of disease. Preliminary investigation of *in vivo* expression of *Helicobacter pylori* genes on contact with gastric epithelium showed that in those in which *iceA* was expressed there was more inflammation of the mucosa. Other genes expressed in *Helicobacter pylori* are urease, catalase and an adhesin (*alpA*) found in studies using differential display PCR or reverse transcription-PCR (RT-PCR). Studies of global expression of *H. pylori* genome combine microarray hybridization with a cDNA–PCR technique called selective capture of

transcribed sequences. These show that many genes were expressed, some of which have been provisionally annotated or identified by sequencing (e.g. *babA* and *alpA*), but the majority of which are of unknown function. Further investigation of this host–pathogen interaction will yield important information on the bioecology of this mucosal-associated organism occupying a unique ecological niche.

The combination of rapid two-dimensional gel electrophoresis with MALDI-TOF mass spectrometry shortens investigative time in the study of proteomics, which can help in the development of novel vaccines. Of the large numbers of potential antigens, a subset may be selected based on criteria such as immunogenicity and abundance (reverse vaccinology) to streamline vaccine development. *In silico* prediction can be made on codon usage, which correlates with protein expression. However, codon use is not the sole criterion of expression, since *in silico* prediction does not robustly correlate with proteomic data. Specific motifs defining outer membrane proteins can also be used as predictors of potential candidates, but again the correlation is not exact.

Use of these techniques during the investigation of the transcriptome and proteome of organisms has predicted antigens that are highly protective in model systems.

Helicobacter genetics

Helicobacter pylori has a high degree of genetic diversity, which has been attributed to horizontal transfer of DNA, frequent recombination, high mutation rate and impaired DNA repair. *Helicobacter pylori* carries plasmids that can undergo conjugation, thereby transferring DNA between cells (**1.17**; from BacMap, *see* **1.16**). Plasmids are usually associated with antibiotic resistance, but in *Helicobacter pylori* generally this does not appear to be the case. *Helicobacter pylori* plasmids appear to replicate by the rolling circle mechanism, which is common in plasmids from Gram-positive bacteria. *Helicobacter pylori* has also been shown to transfer chromosomally encoded antibiotic resistance by conjugation with

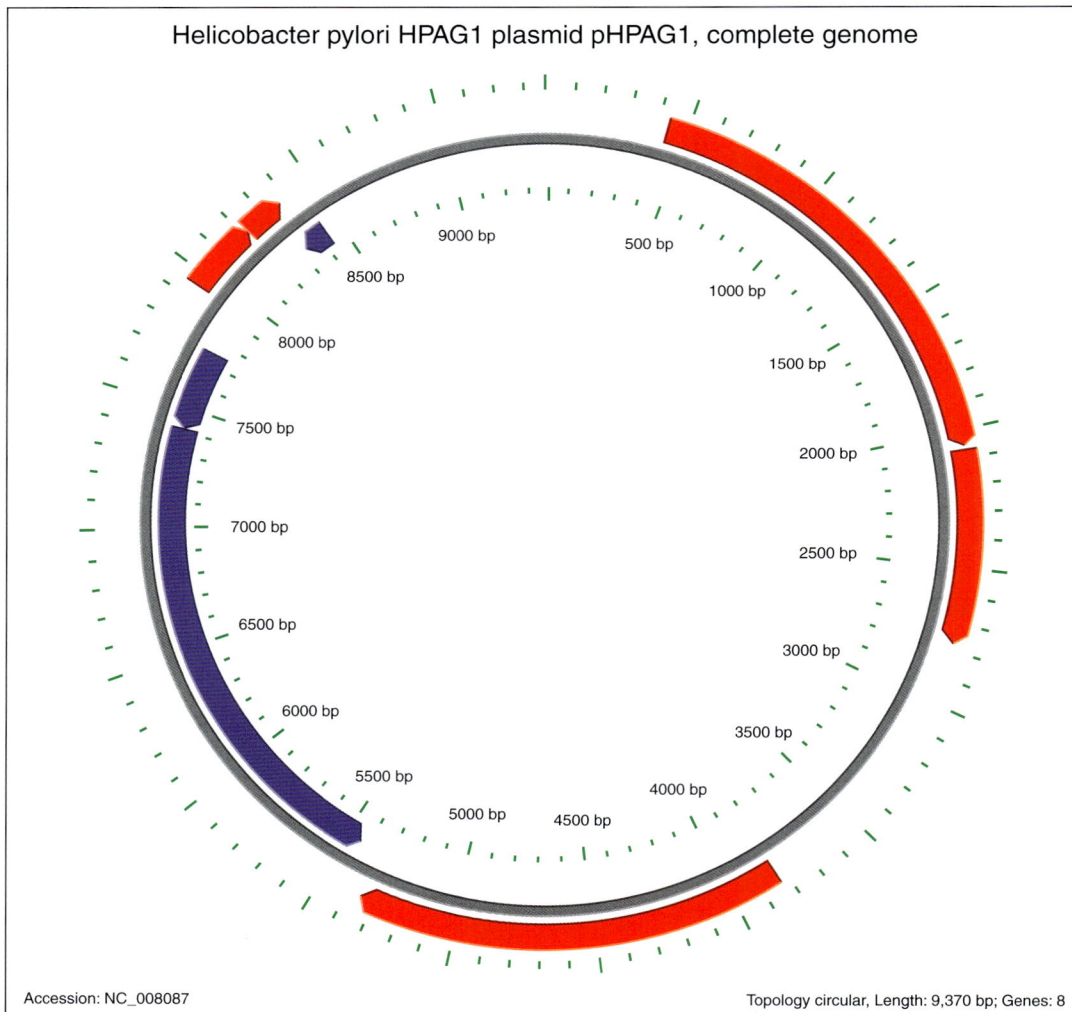

Helicobacter pylori HPAG1 plasmid pHPAG1, complete genome

9000 bp   500 bp
8500 bp   1000 bp
8000 bp   1500 bp
7500 bp   2000 bp
7000 bp   2500 bp
6500 bp   3000 bp
6000 bp   3500 bp
5500 bp   4000 bp
5000 bp 4500 bp

Accession: NC_008087   Topology circular, Length: 9,370 bp; Genes: 8

1.17 Plasmids ranging from 1.8 to 63 kbp have been identified in *Helicobacter pylori* and used as a means of typing and to develop shuttle vectors.

Campylobacter jejuni. Helicobacter pylori is also competent for transformation. Competence occurs in peaks during the growth phase and timing of the peaks appears to be strain dependent. The mechanism of uptake of DNA is related to the type IV secretion system called ComB. The genes *comB2*, *comB3* and *comB4* have been identified and *comB2*, in addition to being part of the transformation unit, is an adhesin. Transformation can occur within 1 minute of exposure to exogenous DNA and double-stranded DNA is a much better substrate compared with single-stranded DNA. In *Helicobacter pylori*, genetic acquisition by transformation has been shown to give a selective advantage when exposed to novel laboratory conditions.

Although *Helicobacter pylori* is deficient in repair mechanisms, UvrD and RecN homologues found in *Helicobacter pylori* are important in repair of DNA damage. The RecG homologue limits recombinational repair by the lack of a typical RecG resolvase leading to varied strains. The main repair pathway in *Helicobacter pylori* appears to be the RuvABC pathway.

Helicobacter taxonomy

Spiral-shaped bacteria have been seen in humans since the time of Anton van Leeuwenhoek (**1.18**) and in the stomach of animals first described in 1881 by Rappin. Leeuwenhoek made improvements to the development of microscopes and is credited with being the first microbiologist. He made several observations of cells, including bacteria, which he called 'animalcules'; his earliest work was published in the *Philosophical Transactions of the Royal Society*.

Subsequently, other studies identified different morphotypes of spiral or helical bacteria in the stomach of dogs (**1.19**). In humans, spiral/helical-shaped bacteria were first noted by Doenges in 1939. A few years after the first isolation of *Helicobacter pylori in* 1983, other larger spiral-shaped bacteria that resisted cultivation were noted and called *Gastrospirillum hominis*—subsequently to be changed to *Helicobacter heilmannii* type 1 and 2. *Helicobacter heilmannii* type 1 is very closely related to "*Candidatus* Helicobacter suis" and *Helicobacter heilmannii* type 2 is closely related to the *Helicobacter bizzozeronii*–*H. felis*–*H. salomonis* group.

Another organism with a distinctive morphotype (spindle-shaped with spiral periplasmic fibres and bipolar flagella), detected in a variety of specimens, in humans and other animals, is *Flexispira rappini*. This belongs to the genus *Helicobacter* and is similar in morphology to other recognized *Helicobacter* species (e.g. *Helicobacter felis*). In the literature, they are called *Flexispira rappini*, *Helicobacter rappini* or *Helicobacter* sp. *flexispira* and so far remain taxonomically uncharacterized.

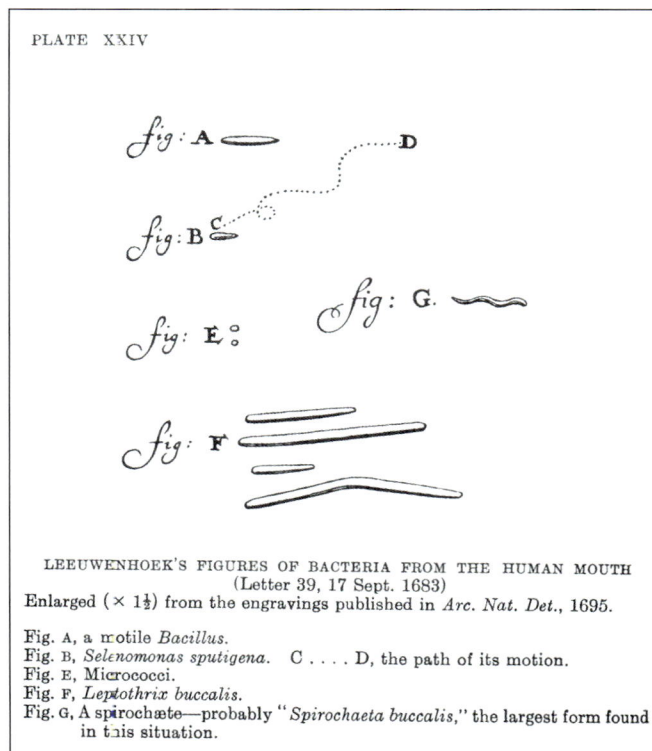

PLATE XXIV

LEEUWENHOEK'S FIGURES OF BACTERIA FROM THE HUMAN MOUTH
(Letter 39, 17 Sept. 1683)
Enlarged (× 1½) from the engravings published in *Arc. Nat. Det.*, 1695.

Fig. A, a motile *Bacillus*.
Fig. B, *Selenomonas sputigena*.   C . . . . D, the path of its motion.
Fig. E, Micrococci.
Fig. F, *Leptothrix buccalis*.
Fig. G, A spirochæte—probably "*Spirochaeta buccalis*," the largest form found in this situation.

1.18 Illustration of a page from the work of Anton van Leeuwenhoek.

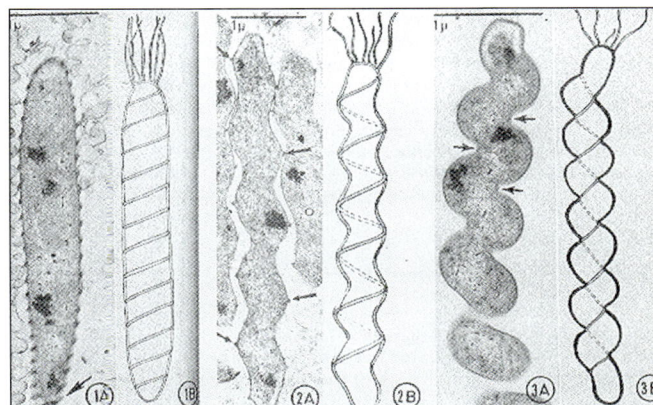

1.19 Illustration from a paper by Lockard and Boler in the *American Journal of Veterinary Research* illustrating spiral-shaped bacteria in the stomach of a dog designated as *Helicobacter heilmannii*. The taxonomic position of *Helicobacter heilmannii* remains unresolved.

The named *Helicobacter nemestrinae*, isolated from a monkey, is now identified as a strain of *H. pylori* and the isolate *H. westmaedii*, isolated from humans, is a strain of *H. cinaedi*. Both *H. cinaedi* and *H. fennelliae* were previously designated as *Campylobacter* spp. but reassigned to the genus *Helicobacter*.

As mentioned, *Helicobacter pylori* was initially known as a *Campylobacter*-like organism, because of its resemblance to *Campylobacter* spp. and its isolation under similar culture conditions. However, several features hinted that it was not a *Campylobacter* sp. as it differed in its flagella morphology and fatty acid profile. Its separation from *Campylobacter* was confirmed by protein profiles, 16S rDNA analysis and DNA–DNA hybridization. The *Helicobacter* genus was proposed in 1989, with *Helicobacter pylori* as the type species.

The discovery of *Helicobacter pylori* as an organism situated on the mucosa of the gastrointestinal tract stimulated a search for other *Helicobacter* species in both humans and other animals. Numerous additions to the genus have now been made, discovered in a range of animal species (*Table 1.3*). These various *Helicobacter* spp. can broadly be divided into two categories: those found exclusively in the stomach (e.g. *Helicobacter acinonychis* and *Helicobacter felis*) and those found principally in the lower intestine and hepatobiliary system (e.g. *Helicobacter hepaticus* and *Helicobacter trogontum*). More recently, a *Helicobacter* sp. has been isolated from dolphins

Table 1.3 Some named *Helicobacter* species

Gastric *Helicobacter* spp.	Lower intestinal *Helicobacter* spp.
H. pylori (human)	*H. cinaedi* (human, hamster, rats, dogs, cats)
H. heilmannii (human, dog, pig)	*H. fennelliae* (human)
H. acinonychis (cheetah)	*H. westmaedii* (strain of *H. cinaedi*)
H. mustelae (ferret)	*H. canis* (dog)
H. felis (cat, dog)	*H. pamatensis* (gulls)
H. bizzozeronii (dog)	*H. muridarum* (rodent)
H. salomonis (dog)	*H. bilis* (rodent)
H. nemestrinae (monkey)	*H. rodentium* (rodent) of *H. pylori*)
H. suncus (shrew)	*H. trogontum* (rodent)
H. suis (pig)	*H. pullorum* (chicken)
H. bovis (cattle)	*H. cholecystus* (hamster)
H. cetorum (dolphins, whales)	*H. rappini* (human, sheep)
	H. hepaticus (rodent)
	H. mesocricetorum (hamster)
	H. canadensis (goose, human)
	H. marmotae (woodchuck)
	H. muricola (rodent)
	H. winghamensis (human)
	H. ulmiensis (human)
	H. aurati (Syrian hamster)
	H. ganmani (rodent)
	H. typhlonius (rodent)
	H. apodemus (rodent)
	H. colifelis (cat)
	H. marmotae (woodchuck)
	H. mastomyrinus (rodent)
	H. equorum (horse)
	H. callitrichis (marmoset)

Several other *Helicobacter* spp. have been recorded without validly published names

(*Helicobacter cetorum*) and two new unnamed *Helicobacter* spp. from harp seals. The interest in the isolation of *Helicobacter* species from a wide range of animals covers several important areas:

- Comparative analysis of closely related species has the potential for increasing the understanding of both host–pathogen interaction and genome evolution.
- As several of these animals can be used as model systems, they are important in understanding the pathogenesis of gastroduodenal disease caused by *Helicobacter pylori* and for the evaluation of vaccine development. Colonization of the human stomach with *Helicobacter pylori* can lead to gastric lymphoma, and similarly colonization of the mouse with *Helicobacter felis* can also lead to lymphoma. Vaccination of mice with *Helicobacter felis* before infection can not only prevent colonization by that strain but also protects

against the development of lymphoma. This exciting development is the first indication that vaccination may be useful against malignancy.

- Some of these animal *Helicobacter* spp. (notably *H. hepaticus* and *H. bilis*) have been linked to the development of liver cancer or inflammatory bowel disease in animals. They are of great interest in relation to what they can reveal about these conditions in humans. In particular, attention has focused on *H. hepaticus*, and recently its whole genome has been sequenced. Additionally, some *Helicobacter* spp. (*H. cinaedi*, *H. fennelliae*) are recognized pathogens in humans, causing colitis primarily in homosexual men.

The genus *Helicobacter* falls within the Epsilonproteobacteria class of the Proteobacteria phylum (rRNA superfamily VI). This class contains a wide diversity

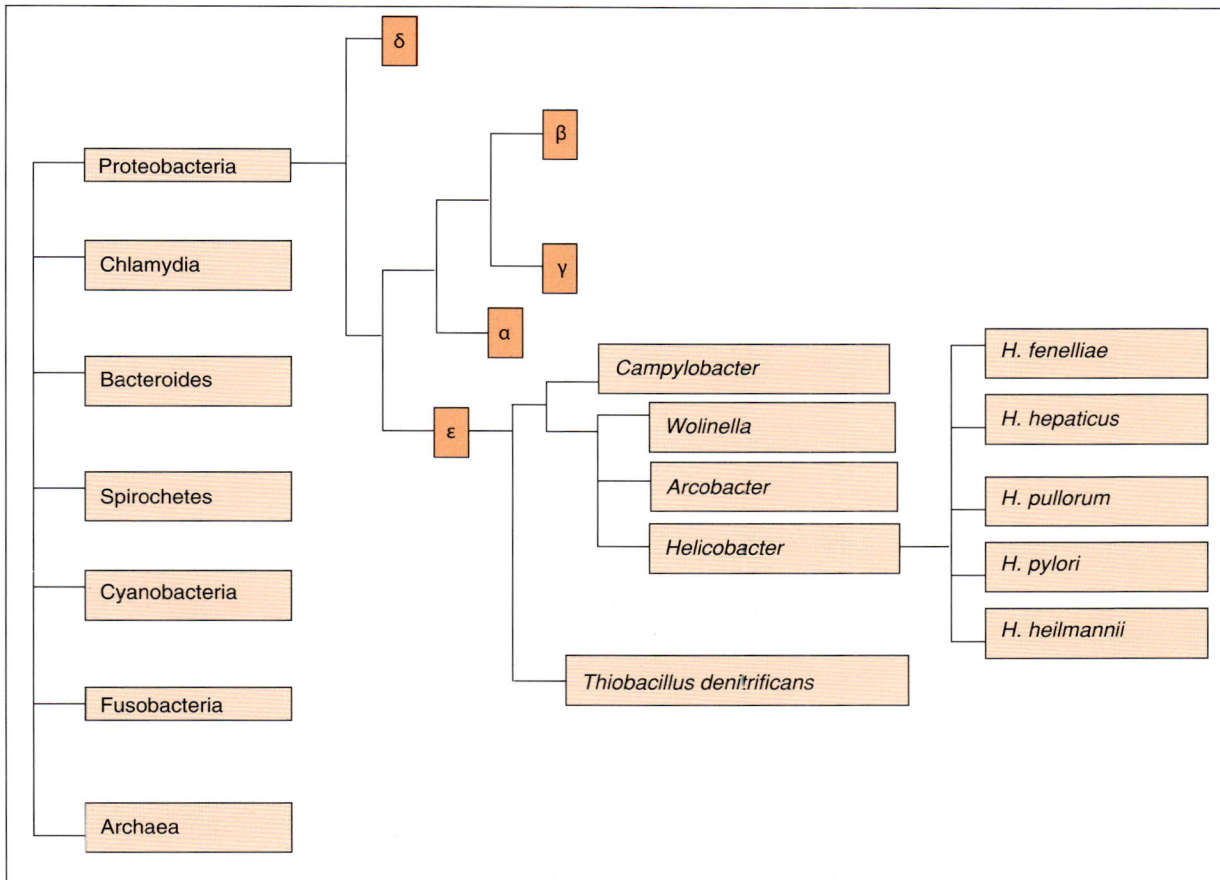

1.20 Schematic illustration of the relationship of *Helicobacter* species to other bacteria. This diagram illustrates the relationship of *Helicobacter* to other Epsilonproteobacteria (*Wolinella*, *Arcobacter*, *Campylobacter*), the phylogeny in relation to other divisions of the Proteobacteria (α, β, γ, δ), and to other major divisions of the microbial kingdom.

of bacteria, including the genera of *Campylobacter*, *Helicobacter*, *Arcobacter*, *Wolinella* (one sp., *Wolinella succinogenes*) and the provisional genus *Flexispira* (*Flexispira rappini*). The taxonomic relationship of *Helicobacter* species to other Epsilonproteobacteria and to other major bacteria divisions is illustrated in **1.20**.

Further reading

Christie PJ. Type IV secretion: intercellular transfer of macromolecules by systems ancestrally related to conjugation machines. *Mol Microbiol* 2001; 40: 294–305.

Fox JG. The non-*H. pylori* helicobacters: their expanding role in gastrointestinal and systemic disease. *Gut* 2002; 50: 273–83.

Goodwin CS, Armstrong JA, Chilvers T, *et al.* Transfer of *Campylobacter pylori* and *Campylobacter mustelae* to *Helicobacter* gen. nov. as *Helicobacter pylori* comb. nov. and *Helicobacter mustelae* comb. nov., respectively. *Int J Syst Bacteriol* 1989; 39: 397–405.

Kusters JG, Gerrits MM, Van Strup JAG, Vandenbroucke-Grauls CMJE. Coccoid forms of *Helicobacter pylori* are the morphological manifestation of cell death. *Infect Immun* 1997; 65: 3672–9.

Marshall BJ, Warren JR. Unidentified curved bacillus on gastric epithelium in active chronic gastritis. *Lancet* 1983; i: 1273–5.

Marshall BJ, Warren JR. Unidentified curved bacilli in the stomach of patients with gastritis and peptic ulceration. *Lancet* 1984; i: 1311–15.

Paley SM, Karp PD. Evaluation of computational metabolic pathway predictions for *Helicobacter pylori*. *Bioinformatics* 2002; 18: 715–24.

Pitson SM, Mendz GL, Srinvasan S, Hazell SL. The tricarboxylic acid cycle of *Helicobacter pylori*. *Eur J Biochem* 1999; 260: 258–67.

Price ND, Papin JA, Palsson BO. Determination of redundancy and system properties of the metabolic network of *Helicobacter pylori* using genome scale extreme pathway analysis. *Genome Research* 2002; 12: 760–9.

Stothard P, Van Domselaar G, Shrivastava S, *et al.* BacMap: an interactive picture atlas of annotated bacterial genomes. *Nucleic Acids Res* 2005; 33: D317–20.

Tomb JF, White O, Kerlavage AR, *et al.* The complete genome sequence of the gastric pathogen *Helicobacter pylori*. *Nature* 1977; 388: 539–47.

Chapter 2

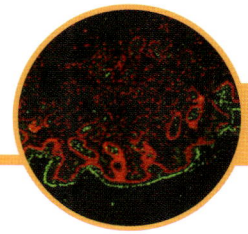

Epidemiology and colonization

Typing of *Helicobacter pylori*

Typing of bacteria is an important aspect of studying the epidemiology of an organism. It allows one to sometimes pinpoint the source of an outbreak, determine routes of infection, determine presence of microevolution and, in the case of *Helicobacter pylori*, to trace the migration of human populations. There are various methods used to type organisms, including phage typing, colicine typing, biotyping, serotyping, antibiotic resistance profiling and molecular methods of typing. With respect to *Helicobacter pylori* the following molecular typing methods have been used: ribotyping, restriction fragment length polymorphism (RFLP) pulse field electrophoresis, polyacrylamide gel electrophoresis (PAGE), random amplification of polymorphic DNA, multilocus enzyme electrophoresis (MLEE) and genome sequencing (*Table 2.1*).

Biotyping

Because of its relative biochemical unreactivity, there is no generally accepted biotyping scheme for *H. pylori*. One scheme has identified four biotypes based on the presence of five enzymes: C4 and C8 esterases; a phosphohydrolase; leucine arylamidase; and acid and alkaline phosphatase. Group I was positive for all, group II lacked esterase, group III lacked esterase and phosphohydrolase, and group IV was only positive for phosphatases. Variations on this biotyping scheme have been used, but overall it is not useful. Another scheme has identified five biotypes.

Serotyping

Examination of the lipopolysaccharide of *Helicobacter pylori* has demonstrated a common core with strain-specific variable chains and the presence of Lewis antigens. Strains can be differentiated on the basis of the expression of Lewis x (Le^x) and or Lewis y (Le^y) epitopes and monoclonal antibodies against the H1 antigen. This typing scheme, however, lacks discrimination power and is rarely used.

Polyacrylamide gel electrophoresis (PAGE)

The bacteria are labelled with ^{35}S-methionine. After ^{35}S uptake in new protein synthesis, the bacteria are lysed. The lysate is then separated and the appropriate fractions subjected to PAGE, the patterns of separated proteins providing a method of typing. The proteomic pattern of 2-dimensional gel separation may also be used to cluster bacteria into clinical associations.

Multilocus enzyme electrophoresis (MLEE)

MLEE uses the relative electrophoretic mobility of a number of enzymes to subdivide bacterial isolates. The net charge on an enzyme, and therefore its mobility through a gel, is determined by the amino acid sequence of the enzyme and thus alleles (where the amino acid is different due to a mutation) can be identified. MLEE is not as discriminatory as DNA sequencing because some amino acids substitutions do not change the charge on the enzyme. In one study of 74 isolates of *Helicobacter pylori* using six housekeeping genes, 73 distinct allelic profiles were generated, emphasizing the highly polymorphic nature of the *Helicobacter* genome.

Restriction fragment length polymorphism (RFLP)

Hydrolysis of whole genomic bacterial DNA with restriction endonucleases and separation of the

Table 2.1 Typing methods and their use for *Helicobacter pylori*

		Description
Typing methods		
Phage typing		Susceptibility to different bacteriophages. Not used for *Helicobacter*.
Bacteriocine typing		Susceptibility to bacteriocines. Not used for *Helicobacter*.
Biotyping		Use of selected biochemical tests to differentiate strains. Biotyping schemes for *Helicobacter* available but limited applicability.
Serotyping		Differentiation of strains based on expression of different antigens. Scheme available for *Helicobacter* based on Lewis antigen. Limited use.
Antibiotic resistogram		Differentiation of strains based on antibiotic resistance. Limited applicability for *Helicobacter*.
Molecular methods		
Protein based	Polyacrylamide gel electrophoresis	Separation of labelled (^{35}S-methionine) or unlabelled total bacterial protein to differentiate strains. Limited applicability for *Helicobacter*.
	MLEE	Typing of strains by separation of different enzymes after gel electrophoresis. Used for genetic analysis of population and typing in *Helicobacter*. Limited use as typing method.
Genomic-based	Pulse field electrophoresis	Use of restriction endonucleases with infrequent targets to generate large DNA fragments and separation by a pulsed field (orthogonal, transverse, inversion, contour clamped). Used for *Helicobacter*.
	RFLP*	Use of restriction endonucleases with frequent targets and separation by gel electrophoresis. Used for *Helicobacter*.
PCR	Ribotyping	Use of 16S and/or 23S labelled probe after restriction endonuclease digestion of DNA, separation by gel electrophoresis and transfer to a membrane. Used for *Helicobacter*.
	rep-PCR	PCR amplification of repetitive extragenic palindromic sequence followed by gel separation. Used for *Helicobacter*.
	ERIC-PCR	PCR amplification of enterobacterial repetitive intergenic consensus sequence followed by gel separation. Used for *Helicobacter*.
	MLVA	Analysis of tandem repeat size and copy number by PCR amplified fragment length polymorphism or sequence data.
	AP-PCR/random amplified fragment length polymorphism	PCR amplification using random generated primers followed by gel electrophoresis. Used for *Helicobacter*.
Sequencing	MLST	Comparison of the DNA sequence of a set of housekeeping genes (e.g. those used in MLEE). *Helicobacter* MLST data base exists at: http://pubmlst.org/helicobacter/
	Pyrosequencing	PCR amplification of target sequence with labelled primer followed by denaturation and DNA synthesis generating adenosine triphosphate producing a chemiluminescent signal.

*Also used with PCR to amplify a target followed by restriction endonuclease, e.g. PCR amplification of ribosomal 16S, 23S or inter 16-23S spacer followed by restriction endonuclease digestion and gel electrophoresis. PCR–RFLP used for *Helicobacter* (N.B. a different ribotyping method). For explanation of abbreviations consult main text or *see* Abbreviations on page viii.

fragments by agarose gel electrophoresis can be used as a typing system for *Helicobacter pylori*. The method of typing is called bacteria restriction endonuclease analysis (BRENDA). Alternatively, a specific part of the genome can be amplified using the polymerase chain reaction and combined with restriction endonuclease analysis (RFLP). When applied to the ribosomal RNA genes it is called ribotyping. Ribotyping can also be performed using labelled probes directed against the ribosome genes following restriction endonuclease activity of whole genome DNA without PCR amplification of ribosome genes.

Several endonucleases can be used and the ones that give the optimal number of fragments that can subsequently be separated are chosen. Enzymes that are used include *Hin*dIII, *Hae*III, *Pvu*II, *Bgl*II, *Cfo*I, *Sma*I, *Ava*I, *Dra*I, *Kpm*I, *Rsa*I, *Sal*I and *Eco*RI, *Sac*I, *Xba*I, *Xho*I, *Bst*EI. When used in BRENDA, the best results were obtained with *Hin*dIII, *Sac*I and *Eco*RI.

One advantage of using PCR–RFLP is that fewer fragments are produced and thus it is easier to compare patterns and discrimination may be increased. Genes that have been used include *ureA*, *ureB*, *ureC*, *flaA* and the 23S rRNA gene.

Pulsed field gel electrophoresis

In pulse field electrophoresis the organism is lysed within a gel to minimize disruption to the genome using a restriction endonuclease that only attacks a small number of targets, which are subsequently separated using a direct current of rapidly changing polarity. This causes the DNA fragments to flex with the changing polarity and the fragments are gradually separated according to molecular size.

rep-PCR, ERIC-PCR, MLVA

Amplification of several repetitive elements (repetitive extragenic palindromic [rep] sequence, enterobacterial repetitive intergenic consensus [ERIC] sequence, and variable number of tandem repeats [VNTR]) relies on the amplification of conserved repetitive regions found at various locations within the bacterial genome of many species of bacteria, including *Helicobacter pylori*. In ERIC, as the name suggests, they were first identified in genomes of *Enterobacteriaceae*; however, they are also found in other bacterial species. Electrophoresis of PCR amplified fragments provides patterns of bands that differentiate the strains.

Random amplified fragment length polymorphism and AP-PCR

Alternatives to using a defined primer sequence for PCR, typing of *Helicobacter pylori* can also be achieved using random sequences as primers. In comparison with PCR–RFLP, different studies have demonstrated superiority for both the techniques.

Pyrosequencing

Pyrosequencing is carried out by synthesizing a complementary DNA strand by sequential addition of the four nucleotides and detecting activity of the DNA polymerase using chemiluminescence. During the reaction pyrophosphate is released and converted to adenosine triphosphate, which activates luciferase and, hence, light is emitted. This method is much more rapid than PCR sequencing but cannot currently sequence long DNA strands.

Epidemiology

It is a reasonable hypothesis that an ancestral *Helicobacter* sp. has been a colonizer of the vertebrate stomach ever since the evolutionary development of the stomach. *Helicobacter pylori* has high genetic diversity, to such an extent that most individuals are colonized by a unique strain. However, as transmission occurs by close contact within cohesive groups (e.g. families), these strains are genetically closely related. Populations of ethnically related groups also show degrees of genetic similarity within *Helicobacter pylori*. Thus, by genetic analysis of the isolates in respect of the vacuolating cytotoxin A (*vacA*) and cytotoxin-associated gene A (*cagA*) regions, the migration pattern of human populations can be followed. Polymorphisms within the leader sequence of *vacA* (s1a, s1b and s1c; *see* also Chapter 1) are predominant in different geographical regions of the world and linked to different ethnic groupings. These polymorphisms can be used as surrogate markers for human migration patterns. The s1a sequence is found mainly in North America and Europe, and relates to the flow of colonizing populations from northern Europe to North America; s1b is found mainly in Spain and South America, reflecting the colonization by southern Europeans of South America; and s1c is found mainly in the Far East.

Variation occurs in the 3′ end of the *cagA* region and, so far, four types (A–D) have been identified. In addition, the sequence in this region of the pathogenicity island varies, with one sequence being found principally in strains isolated from Western countries and one from Asian countries. Ethnicity also accounts for differences in colonization (e.g. Polynesians and European New Zealanders are colonized by genetically different strains testifying to race-specific lineages of *Helicobacter pylori*). Additionally, in the USA, ethnicity contributes to the different colonization rates between caucasian, hispanic and black people when other recognized confounding factors are taken into account. Even populations that have lived closely together for considerable periods of time can be distinguished by *Helicobacter pylori* typing. In the Himalayan region of India, where Buddists and Muslims coexist, each religio-ethnic group is colonized by a different *Helicobacter* population.

A more complete analysis of population structure of *Helicobacter pylori* from 370 strains, representing 27 geo-ethnic groupings and using 1418 polymorphic sequences, has defined five populations and subpopulations, as shown in **2.1**: Europe 1 (Europe, North Africa, Central Asia); Europe 2 (Global distribution); Africa 1 (West Africa, South Africa, North and South America);

Africa 2 (South Africa); East Asia (East Asia, New Zealand, North Canada, Amerind, Maori and East Asia subpopulations). The East Asian subpopulation is found almost exclusively in East Asian countries; the Maori subpopulation exclusively in Polynesians from New Zealand; and the Amerindian subpopulation in native North and South Americans. Apart from modern European isolates, all other isolates derived over 85% of their nucleotides from the putative ancestral type, whereas modern European isolates were an equal admixture of ancestral Europe 1 and 2 types (**2.1**).

Helicobacter pylori infects over 50% of the world population and molecular studies have shown that specific polymorphisms are located in different regions of the world and that the distribution of these polymorphisms follows known human migration patterns. Not only are different polymorphisms located in different regions of the world but the distribution of colonization by *Helicobacter pylori* is not equal within this population. Sero-epidemiological studies have identified geographical, ethnic (**2.2**) and social (**2.3**) differences associated with colonization. Two main sero-epidemiological patterns can be identified. In more developed countries (Europe, North America, Australia) the seroprevalence increases with increasing

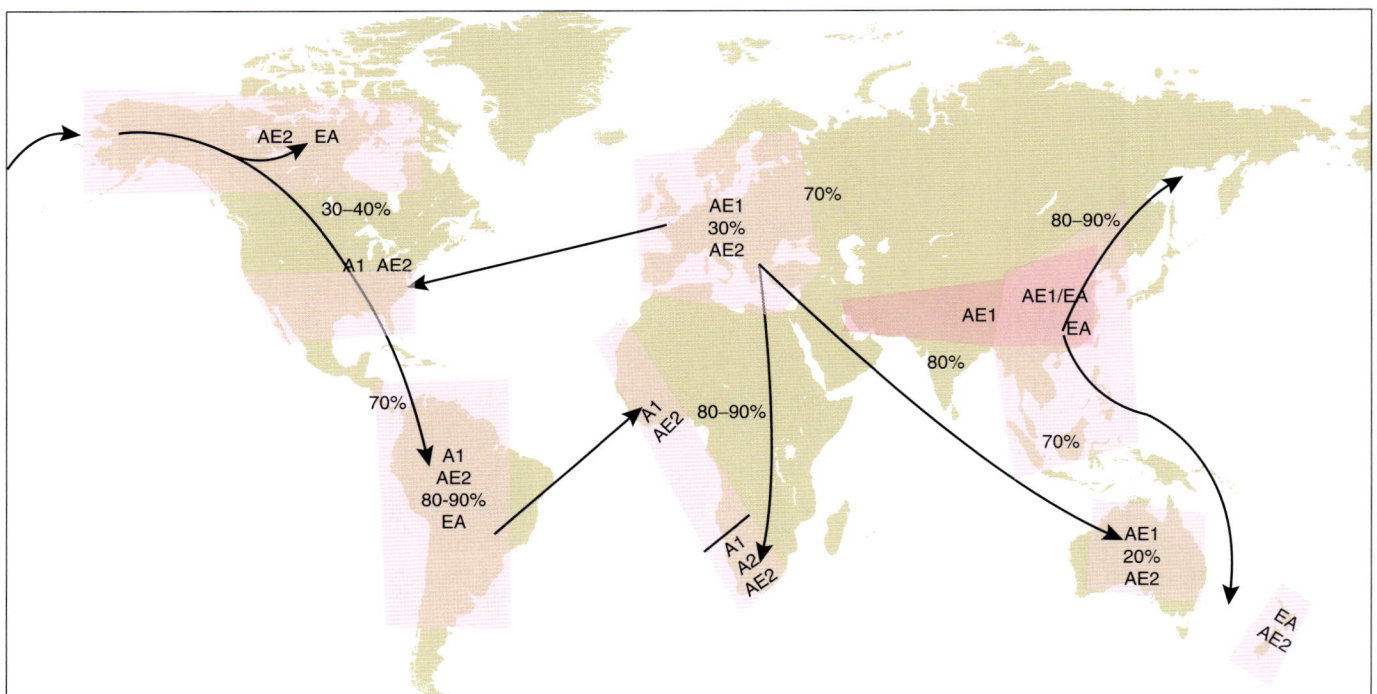

2.1 Predominant composition of ancestral *Helicobacter pylori* nucleotides in modern isolates, with suggested routes of human migration. A1 = Africa 1; A2 = Africa 2; AE1 = ancestral Europe 1; AE2 = ancestral Europe 2; EA = East Asia.

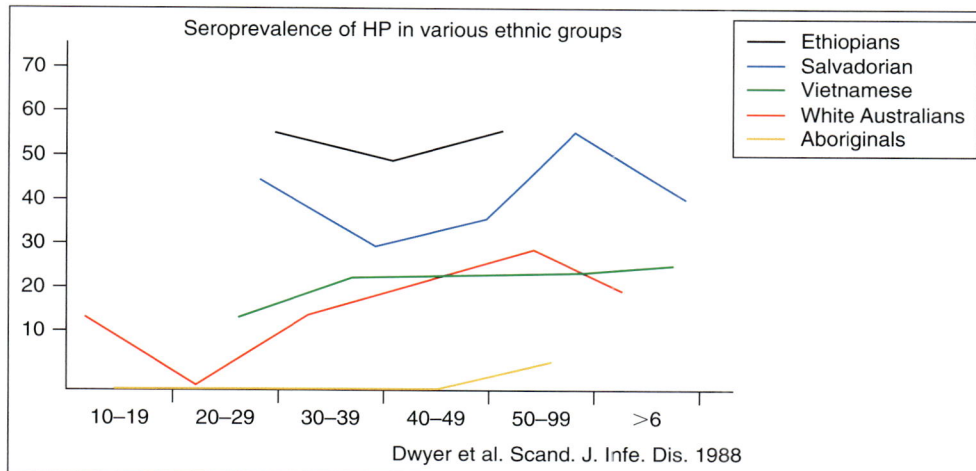

Seroprevalence of HP in various ethnic groups

Dwyer et al. Scand. J. Infe. Dis. 1988

2.2 A study from Australia indicated seroprevalence differences between different ethnic groups. Remarkably, the Aboriginals had the lowest prevalence rate, the organism being virtually absent in this racial group. Numerous other studies from different geographic locations have also demonstrated ethnic differences, which are probably partly genetic, and partly environmental, e.g., standards of public sanitation.

age, rising from about 5% in the first decade to 50–60% in the sixth decade; there is also a direct association between seroprevalence and lower social class. In less developed countries (South America, Africa, Middle and Far East), the prevalence may be as high as 60–90% (depending on the country) in the first decade with little increase with age. The distribution of *Helicobacter pylori*

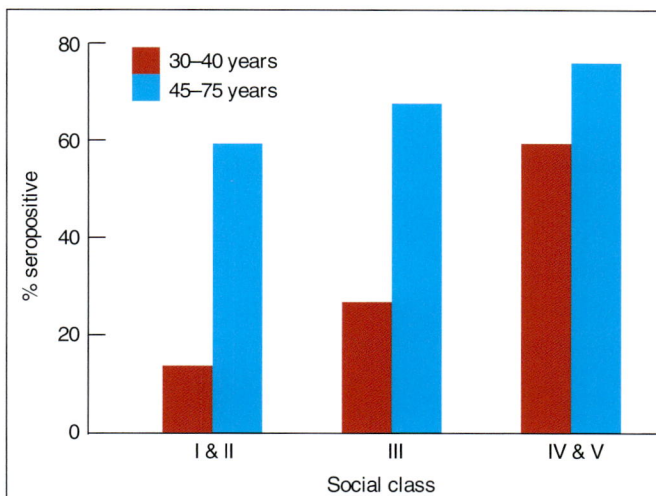

2.3 Higher social class in society equates to a lower prevalence of *Helicobacter pylori*, and vice versa. In most countries social class is a representation of education level, occupation and income. Transmission of *Helicobacter pylori* occurs in childhood and in conditions of overcrowding and poor hygiene. Conditions for the transmission of the organism occur less frequently in the higher social classes.

around the world shows that in industrialized countries the prevalence is low (about 30%) compared with less industrialized countries (about 80–90%). This variation is related to the volume of transmission, with low levels of acquisition in Europe, Australia and North America, and high levels elsewhere. Infection is acquired in childhood and age of acquisition depends upon the overall prevalence of *Helicobacter pylori* in the country. In studies on the age of seroconversion, in China the peak seroprevalence rate was at 5 y, but in Ethiopia the age of maximum seroconversion was 2–4 y, with 60% becoming seropositive by 4 y of age and virtually 100% by the age of 10 y. On the other hand, in Sweden the age of maximum seroconversion was 9–10 y, with 20% of children becoming seropositive by the age of 10 y. In Brazil, in a slightly different study, the reinfection rate in children cleared of *Helicobacter pylori* was recorded as 3.7%/month but in adults the reinfection rate was 1.1%/month indicating higher transmission occurs in children. In industrialized countries the acquisition rate is even lower with a value of 0.3–0.5%/y. These differences in age of acquisition relate to social conditions and public health infrastructure. In industrialized countries the low rate in childhood and high rate in the elderly can be explained by improving social standards of housing (with less overcrowding), potable water supplies and sewage disposal. The high rate in the elderly can be explained as a cohort effect, reflecting the housing and public health standards when they were children (**2.4**).

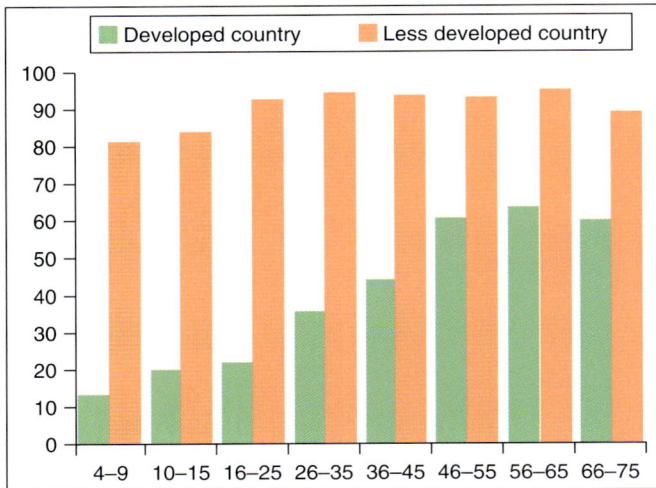

2.4 Histogram showing the age distribution for seroprevalence of *Helicobacter pylori* in developed and less developed countries.

In addition, the reinfection rate depends upon the geographical location. For adults in industrialized countries the acquisition of *Helicobacter pylori* following a previous infection is 1–2%/y. In some less industrialized areas the reinfection rate may be as high as 70%.

The source and route of infection of *Helicobacter pylori* is not known with any certainty, but there are three potential sources of infection:

1. Animals.
2. The environment.
3. Another human.

The most important source of infection is transmission from one human to another. The exact route is unknown, but the organism is usually acquired in childhood from either a parent or a sibling. The second most likely source is from the environment (contaminated water or food in the community and endoscopes in the hospital environment) but this usually only occurs in those countries with a poor public hygiene infrastructure. Acquisition of *Helicobacter pylori* from animals is probably very rare and little solid evidence supports this as a source of infection (**2.5**).

Helicobacter sp. are found in a wide range of animals (**2.6**), including land mammals, birds and cetaceans. Some evidence is suggestive of sheep as a source of *Helicobacter pylori* in humans. On the whole, however, animals as a routine source of human infection with

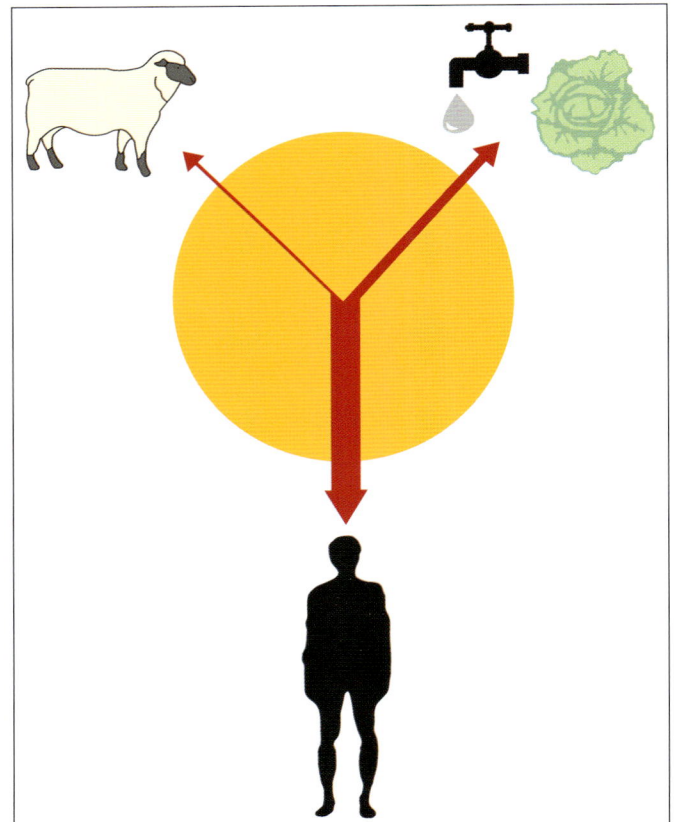

2.5 The relative importance of infection acquired from animals, the environment or directly from another human.

Helicobacter pylori is unproven, the evidence being circumstantial. Other animals, such as dogs and poultry, may be the source of infection for *Helicobacter* spp. other than *Helicobacter pylori*. Ferrets and mice, which are colonized by *Helicobacter mustelae* and *Helicobacter muridarum* respectively, have been used as animal models of infection with *Helicobacter pylori*.

There is, however, better evidence that environmental reservoirs such as contaminated water may act as a source of infection. This is based upon seroprevalence studies from Peru and Chile demonstrating an association between infection and exposure to potentially contaminated water and food supplies. Additionally, *Helicobacter pylori* can be detected in faeces; can survive in water for several days; and detection of presumed *Helicobacter pylori* DNA has been reported from sewage and drinking water, thus completing a biologically plausible route of infection. Figure **2.7** shows the possible routes of acquisition of *Helicobacter pylori* from the environment by the use of human manure,

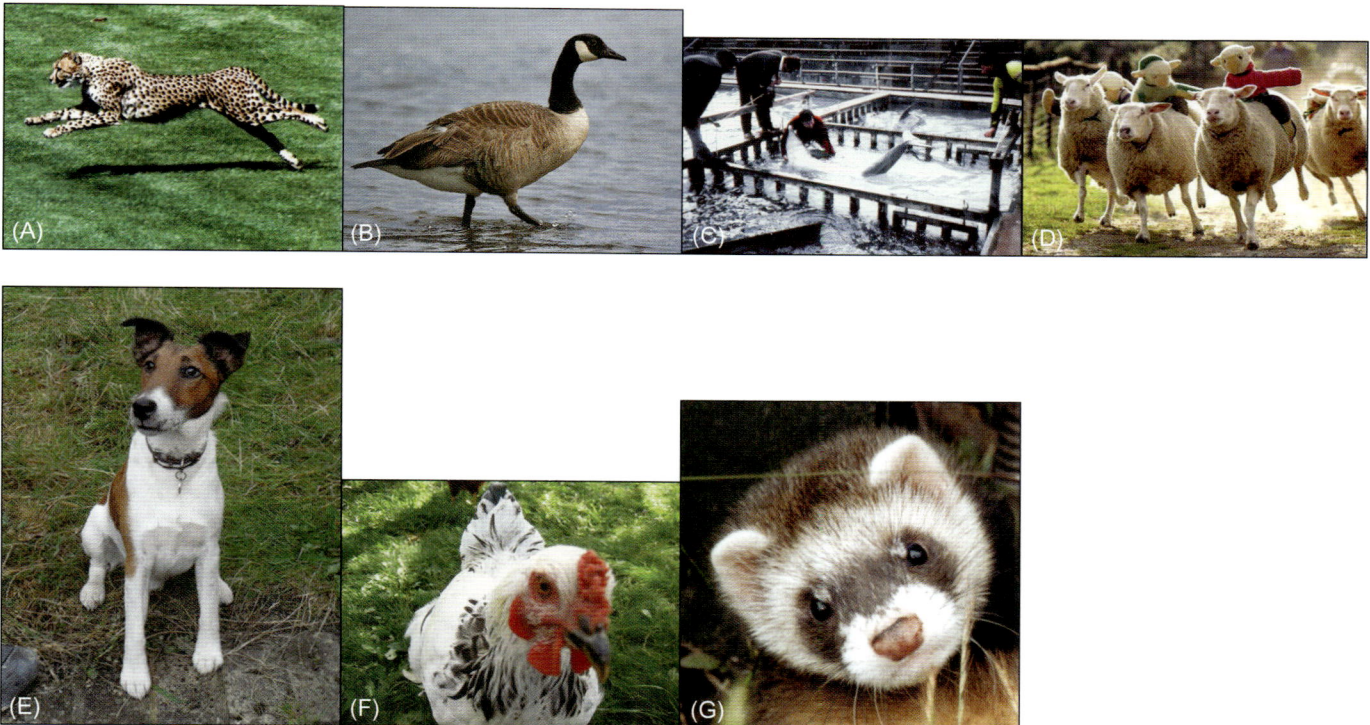

2.6 (A) Cheetah: Spiral bacteria were first seen in captive cheetahs in 1991 (one morphologically similar to *Helicobacter pylori*, the other to *Gastrospirillum hominis*). *Helicobacter acinonychis* (*acinonyx*) was isolated as a separate species from cheetahs with gastritis in 1993, and, morphologically resembles *Helicobacter pylori*. Taxonomic analysis using 16S sequence data place it closest to *Helicobacter pylori*, followed by *Helicobacter felis* and *Helicobacter mustelae*. Gastritis is common in captive cheetahs but rare in wild animals and the role of *Helicobacter acinonychis* in relation to gastritis is questionable. Although *Helicobacter acinonychis* is genetically closely related to *Helicobacter pylori*, the two hosts (i.e. *Acinonxy jubilatus* and *Homo sapiens*) are not. Vertebrate species more closely related to *Homo sapiens* are colonized by more distantly related *Helicobacter* sp., which suggests a species jump in some direction between humans and cheetahs. Genomic sequence analysis of the two *Helicobacter* sp. suggests the jump occurred about 200 000 years ago from humans to cheetahs, presumably postprandially. **(B)** Canada goose: *Helicobacter* sp. have been isolated from sea-birds (e.g. geese, terns, gulls), and land birds (e.g. sparrows). Sea-birds are also known to carry *Campylobacter*, *Salmonella*, *Aeromonas* and *Plesiomonas* spp. and may pose a zoonotic risk to humans. Contamination of European beaches with these organisms may affect the grading of the beach. A *Helicobacter* sp. isolated from gulls has been designated *Helicobacter pamatensis*. An isolated species from the European Canada goose (*Branta canadensis*) and barnacle goose (*Branta leucopsis*) has been designated *Helicobacter canadensis* and has been isolated from several cases of humans with diarrhoea. Different *Helicobacter* spp. have been isolated from 40% of a flock of 97 American Canada geese and designated *Helicobacter anseris* (from 20 geese) and *Helicobacter brantae* (from seven geese). **(C)** A dolphin being prepared for endoscopy: as part of an investigation into the seroprevalence of *Helicobacter pylori* in zoo workers, in 1986 the authors (DV, JH) attempted to isolate *Helicobacter pylori* from Smartie, a female dolphin with an ulcer. Unfortunately, the diameter of the colonoscope was too wide to pass from the first part of the dolphin's stomach into the second part and the attempt was aborted. Happily, Smartie recovered from her ulcer with one ranitidine given with the last fish at night. More recently, a dead dolphin was found on a beach in California and microbiological investigation of the stomach revealed a new species: *Helicobacter cetorum*. The seroprevalence of *Helicobacter pylori* in zoo workers and matched controls who did not have contact with zoo animals was identical. *Helicobacter* sp. similar to *Helicobacter cetorum* have also been isolated from other sea animals, including fur seals and sea lions, and other novel isolates have also been identified. **(D)** Sheep: Devon's racing rams (photo courtesy of Rick Turner). Two studies, one in Sardinian shepherds and one in Polish shepherds, have shown the shepherds are more likely to be *Helicobacter pylori* seropositive compared with matched populations (Sardinia 98% compared with 43%, Poland 97% compared with 65%, respectively) and the suggestion is that sheep may be a vehicle for transmission through consumption of their milk. *Helicobacter pylori* has been detected in 60% ($n = 63$) of milk samples and 30% ($n = 20$) of sheep gastric tissue samples by using PCR and isolation by culture. Conversely, in a study from Turkey, in 440 raw sheep milk samples, cultured *Helicobacter pylori* was not isolated. In a study from southern Italy, 400 raw milk samples from cows, sheep and goats were investigated by PCR and culture, and although *Helicobacter pylori* was detected in 34%, the cultures were negative. Only tenuous evidence supports animals as a source of infection. Original studies on the seroprevalence of

(**2.6** *continued*) *Helicobacter pylori* in abattoir workers demonstrated a higher seroprevalence in those who had contact with the animals compared with matched controls that worked in the abattoir but were not involved in animal processing. A study on vegans compared with meat-eaters did not show any difference in the seroprevalence rate. Similarly, seroprevalence of *Helicobacter pylori* is high in Muslim countries, suggesting that pigs, at least, are not a source of infection. In a study in Colombia, where contact with animals as a food source or as pets is high, there was an apparent protective effect of this contact on seroprevalence rates except for contact with sheep, where there was a higher prevalence. Evidence of animals being a source of infection derives principally from the isolation of *Helicobacter pylori* from a colony of laboratory cats. Subsequent work did not detect *Helicobacter pylori* in cats in general and cat owners are not more frequently serologically positive than non-cat owners. It is more than likely those cats were infected by humans. The most likely explanations for most of these apparent associations between seroprevalence in humans and animal contact are infection by non-pylori *Helicobacter* from the animals, albeit transient, and the cross-reaction between animal *Helicobacter* sp. and antigens of *Helicobacter pylori* used in the assay. (**E**) Dog: several *Helicobacter* sp. have been isolated from the canine (and feline) stomach and reported in various studies: *Helicobacter cynogastricus, Helicobacter bizzozeronii, Helicobacter felis, Helicobacter canis, Helicobacter salomonis, Helicobacter baculiformis, Helicobacter bilis, Helicobacter cinaedi* and *Helicobacter heilmannii*. None of these species appear to be related to either gastritis or diarrhoea in the animals. *Helicobacter canis* is most closely related *Helicobacter cinaedi* and *Helicobacter fennelliae*, both recognized pathogens of humans. *Helicobacter felis, Helicobacter bizzozeronii, Helicobacter heilmannii* type I and *Helicobacter salmonis* form another closely related, morphologically distinct group. In addition to *Helicobacter pylori*, bacteria with a morphology similar to *Helicobacter heilmannii* (large spiral shaped) have been found in association with gastritis, peptic ulcer, mucosal-associated lymphoid tissue lymphoma and bacteraemia in humans. The organisms have been identified in various studies as *Helicobacter bizzozeronii, Helicobacter felis, Helicobacter salomonis, Helicobacter suis* and "*Candidatus* Helicobacter heilmannii". Overall, such organisms represent about 0.1–2.0% of all cases, and in a study of over 500 Bulgarian children, *Helicobacter heilmannii* occurred in 0.3% of cases. Infections are likely to be acquired after close contact with animals, particularly domestic pets. A questionnaire study of 177 patients with *Helicobacter heilmannii* compared with 485 patients with *Helicobacter pylori* infection demonstrated an epidemiological link between infection and close contact with either dogs, cats, cattle or pigs. Case reports also implicate close contact with dogs as the source and in some cases the pet was examined and the same organism isolated from the canine stomach as the patient. (**F**) Poultry: *Helicobacter pullorum* is found in 60–100% of chickens as part of their normal flora but has also been isolated from the liver of chickens with evidence of hepatitis. It has also been detected in human cases of gastroenteritis, bacteraemia and hepatitis, particularly in association with hepatitis C virus infection. A study of 531 patients with gastroenteritis compared with 100 asymptomatic individuals demonstrated *Helicobacter pullorum* in 4.3% of symptomatic patients and 4% of healthy individuals, raising questions of its pathological aetiology in this context. Additionally, *Helicobacter pullorum* (and *Helicobacter canadensis*), if detected in intestinal biopsies, has been associated with cases of Crohn's disease compared with controls (odds ratio [OR] 2.88), raising further questions of their aetiological significance. So far, an epidemiological link between gastroenteritis associated with *Helicobacter pullorum* and contact with chickens is lacking. (**G**) Ferret: these are naturally colonized by *Helicobacter mustelae*. Although not a recorded source of infection, ferrets are used as an animal model of human infections with *Helicobacter pylori* for investigating pathophysiological mechanisms, therapeutic regimens and the development of vaccines. Ferrets also develop mucosal-associated lymphoid tissue lymphoma and gastric adenocarcinoma after natural infection with *Helicobacter mustelae* and thus provide a useful model for studying the pathogenesis and treatment of these conditions. Such models have helped us to understand the normal physiological defence mechanisms of the stomach, pathological processes following infection with *Helicobacter*, and the action of non-steroidal anti-inflammatory drugs. Other animals used to study *Helicobacter pylori* pathogenesis and treatment are mice, monkeys, pigs and Mongolian gerbils, the latter particularly in relation to the development of gastric cancer.

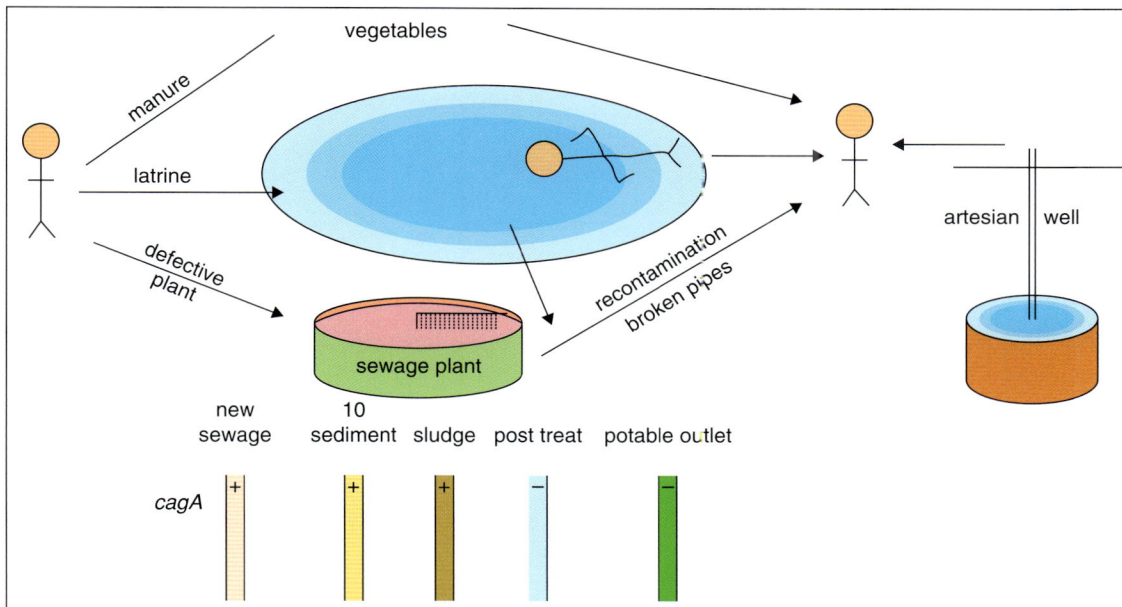

2.7 Potential environmental routes of *Helicobacter pylori* transmission.

swimming in contaminated rivers, consumption of contaminated vegetables, inadequate sewage treatment and contaminated water from artesian wells. The figure also illustrates the presence of *Helicobacter pylori* at various stages during sewage treatment by the detection of *cagA* using PCR undertaken by one of the authors (JH: unpublished).

There is more evidence that contaminated water may act as a source of infection. In South America, some seroprevalence studies have shown that individuals using the municipal water source are more likely to be positive than those using an artesian well. This suggests that faecally contaminated public water in some countries may be a risk for colonization. In a study in Colombia of children aged <10 y, consumption of raw vegetables, drinking water from a stream and swimming in a river were risk factors for colonization by *Helicobacter pylori*. Similar studies in Peru and Chile demonstrated that a piped municipal water source was a risk factor (OR 12.0), along with consumption of raw vegetables probably irrigated with human sewage (OR 3.0). However, in China, consumption of water known to be contaminated by faecal organisms was not a risk factor for colonization by *Helicobacter pylori*. These apparently conflicting results may be explained by co-variables that may not have been taken into account in the studies. The suggestion that raw vegetables or

environmental water could act as a source of infection is supported by survival of *Helicobacter pylori* in artificially contaminated food or water for days, or even months if refrigerated. The organism survives and can be cultured only for a relatively short time (a few hours) but can still be detected, using PCR, after some months. The organism changes into a viable but non-culturable coccoid form. In addition, the detection of *Helicobacter pylori* DNA by PCR from streams and water distribution systems adds credence to environmental sources for *Helicobacter pylori*. Whether this coccoid form can act as an infectious form or whether it is a degenerate form is still open to debate. Additionally, experiments showed that *Helicobacter pylori* can survive on the surface and in the gastrointestinal tract of flies that had been artificially contaminated. However, there is no convincing evidence that flies act as a vector for the transmission of *Helicobacter pylori*.

The most likely source of infection is from another infected human with acquisition occuring in childhood. Under natural circumstances, transmission could be by either of two routes: oral–oral or faecal–oral. It is worth pointing out, however, that there may be multiple routes of transmission, which may vary in importance according to geographic and socio-demographic factors. Several risk factors have been identified as contributing to infection with *Helicobacter pylori* (*Table 2.2*).

Table 2.2 Risk factors associated with *Helicobacter pylori* infection in the human

Increased risk of infection	No effect on risk of infection
Living in an institution	Sexual contact
Member of a submarine crew	Sex (gender)
Living in military barracks	Smoking
Attending a daycare centre	Alcohol consumption
Birth order	Occupation as a dentist
Number of siblings	
Sharing a bed with a sibling	
Lack of hot water supply	
Social class as a child	
Educational level	
Occupation as an endoscopist	

Sero-epidemiological studies have identified socio-economic and demographic factors which indicate that close personal contact is important in the transmission cycle and that infection most commonly happens in childhood. These demographic factors, such as social class (higher in Social Class IV and V compared with I and II) reflect the childhood living conditions and overcrowding in areas of social deprivation with poor public hygiene infrastructure. Two factors that are strongly correlated with seropositivity are lack of a fixed hot water supply and domestic overcrowding in childhood. During childhood, risk factors for acquisition of *Helicobacter pylori* have been reported in some studies to include: number of siblings in the household, birth order, sharing a bed with a sibling, and having a father of low socio-economic status. Additional evidence that overcrowding is important in the transmission of *Helicobacter pylori* derives from sero-epidemiological studies of institutions such as orphanages, psychiatric institutions, military barracks, submarine crews and families, which all support a role of person-to-person transmission of *Helicobacter pylori* facilitated by social overcrowding and lack of social hygiene. Studies of seropositivity of *Helicobacter pylori* in adults demonstrate that higher colonization rates were associated with low educational level and low socio-economic class, but no correlation was noted with alcohol consumption or smoking.

Helicobacter pylori has been detected in oral secretions, gastric juice and faeces. Several studies have investigated the presence of *Helicobacter pylori* in oral secretions and dental plaque. The results have been contradictory, with some studies demonstrating 100% colonization while other studies could not detect the organism. Similarly, while *Helicobacter pylori* has been cultured from faeces (in Africa), other studies have been unable to culture the organism. *Helicobacter pylori* DNA can, however, be detected in faeces, although the role of faeces in transmission has not been confirmed. The opportunity for transmission occurring under conditions of overcrowding would be high if this were associated with an absence of basic hygienic standards, as may happen in childhood, or if there were a lack of adequate sanitary facilities. There is no strong evidence to support either the oral or faecal route as the primary one and both may be relevant depending on other factors. Although the oral route (via oral secretions or vomit) is a more direct one and is consistent with direct person-to-person transmission, the faecal route may, in addition to direct faecal–oral spread occurring within a family unit, be spread indirectly via faecally-contaminated food or water from a contaminated river source. Several studies on the seroprevalence of *Helicobacter pylori* in dentists do not support infection from contamination by oral secretions, but a prospective longitudinal study examining the seroconversion rate over a 6-year period indicates that being a dental professional carries a relative risk (RR) of infection of 2.6. Other seroprevalence studies have tried to link the seroprevalence of *Helicobacter pylori* to that of known faecally transmitted organisms, such as hepatitis

A and *Giardia* sp. Although conflicting results have been reported, most studies did not show an association and, by implication, did not support a faecal–oral route of transmission.

A mathematical model representing the transmission of *Helicobacter pylori* that is linked to the known trends of peptic ulcer disease and gastric cancer, and taking into account susceptibility, age and disease progression, indicates that the transmission of *Helicobacter pylori* has over time decreased to such an extent that it may disappear naturally within the next century. A model incorporating the various potential sources and routes of transmission of *Helicobacter pylori* suggests that the decline in transmission in industrialized countries is largely due to the elimination of environmental reservoirs by enhanced public hygiene infrastructure in these countries. The consequence of the loss of these environmental reservoirs is to eliminate direct transmission from the environment and to diminish the pool of genetic material and, hence, microbial diversity by horizontal transfer of DNA. Finally, a longitudinal study has demonstrated that type I strains (*cagA* positive) are becoming less frequent in the younger age groups, which can be interpreted as an evolutionary change in *Helicobacter pylori* to a more commensal existence with loss of virulence properties.

Colonization and persistence

Helicobacter pylori enters the body via the mouth. A number of virulence characteristics are specifically linked to the ability to colonize the stomach. Once in the stomach, *Helicobacter pylori* can only survive for a short time before it is killed by the acid. The bacterial enzymes urease, carbonic anhydrase and superoxide dismutase are important in maintaining viability of *Helicobacter pylori* during its brief residence in the stomach lumen. The enzyme urease is important in regulating the periplasmic pH of *Helicobacter pylori* and along with periplasmic carbonic anhydrase, which converts the CO_2 (produced from the hydrolysis of urea by urease) to HCO_3 thus maintaining viability of the organism. This buffering capacity allows sufficient time for *Helicobacter pylori* to penetrate the mucus layer where it remains or localizes at the surface of the gastric epithelial cell. The spiral shape, motility, production of phospholipases and production of NH_4^+ by urease all contribute to colonization. The physical attributes of shape and motility facilitate penetration of the viscous mucus layer protecting the epithelial cells; the phospholipase and NH_4^+ affect the tertiary structure of the mucus, making it thin and watery allowing the *Helicobacter* to penetrate the mucus layer very quickly. Superoxide dismutase will protect the organism from peroxide radicals during the inflammatory response.

Helicobacter pylori can only adhere to mucins and gastric tissue, which is found in the stomach or as islands of gastric metaplasia in the first part of the duodenum. Binding to mucins is dependent on the mucin type, charge and pH. Many adhesins have been identified, but the principal adhesin is BabA, which binds to the Lewis b blood group antigen (Le^b) expressed on gastric tissue. Sialyl Le^b (SLe^b) is expressed during inflammation and binds to SabA (**2.8**). The best characterized adhesin for *Helicobacter pylori* is BabA – a 75 kDa adhesion molecule that mediates the attachment of *Helicobacter pylori* to SLe^b (α-1,3/4-difucosylated) blood group antigens on human gastric epithelial cells. Although three *bab* alleles have been identified (*babA1*, *babA2* and *babB*), only the *babA2* gene product is necessary for Le^b binding activity. The gene *babA1* has a small deletion and is silent (i.e., not normally expressed) but is important in recombining with *babA2* and is involved in the meta-stability of expression (and therefore binding) of BabA. Mutation in the *babA2* gene leads to loss of binding in human gastric tissue as well as α-1,3/4-fucosyltransferase-expressing transgenic mice. In addition to BabA, the SabA protein, is important for adhesion. SabA is encoded by the *sabA* gene of *Helicobacter pylori* and was found to interact with the sialylated Le^x antigen (SLe^x), which is expressed after chronic inflammation induced by the *Helicobacter pylori* flora adherent to BabA. The proportion of *sabA* carrying strains differs between population groups. In Taiwan, for instance, *Helicobacter pylori* isolates are 100% BabA-positive, but only 31% of them express SabA. On average, SabA adhesin is present in about 40% of *Helicobacter pylori* strains and is subjected to phase variation. The interaction between gastric SLe^x and SabA of *Helicobacter pylori* determines the colonization density of patients who do not express gastric Le^b or who express it weakly. Other adhesins, including AlpA, AlpB and HopZ have also been identified. Le^b expression in children is reduced compared with adults and other

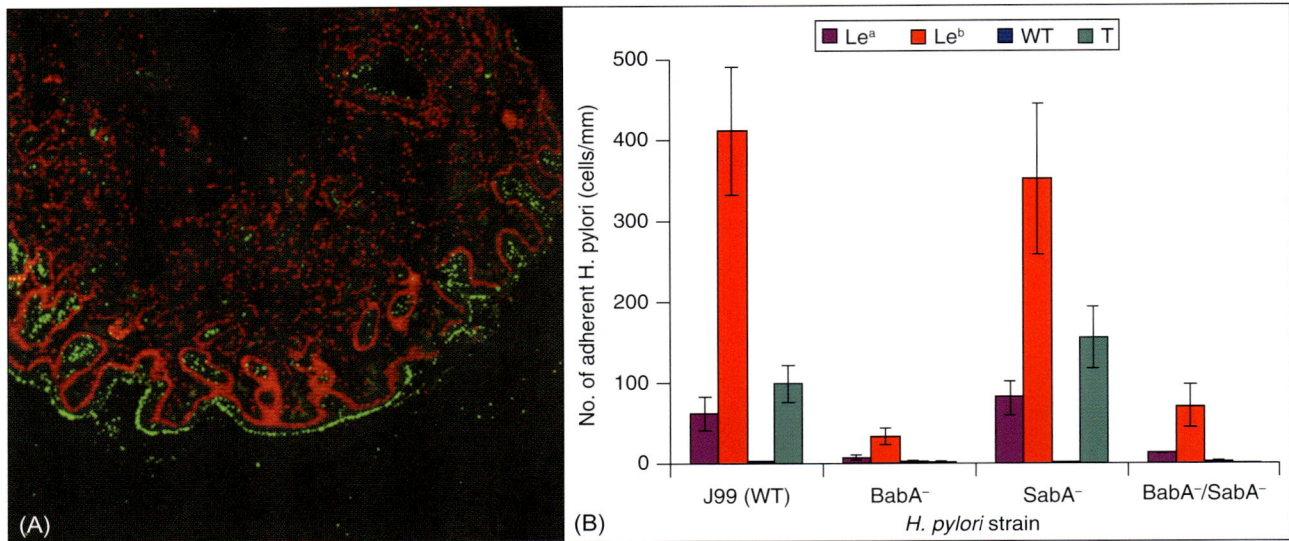

2.8 (A) Section of human stomach showing adhesion of fluorescein isothiocyanate-labelled *Helicobacter pylori.* (B) Histogram showing the relative binding of *Helicobacter pylori* adhesin mutants to human and animal stomach sections. J99(WT) = strain lacking mutant *babA*, *sabA* or both mutations; T = transgenic mouse; WT = wild-type mouse.

adhesions may be important. The organism only binds to specific cell types (i.e. surface mucosal cells but not neck or parietal cells). The organism is found mainly in the antrum of the stomach but can spread to all parts of the stomach. The location of inflammation and resultant pathological changes have a bearing upon the clinical outcome (**2.9**). *Helicobacter pylori* is found principally in the antrum of the stomach and first part of the duodenum, where it is associated with duodenal ulcer formation and a high level of stomach acid. When the organism spreads to the fundus of the stomach, giving rise to a pan-gastritis, stomach acid is reduced and this is associated with gastric ulcer and cancer. The majority of infections, however, remain asymptomatic.

Genetic analysis of isolates from a single individual demonstrate a diversity that can either represent infection with multiple isolates or the micro-evolution of a single infecting strain. Molecular studies of whole genome micro-array data of independent isolates from the same individual have demonstrated that a high degree of heterogeneity exists in closely related strains, suggesting that infection occurs not by a single strain but by a multiple of closely related strains. The average divergence reported from several studies occurs in 4–7 loci. Additionally, however, studies of experimentally infected volunteers could not demonstrate any divergence over a relatively short period of about three

months, although evidence for micro-evolution over longer time periods does exist.

The polymorphism that exists both within the host and the bacterium for Lewis antigen expression allows a mathematical model to be developed for phenotypic

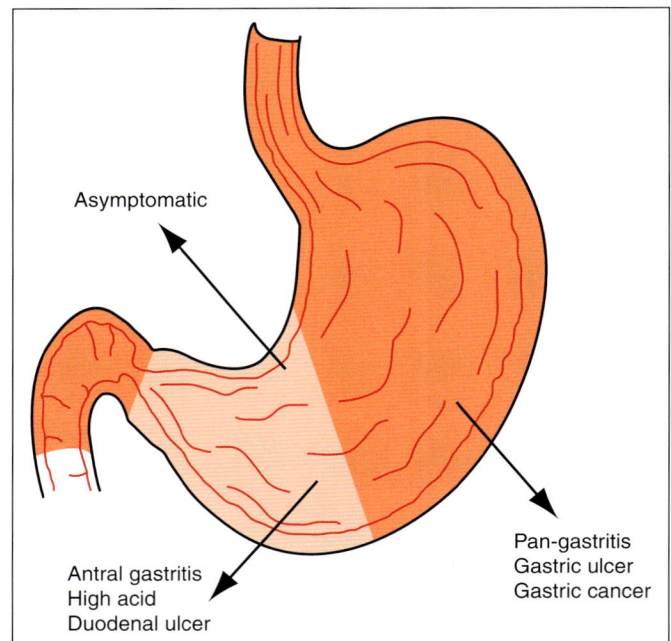

2.9 Regions of the stomach colonized by *Helicobacter pylori* and clinical outcome.

evolution during infection. It is hypothesized that, because of variable expression of Lewis antigens in the infecting strain, this is a characteristic amenable to selection by the host, which may have significance for topographical localization of different clades within the stomach or even differences in clinical outcome. The dynamics of this host–pathogen interaction can be expressed by a further mathematical model invoking microbial populations within the mucus layer and on the epithelial cell surface, and feedback systems of nutrient and effector concentration. This model can explain the steady state, microbe loss, competition and transient perturbation, and also affirm the importance of adhesion. The latter clearly implies that interference with microbial adhesion would be a suitable target for therapeutic agents.

Although *Helicobacter pylori* is regarded as a surface pathogen, it can also be found in an intracellular location (**2.10**). Several studies have demonstrated the presence *in vivo* of *Helicobacter pylori* in an intracellular location in gastric epithelial cells; that the integrity of the organism is maintained within this location; and that it is viable as confirmed by the presence of *Helicobacter pylori* mRNA.

The organism is also taken up by macrophages, and evidence of the organism can be found in regional lymph nodes localized to macrophages or dendritic cells. The organism has also been detected *in vitro* in epithelial cell monolayers and it has been demonstrated that the organism can penetrate and transit across an epithelial cell monolayer or repopulate the epithelial surface again. Analysis of the genome of *Helicobacter pylori* has further indicated that it possesses genes, homologous to those in known intracellular pathogens, that are involved in the invasion process (e.g. *invA*, which has 40% homology with *Salmonella typhi invA*). Similar homologues have also been identified for other genes important in intracellular survival (e.g. the superoxide dismutase of *Helicobacter pylori* has considerable sequence homology with that of *Coxiella* and *Legionella*). The clinical significance of these findings is unclear but it may be a way for the organism to be sequestered during chemotherapy and, in some cases, to be linked to relapses.

Further reading

Azevedo NF, Guimaraes N, Figueiredo C, Keevil CW, Vieira MJ. A new model for the transmission of *Helicobacter pylori*: role of environmental reservoirs as gene pools to increase strain diversity. *Crit Rev Microbiol* 2007; 33: 157–69.

Begue RE, Gonzales JL, Correa-Gracian H, Tang SC. Dietary risk factors associated with the transmission of *Helicobacter pylori* in Lima Peru. *Am J Trop Med Hyg* 1998; 59: 637–40.

Colding H, Hartzen SH, Roshanisefat H, Andersen LP, Krogfelt KA. Molecular methods for typing *Helicobacter pylori* and their applications. *FEMS Immunol Med Microbiol* 1999; 24: 193–9.

Falush D, Wirth T, Linz B, *et al*. Traces of human migration in *Helicobacter pylori* populations. *Science* 2003; 299: 1582–5.

Nayak AK, Rose JB. Detection of *Helicobacter pylori* in sewage and water using a new quantitative PCR method with SYBR green. *J Appl Microbiol* 2007; 103: 1931–41.

Parsonnet J, Shmuely H, Haggerty T. Faecal and oral shedding of *Helicobacter pylori* from healthy infected adults. *JAMA* 1999; 282: 2240–5.

Sachs G, Kraut JA, Wen Y, Feng J, Scott DR. Urea transport in bacteria: acid acclimation by gastric *Helicobacter* spp. *J Memb Biol* 2006; 212: 71–82.

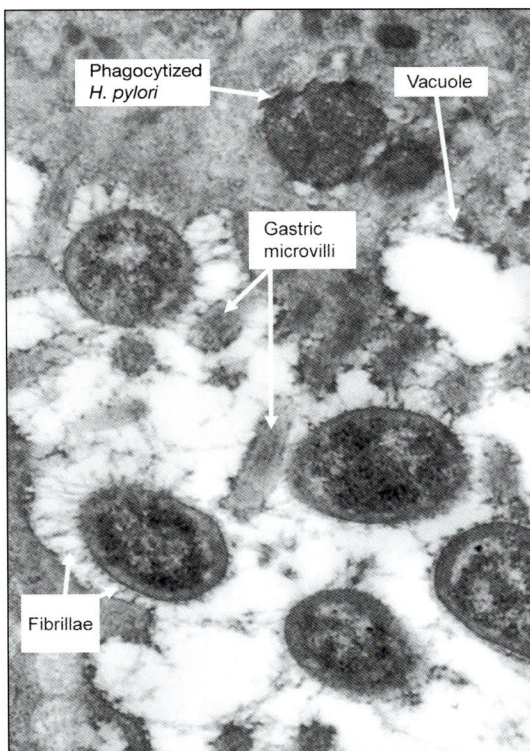

2.10 Electron micrograph of intracellular *Helicobacter pylori*.

Weyermann M, Rothenbacher D, Brenner H. Aquisition of *Helicobacter pylori* infection in early childhood: independent contributions of infected mothers, fathers and siblings. *Am J Gastroenterol* 2009; 104: 182–9.

Whary MT, Fox JG. Natural and experimental *Helicobacter* infections. *Comp Med* 2004; 54: 128–58.

Yamaoka Y. Roles of *Helicobacter pylori* BabA in gastroduodenal pathogenesis. *World J Gastroenterol* 2008; 14: 4265–72.

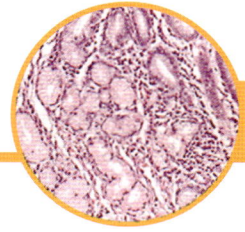

Chapter 3

Clinical features

Anatomy of the oesophagus and stomach

The oesophagus is a muscular tube connecting the pharynx to the stomach, the proximal margin of which is the upper oesophageal sphincter. The oesophagus extends distally for 18–26 cm within the posterior mediastinum as a hollow muscular tube to the lower oesophageal sphincter (**3.1**), which is a focus of tonically contracted, thickened, circular smooth muscle 2–4 cm long, that lies within the diaphragmatic hiatus.

The stomach is a dilated sac continuous with the oesophagus at the proximal end and the first part of the duodenum at the distal end. It acts as both a reservoir for food and a digestive organ. From the outside toward the lumen, the stomach wall (**3.2**) consists of three main layers: muscle, submucosa and mucosa comprising muscularis mucosae, lamina propria and epithelium. The external muscular layer (muscularis externa) comprises outer longitudinal, middle circular and inner oblique layers of muscle covered by the serosa. Beneath this muscle layer is the submucosa consisting of connective tissue (collagen and elastin fibres, blood vessels and nerve plexus). Beneath this is the muscularis mucosae comprising: a thin layer of circular and longitudinal muscle fibres; the lamina propria, a connective tissue framework supporting the gastric glands and consisting of collagen, nerves, capillaries and lymphoid tissue; and, finally, the surface epithelial layer, which is principally columnar epithelial cells with mucus-secreting cells and other specialized secretory cells.

The epithelial layer is invaginated to form gastric glands that open on to the lumen surface as gastric pits.

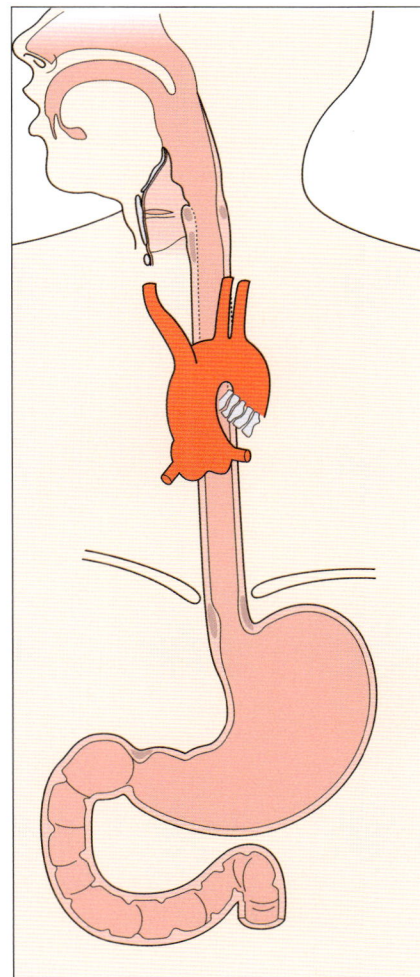

3.1 Anatomy of the stomach. Owing to its shape it has a greater and lesser curvature. The inner surface of the stomach is covered in folds called rugae, which when distended flatten out to a smooth surface.

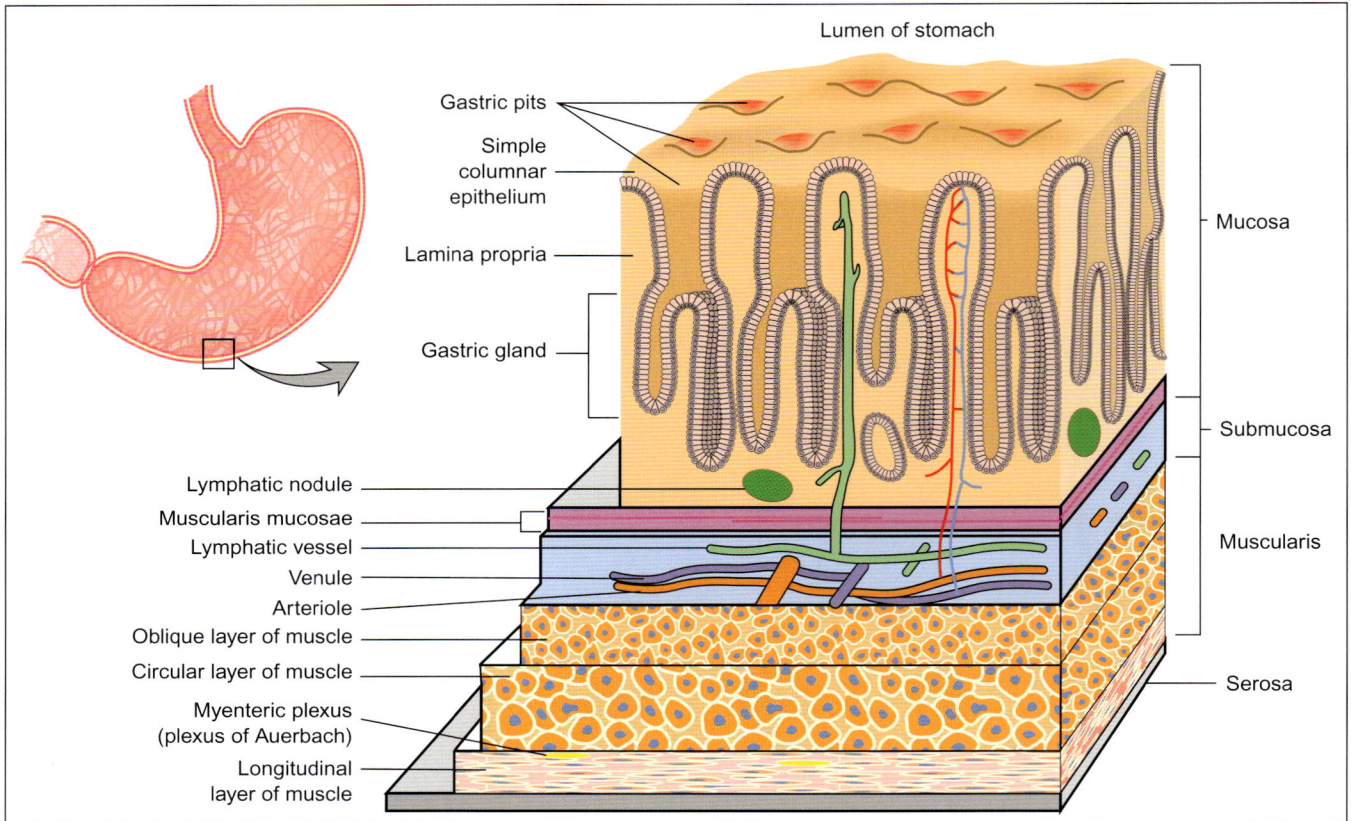

3.2 Structure of the stomach wall.

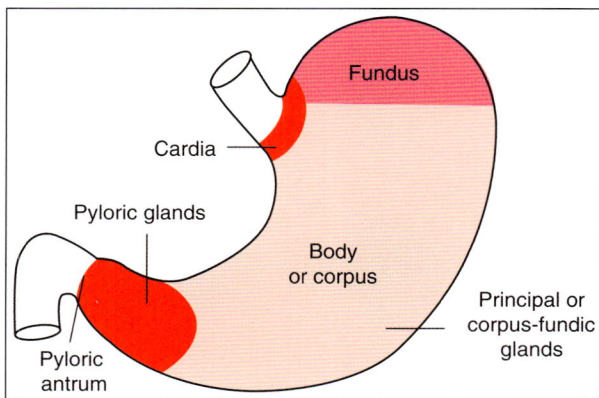

3.3 Regions of the stomach. The stomach is divided into the cardia (containing the cardiac glands), body, fundus, antrum and the pylorus as indicated. The gastric glands vary in histology according to the region of the stomach.

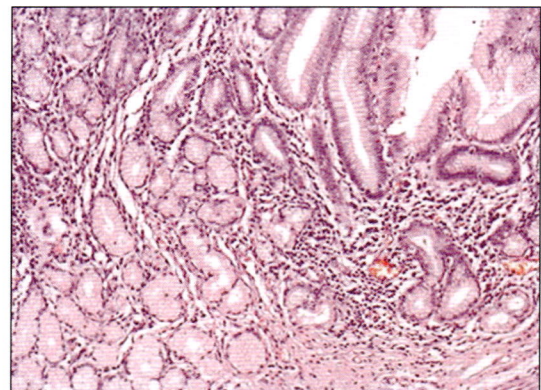

3.4 Cardiac glands. Cardiac glands are simple tubular glands that may also branch and consist of mucus-secreting cells.

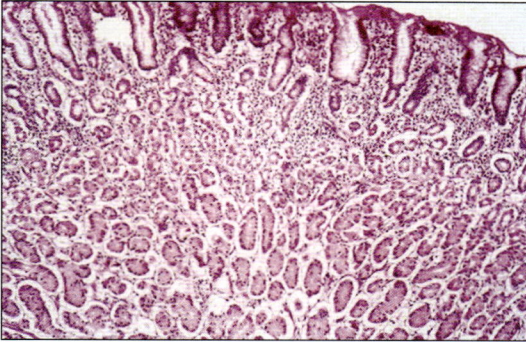

3.5 Fundic glands. These glands are found in the body and fundus of the stomach. They have three regions: a deep base, a neck region and an upper isthmus region opening into the gastric pits. They consist of five types of cells: mucous neck cells; chief cells, which are the most numerous and secrete pepsinogen; parietal (oxyntic) cells, which are found deeper in the glands and secrete hydrochloric acid and intrinsic factor; neuroendocrine cells, which are scattered in all areas of the gland and secrete gastrin (G cells), somatostatin (D cells), vasoactive intestinal peptide (VIP) cells and enterochromaffin cells secreting serotonin; and stem cells, the least numerous, which are undifferentiated cells replenishing the other cell types every 3–4 days.

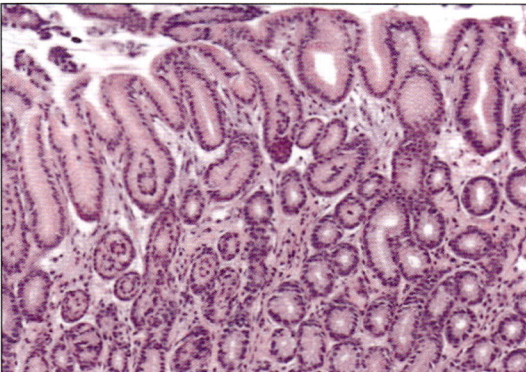

3.6 Pyloric glands. These glands are coiled rather than straight and consist principally of mucus-secreting cells and G cells with very few parietal cells. Several open on to deep gastric pits.

The arrangement of the gastric glands varies according to the region of the stomach (**3.3**, **3.4**, **3.5**, **3.6**).

Intragastric conditions

Peptic ulcer disease

An association between *Helicobacter pylori* and gastritis was first noted by Warren in 1983 and the suggestion

was made that *Helicobacter pylori* (then designated as *Campylobacter*) may be the causal agent of both gastritis and ulceration. It is now recognized that *Helicobacter pylori* is the major causal factor for peptic ulcer disease. Most persons colonized by *Helicobacter pylori* will remain symptom free. About 20% will go on to develop peptic ulcer disease. *Helicobacter pylori* is the principal cause of peptic ulcer disease (gastric or duodenal ulcer), the other major cause being consumption of non-steroidal anti-inflammatory drugs (NSAIDs). Following on from the original observations of Warren, then Warren and Marshall, many studies have demonstrated an association between the presence of duodenal or gastric ulcer and colonization by *Helicobacter pylori*. The prevalence of *Helicobacter pylori* in cases of peptic ulcer disease is over 90%. Failure to detect *Helicobacter pylori* either by histology, culture or polymerase chain reaction (PCR) can be accounted for by the patchy distribution in the stomach. Other confounding factors that may mitigate detection of the organism in gastric ulcer disease may be the presence of gastric atrophy or the development of areas of intestinal metaplasia, both of which can lead to loss of binding sites and therefore loss of the organism.

The principal lines of evidence supporting a causal role for *Helicobacter pylori* in peptic ulcer disease are:

1. The statistical correlation by the presence of the organism and disease.
2. Self-inoculation: although this only relates the development of inflammation and not ulceration.
3. The use of animal models that mimic human disease, particularly the Mongolian gerbil or the rhesus monkey. Additionally, other *Helicobacter* spp. associated with other animals lead to similar clinical presentation of inflammation and ulceration.
4. Biologically plausible mechanisms of disease production.
5. The effect of eradication of *Helicobacter pylori*.

The causal link between *Helicobacter pylori* and peptic ulceration is supported by the correlation between eradication of *Helicobacter pylori* using antibiotics and the resolution of ulceration, and the correlation between the relapse rate of ulceration and eradication of the organism. In 100 patients who were given only antibiotics the ulcer healing rate was 100% at 3 months compared with 63% for a control group. Ulcer healing occurred in 87% of those that had the *Helicobacter* eradicated compared with 42% in which eradication was unsuccessful. Successful eradication of *Helicobacter pylori* is strongly correlated with a low ulcer relapse rate. Several studies have confirmed this association. After a follow-up period of 1 y, in 39 patients in whom *Helicobacter pylori* was not eradicated, 86% had gastritis and 76% had an ulcer relapse; this compared with 10 patients in whom *Helicobacter* had been eradicated, where none had gastritis and only one patient relapsed. In a similar study, 3% of 69 patients relapsed after eradication of the organism compared with 16% of 36 patients in whom *Helicobacter pylori* had not been eradicated. In a study of 169 asymptomatic blood donors followed up for 10 y, the presence of *Helicobacter pylori* was strongly correlated to the incidence of dyspeptic symptoms and peptic ulcer disease (1.839/100 person years) compared with *Helicobacter* negative subjects (0.163/100 person years) ($P = 0.003$) (**3.7**).

Cancer

The International Agency for Research on Cancer published a monograph in 1994 identifying *Helicobacter pylori* as a class I carcinogen, linking long-term colonization by *Helicobacter pylori* as the principal cause of distal gastric adenocarcinoma (**3.8**) and mucosal associated lymphoid tissue (MALT) lymphoma (**3.9**). The Laurén system of classification for gastric cancer divides it into intestinal or diffuse—the former relates to environmental factors such as salted fish, alcohol consumption and smoking, while the diffuse type has a primary genetic basis due to E-cadherin mutations. Several studies have demonstrated an association between colonization with *Helicobacter pylori* and distal gastric adenocarcinoma. Long-term colonization by

Helicobacter pylori increases the risk of developing gastric cancer about sixfold. Despite the current decline in the prevalence of *Helicobacter pylori*, it still remains a common carcinoma globally. *Helicobacter pylori* is epidemiologically associated with both intestinal and diffuse types; the intestinal histological type because

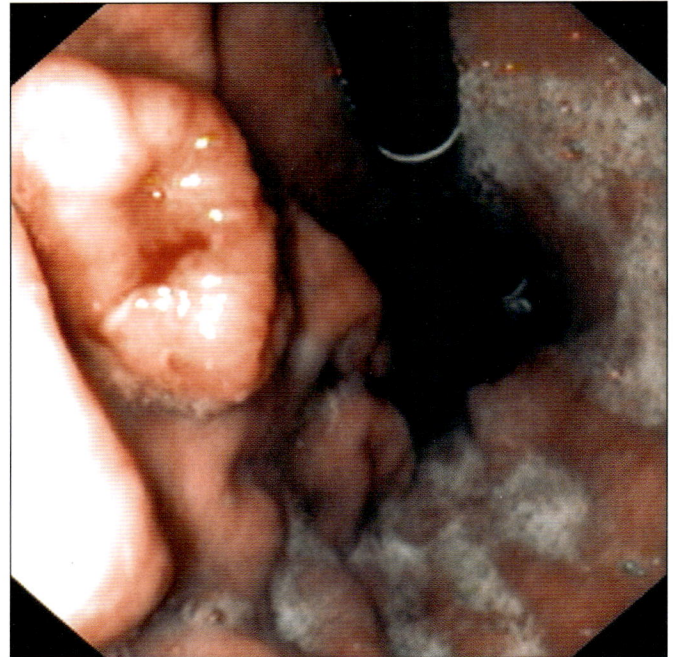

3.8 Endoscopic appearance of gastric adenocarcinoma.

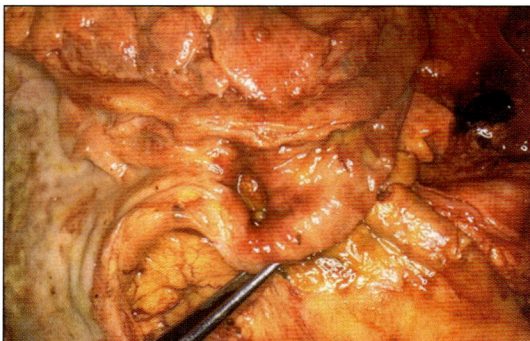

3.7 Macroscopic view of a peptic ulcer.

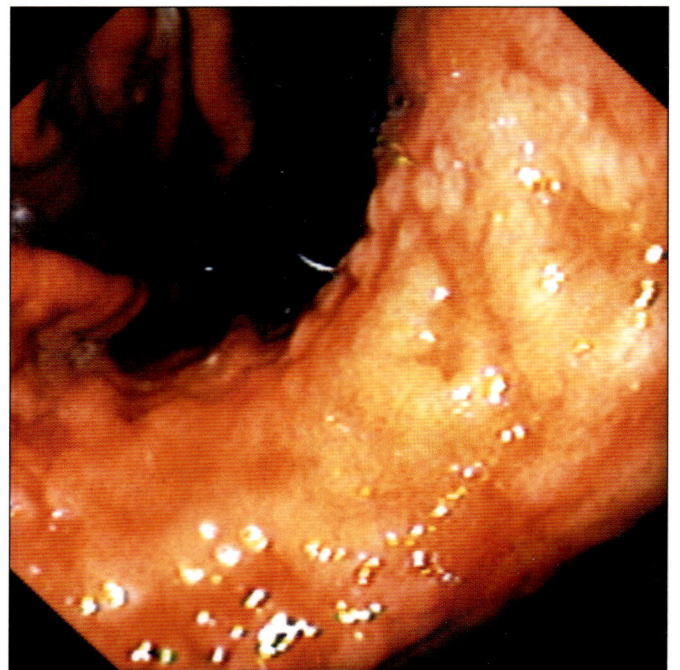

3.9 Endoscopic appearance of MALT lymphoma.

of gastric atrophy induced by the organism, the diffuse histological type by reason of the inflammation induced by *Helicobacter pylori*. Gastric cancer of the cardia is of two types: one associated with *Helicobacter pylori* and gastric atrophy, the second not associated with gastric atrophy or *Helicobacter pylori* and more akin to oesophageal carcinoma.

Gastric cancer occurs more frequently in people of low socio-economic class and there are geographical variations in rates of gastric cancer, with low rates in Europe and high rates in Japan, Korea, China and South America. Geographical variation in severity of gastric atrophy showed the highest scores in Japan and the lowest in Europe, which correlated with prevalence of gastric cancer. Populations known to be at risk of developing gastric cancer, with some notable exceptions, have high prevalence rates of *Helicobacter pylori*. In China, the prevalence rate between the different regions can vary from 3 to 69/1000 population. In a study of 1882 men aged between 35 and 64 y from 46 rural provinces of China, there was a correlation of 40% between the prevalence of *Helicobacter pylori* and gastric cancer. In a longitudinal study of 5908 Japanese Americans living in Hawaii, there were 109 cases of gastric carcinoma identified over a period of 20 years. Stored sera from this study were tested for antibodies to *Helicobacter pylori* and 94% of these patients were seropositive compared with 76% for matched controls. In addition, the higher the level of the antibody titre, the closer the correlation with gastric cancer. A similar longitudinal study of 22000 subjects in the UK demonstrated that 69% of 29 subjects who developed gastric cancer were seropositive for *Helicobacter pylori* compared with 47% who did not have gastric cancer. The median antibody titre in those with gastric cancer was higher in subjects who developed cancer compared with the control population (90 µg/ml vs 3.6 µg/ml). *Helicobacter pylori* had an odds ratio (OR) of 2.7 as a risk factor for the development of gastric cancer. In a longitudinal study of 128992 persons in the USA, 109 were identified as developing gastric adenocarcinoma, 84% having suffered a previous *H. pylori* infection (overall OR 3.6; OR 18.0 for women; and OR 9.0 for blacks). In an American study of 169 persons in New Orleans, a region that has a prevalence of gastric cancer of 28.5/100000 population, the seroprevalence of *Helicobacter pylori* was 71%.

Only distal adenocarcinoma is strongly associated with colonization by *Helicobacter pylori*. In a study of 379 patients with gastric cancer of all types, the prevalence of *Helicobacter pylori* was lowest in patients with cancer of the cardia (50%) or of the diffuse type (56%) (combined OR 0.69) compared with non-cardia cancers (63%) or intestinal type (70%) (combined OR 3.39). In some studies, a lower correlation between *Helicobacter pylori* and intestinal-type gastric adenocarcinoma has been demonstrated, which can be explained by the higher prevalence of gastric atrophy and intestinal metaplasia, both of which lead to the loss of binding sites for *Helicobacter pylori*. Not all studies have demonstrated an association between colonization by *Helicobacter pylori* and gastric cancer. In a study from Korea there was no such association and other explanations such as environmental factors, host factors or bacterial strain types may have an influence.

The gastrointestinal tract is a major immune organ with approximately 10^{10} immune cells per metre of intestine, making it a significant part of the MALT. Lymphoid tissue is normally absent in the stomach, but colonization by *Helicobacter pylori* leads to infiltration of the lamina propria and epithelial layer with neutrophils and the appearance of lymphocytes organized into lymphoid follicles in the subepithelial layer of the stomach. The appearance is of active chronic superficial gastritis. Occasionally there is infiltration of the epithelial layer by T cells giving rise to a nodular appearance called lymphocytic gastritis. The lymphocytes associated with active chronic gastritis are largely B cells and these are the basis of MALT lymphoma. The universal appearance of lymphoid follicles in association with *Helicobacter pylori* suggests the possibility that it may be linked to the appearance of MALT lymphoma. The evidence for the causal association of *Helicobacter pylori* and MALT lymphoma is similar to that linking the organism to gastric adenocarcinoma or peptic ulcer disease. There are geographical associations between the prevalence of *Helicobacter pylori* and MALT lymphoma, and patients with MALT lymphoma have high seroprevalence rates for *Helicobacter pylori*. A study of 230593 individuals has demonstrated that colonization by *Helicobacter pylori* is a risk factor (OR 6.3) for the development of MALT lymphoma. Additionally, as further evidence of a causal association, the eradication of *Helicobacter pylori* can lead to regression of early stage lymphoma.

The Asian and African enigma

However, in some geographic areas the prevalence of *Helicobacter pylori* cannot be linked to some clinical outcomes leading to a series of geographical 'enigmas'. Studies in the Americas and Europe demonstrate a correlation between high rates of colonization by *Helicobacter pylori* and both peptic ulcer disease and gastric cancer. In Colombia, in regions of high gastric cancer risk, the seroprevalence of *Helicobacter pylori* is 93% compared with 63% in low gastric cancer risk areas. Similarly, in New Orleans, where black adults have a high gastric cancer rate, the seroprevalence of *Helicobacter pylori* is 70%, this compared with white adults with a low gastric cancer risk and a seroprevalence of 43%. Other studies have confirmed this in Europe. However, several studies have shown an apparent disconnect between the high rates of colonization by *Helicobacter pylori* and low rates of *Helicobacter pylori*-related diseases, particularly gastric cancer. These disconnects are known as the African and Asian enigma. In Africa, where colonization by *Helicobacter* is high (>90%) and infection is children occurs at an early age, the prevalence of *Helicobacter*-related diseases has been reported to be low. Two studies cast doubt on this. In one study, across 17 countries in Africa between 1972 and 2001 of 20 531 persons, and a second retrospective review of eight sero-epidemiological studies and 21 prospective endoscopic studies, the prevalence of *Helicobacter pylori*-related duodenal ulcer was reported as 21–26%, that of gastric ulcer as 3.4–7% and that of gastric cancer as 2.4–3.4%. These figures are similar to those found in Europe and America, and the conclusion of both studies was that the African enigma does not exist. Anomalous results have also been reported. In Burkina Faso, where *Helicobacter pylori*-related disease is reported as low, a sero-epidemiological study demonstrated a high rate of colonization by *Helicobacter pylori* in children, yet counter to virtually all other studies, a falling seroprevalence rate in adults. These results have yet to be confirmed. A study from the Gambia reported high seroprevalence rates of *Helicobacter pylori* but low prevalence for gastric atrophy and intestinal metaplasia, both of which are precursors of gastric cancer.

The Asian enigma is similarly due to a high prevalence of *Helicobacter* with a low prevalence of related disease. The seroprevalence of *Helicobacter pylori* in India, Bangladesh, Pakistan and Thailand ranges from 55% to 90% and is higher than that in Japan and China (44–55%), yet the incidence of gastric cancer ranges from 1.3 to 10.6/100 000 people, whereas in China and Japan it is in the order of 80–115/100 000 people. In India, endoscopic and serological studies have also demonstrated that prevalence of *Helicobacter pylori* in non-ulcer dyspepsia compared with gastric cancer is equivalent for the rapid urease test (RUT) (46% vs 38%), serology (84% vs 78%) and histology (55% vs 64%). In Malaysia, three ethnic populations coexist: Chinese, Malay and Indian. In one study of 1060 consecutive patients, the seroprevalence according to ethnic group was 16% (Malay), 48% (Chinese) and 61% (Indian). However, peptic ulcer disease rates are higher in the Chinese compared with the Indian ethnic group, with the Malay group having the lowest rate of colonization and peptic ulcer disease. In a further study of 7000 persons, the seroprevalence of *Helicobacter pylori* was 27% (Malay), 46% (Chinese) and 48% (Indian)—the gastric cancer rates were high for the Chinese group, but low for the other two, illustrating a disconnect between *Helicobacter pylori* and gastric cancer for the Indian population. These geo-ethnic differences may be explained by host genetics, diet, *Helicobacter* strain variation or some other environmental factor (*Table 3.1*).

Functional dyspepsia

The role of *Helicobacter pylori* in functional dyspepsia (FD) is controversial, but it may be that a subset of

Table 3.1 Enigmas: showing relationship of prevalence of *Helicobacter pylori* and gastric cancer

	USA	Europe	Africa	India	Malaysia (Indian)	Malaysia (Malay)	Malaysia (Chinese)
Helicobacter pylori	Low	Low	High	High	High	Low	High
Gastric cancer	Low	Low	Low	Low	Low	Low	High

individuals who have FD do benefit from eradication of the organism. FD is a frequent cause for attendance at gastroenterology clinics, consuming a great deal of time and resources. It occurs in about 40% of individuals—in an endoscopic study of 346 patients, about two-thirds had a specific disease identified to account for the symptoms; the remainder did not have any abnormality to account for the symptoms. An additional issue is that symptoms of dyspepsia or heartburn are variable, subjective and difficult to quantify and, in the absence of a specific test, it remains a diagnosis of exclusion. Quantification of the condition is necessary in order to determine if any improvement has occurred and to correlate this with any treatment given. There have been several attempts to define FD. The Rome I and II definitions defined it as 'pain or discomfort centred in the upper abdomen in the absence of organic disease that could explain the symptoms' (**3.10**). The problem with this definition is that 'discomfort' is itself hard to define: does it include mild pain, a feeling of fullness, bloating, burning or belching? Both the Rome I and II definitions recognized subgroups of reflux-like (hearburn), ulcer-like (pain) and dysmotility-like (discomfort) symptoms. The Rome II definition excluded reflux symptoms (heartburn) linking it to gastro-oesophageal reflux disease (GORD). The Rome II definition excluded irritable bowel syndrome as a cause, by dissociating dyspepsia from defecation. The Rome III definition of FD reduced the number of symptoms to four:

1. Epigastric pain.
2. Postprandial fullness.
3. Early satiation.
4. Epigastric burning.

Other symptoms commonly complained of, such as nausea, belching or bloating, may arise from other regions of the body and are not considered cardinal symptoms of FD. The four symptoms can be divided into two main groups: meal-induced symptoms characterized by postprandial fullness and early satiety (postprandial distress syndrome); and meal-unrelated symptoms characterized by epigastric pain and burning (epigastric pain syndrome). The overlap with symptoms of GORD and irritable bowel syndrome remains unresolved.

An important and as yet unresolved issue is the relationship between colonization by *Helicobacter pylori*

and FD. Although it is evident that *Helicobacter pylori* is linked to gastritis, the role of this in producing upper gastrointestinal symptoms is not clear, as the majority of individuals colonized by *Helicobacter pylori* are asymptomatic. Several studies have shown that *Helicobacter pylori* is present in 50–60% of patients with FD, but in some studies the prevalence has been two to three times the rate of carriage compared with a control population, and in one study a prevalence of 87% was recorded. Other studies, however, have not found an association between colonization by *Helicobacter pylori* and FD. The major problem with comparing these studies is the problem of comparing the subject populations between the studies because of the difficulty in defining FD. An alternative approach is to determine the effects of eradication of *Helicobacter pylori* on symptoms of dyspepsia. Two multinational studies of symptom improvement after eradication of *Helicobacter pylori*, the OCAY (Omeprazole plus Clarithromycin and Amoxicillin Effect One Year after Treatment) and ORCHID (Optimal Regimen Cures Helicobacter Induced Dyspepsia) studies in a total of 718 patients demonstrated that, over a 12-month period, 21–26% of patients had a sustained improvement of symptoms. This improvement occurred in the ulcer-like and reflux-like subgroups with no effect seen in the dysmotility subgroup. A systematic review in 2006 analysed 21 randomized controlled clinical trials of different eradication regimens and concluded that a statistically significant improvement in symptoms occurred with eradication of *Helicobacter pylori*. Other benefits may accrue from eradication of *Helicobacter pylori* in this setting: a reduction in the progression to ulceration, which may occur in some patients; a reduction in the complication rate if ever given NSAIDs, and possibly a reduction in the progression to atrophic gastritis (AG) and gastric cancer, although the latter has not been proven. Current thinking in relation to FD is a disturbance of nociception by the enteric nervous system involving the spinal reflex and the brain–gut–endocrine axis. Similarly, the role of *Helicobacter pylori* in recurrent abdominal pain in children is controversial.

Oesophagitis

The experimental results on the relationship between *Helicobacter pylori* and GORD, oesophagitis,

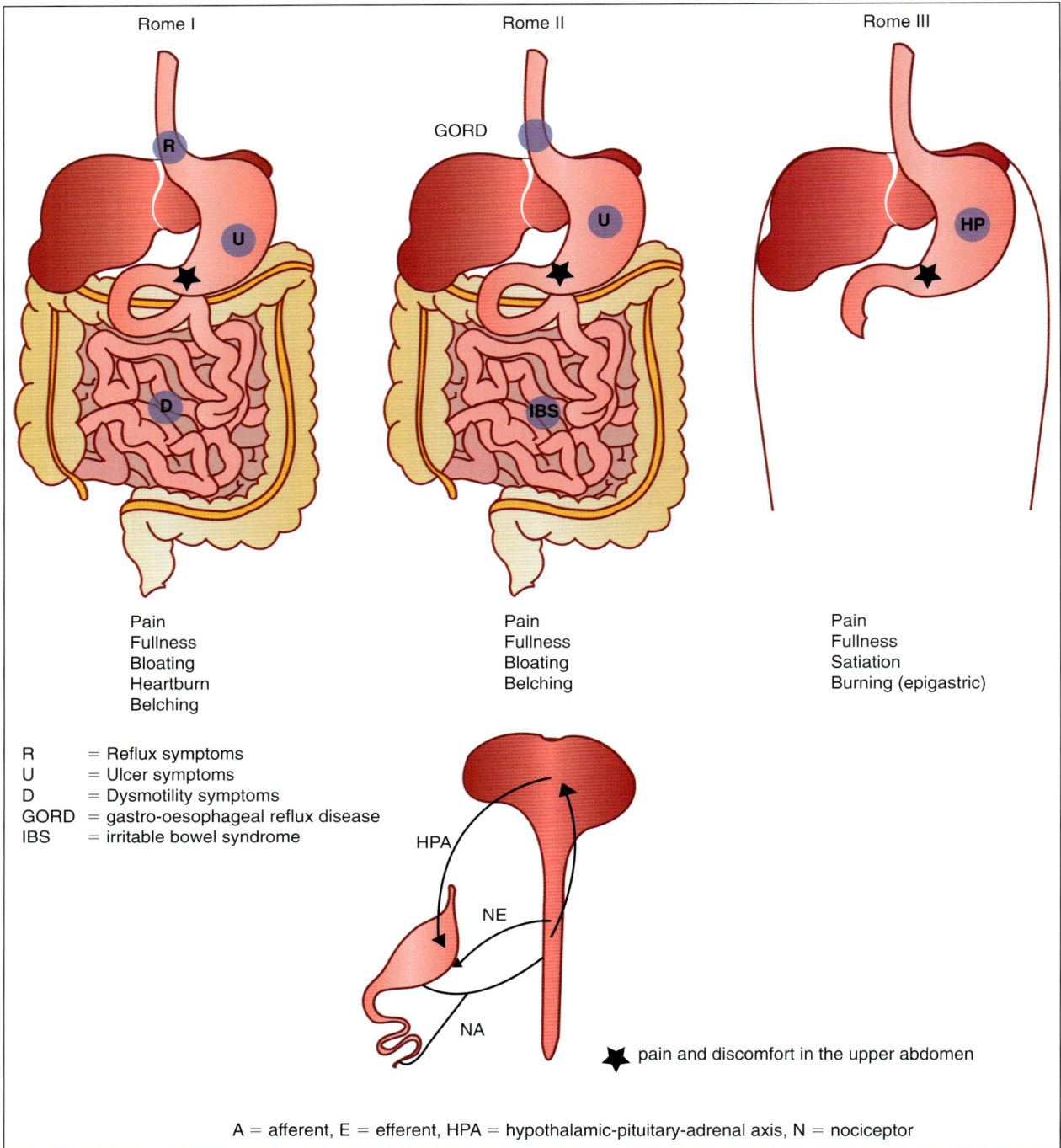

Rome I	Rome II	Rome III
Pain	Pain	Pain
Fullness	Fullness	Fullness
Bloating	Bloating	Satiation
Heartburn	Belching	Burning (epigastric)
Belching		

R = Reflux symptoms
U = Ulcer symptoms
D = Dysmotility symptoms
GORD = gastro-oesophageal reflux disease
IBS = irritable bowel syndrome

★ pain and discomfort in the upper abdomen

A = afferent, E = efferent, HPA = hypothalamic-pituitary-adrenal axis, N = nociceptor

3.10 Symptoms and suggested pathophysiology of functional dyspepsia.

Barrett's oesophagus and oesophageal carcinoma are contradictory, making any relationship uncertain.

Helicobacter pylori infection can lead to both an increase or decrease in the acid content of the stomach depending upon the topographical location of the gastritis and its effect upon acid production. As acid is an important determinant of reflux disease, and complications caused by inflammation (including Barrett's oesophagus (**3.11**) and oesophageal adenocarcinoma), there are three possible associations between *Helicobacter pylori* and symptoms of reflux disease and oesophagitis. *Helicobacter pylori* may be *ab initio* causal; or it may exacerbate already existing disease caused by something else; or it may protect from oesophageal disease. However, the evidence for any association between colonization by *Helicobacter pylori* and reflux disease is contradictory and split along geographical lines with most evidence for an association coming from studies in the East and most evidence against coming from the West. In one study of 93 patients with both symptoms and endoscopic evidence of inflammation, there was no significant correlation between presence of the organism and degree of oesophagitis. A histological study of 71 patients with oesophageal columnar epithelium could not demonstrate any difference in *Helicobacter pylori* prevalence. In a similar study of 108 subjects, which included asymptomatic controls, colonization by *Helicobacter pylori* was not more common in patients (36%) compared with controls (36%). A systematic endoscopic survey of 135 dyspeptic patients demonstrated an association between inflammation in the cardia, fundus and antrum of the stomach, which occurred in 91% of subjects. Oesophagitis was found in 37% and was correlated with reflux symptoms but neither symptoms nor inflammation were correlated with gastritis. In 2004, in a prospective study of 1000 dyspeptic multi-ethnic patients from Malaya, 38% were diagnosed with GORD, of whom 13% had oesophagitis, the remainder being diagnosed as non-erosive reflux disease. There was no association between any of these conditions and colonization by *Helicobacter pylori*. A similar study in Iran could not demonstrate any difference between patients with GORD compared with matched controls in relation to colonization by *Helicobacter pylori* and nor could a population-based study in Norway where 472 patients with GORD were compared with 472 control individuals from a population of 65 363. In the Norwegian study, the prevalence of *Helicobacter pylori* was similar in both groups, as was the *cagA* status of the infection strain. Similarly, there was no difference detected in the strain type of *Helicobacter pylori* for the virulence markers *cagA*, *vacs1*, *icsA1* between patients with duodenal ulcer or GORD, indicating that these were not protective for the development of reflux disease. On the other hand, a systematic review of 20 studies showed that there was a lower prevalence of *Helicobacter pylori* in patients with GORD compared with those without GORD and this effect was most marked from the studies in the East. A further meta-analysis of 24 studies demonstrated an association between lack of colonization by *Helicobacter pylori* and GORD. In the stomach, *Helicobacter pylori* is associated with intestinal metaplasia and the question arises whether it is also associated with Barrett's oesophagus in association with GORD. A study of 288 patients with Barrett's oesophagus compared with 217 patients with GORD found *Helicobacter* in 32% of the former and 44% of the latter. When the patients with Barrett's oesophagus were analysed according to the degree of dysplasia or the presence of adenocarcinoma, *Helicobacter pylori* was found at a much lower frequency in severe disease compared with mild disease. In a study including 2201 patients, 297 were diagnosed with GORD and 1192 with Barrett's metaplasia. Although there was no difference in the prevalence of *Helicobacter pylori* in relation to GORD with or without Barrett's metaplasia or neoplasia (53%, 51% and 47% respectively), the prevalence of *Helicobacter pylori* in patients with GORD was less than that in the control group with FD. In a study of 318 patients with Barrett's oesophagus, 312 patients with GORD and 299 control subjects, there was a strong negative relationship between *Helicobacter pylori*, *cagA* status and Barrett's oesophagus.

These analyses suggest that colonization by *Helicobacter pylori* may have a protective effect against

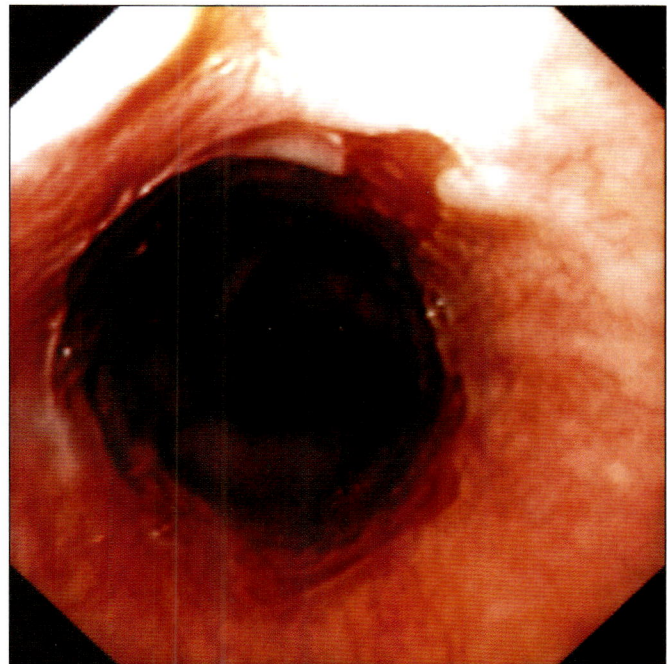

3.11 Endoscopic view of Barrett's oesophagus.

the development of GORD and its severe complications. However, the conflicting nature of these results suggests that other factors may be important in the development of GORD or there may be specific subgroups of patients with GORD that have different associations with *Helicobacter pylori*.

Because of (a) the studies demonstrating a negative association between colonization by *Helicobacter pylori* and reflux disease and its complications; (b) the importance of acid load in the pathogenesis of reflux disease; and (c) the fact that infection with *Helicobacter pylori* can lead to gastric atrophy with hypochlorhydria, it has been suggested that eradication of the organism can lead to an increase in oesophagitis and reflux symptoms. A counter argument is that eradication of *Helicobacter pylori* simply reveals an already existing reflux disease rather than causing it. Epidemiological evidence shows that the incidence of GORD is increasing in industrialized countries along with a falling prevalence of *Helicobacter pylori*, so a reasonable question is whether the one is related to the other. In a placebo-controlled multicentre study of 242 patients with duodenal ulcer before the study, 53% reported heartburn. At follow-up, 35% in which *Helicobacter pylori* had not been eradicated still had heartburn and in those in which *Helicobacter pylori* had been eradicated, 25% had heartburn. Of those who did not have heartburn before the study (47%), 20% developed heartburn at follow-up but there was no correlation with *Helicobacter* status. In a study of 70 patients with GORD treated with a proton pump inhibitor and antibiotics if *Helicobacter pylori* positive, of those in which *Helicobacter* had not been eradicated, relapse of symptoms occurred at 54 days compared with 100 days for those in which the organism had been eradicated. In the *Helicobacter pylori* negative group, relapse occurred at 110 days. This study therefore does not support the suggestion that the presence of *Helicobacter pylori* is protective for GORD, but advocates its eradication as it is directly symptom related. In 255 patients with duodenal ulcer who were followed up for 12 months following treatment, there was a reduction from 44% to 21% of patients with GORD when *Helicobacter pylori* had been eradicated but no association with reflux oesophagitis. A study from China involved 236 patients with GORD who were followed up while on acid suppressive maintenance treatment with half the patients also given a course

of *Helicobacter pylori* eradication therapy. The results demonstrated that eradication of *Helicobacter pylori* was associated with an increased risk of treatment failure for GORD and the majority of patients were infected with CagA-positive strains. In the European prospective study on GORD (ProGORD), results from 6215 patients (half with erosive reflux disease and half without) showed a complex relationship between symptoms, healing of inflammation and the status of *Helicobacter pylori* colonization. The presence of the organism enhanced the healing of erosive gastritis, but only in those patients with Barrett's oesophagus. The explanation for this may be an enhanced acid suppression due to concomitant proton pump inhibitor and presence of *Helicobacter pylori*. In patients with gastric ulcer a study demonstrated that there was no difference in the incidence of GORD after eradication of *Helicobacter pylori* compared with a control group in which *Helicobacter* had not been eradicated.

Symptoms of reflux disease ('heartburn') occur in about 40% of individuals, whereas inflammation only occurs in about 2%, making this a very common condition often dealt with in primary care.

Chronic infection

Helicobacter pylori is a good example of a 'slow' infection, as infection occurs in childhood but related diseases occur in adulthood. Ulcer disease presents with epigastric pain, heartburn or dyspepsia, or may be totally asymptomatic. Anaemia (due to blood loss from the ulcer) and weight loss may also occur, plus signs and symptoms of perforation (acute abdominal pain, abdominal rigidity and guarding, rebound tenderness and shock). Clinical presentation of carcinoma is very non-specific and is usually associated with gastric ulcer rather than duodenal ulcer. It presents with abdominal pain or a mass with so-called 'alarm symptoms' (i.e. weight loss and anaemia). Gastric cancer originating at the cardia (gastro-oesophageal junction) does not appear to be related to colonization by *Helicobacter pylori*.

Acute infection

A syndrome associated with acute infection by *Helicobacter pylori* in adults who have either swallowed the organism or who have been iatrogenically infected during pH measurements, includes severe cramping epigastric pain, headache, nausea and vomiting.

In children, acute haematemesis may occur. Most infections, however, may pass unnoticed.

Extra-gastric conditions

Helicobacter pylori is also suggested as a causal agent for extra-gastric gastrointestinal conditions, including lower gastrointestinal and pancreatohepatobiliary diseases. In all these cases, the relationship between colonization by Helicobacter pylori and various diseases is not as clear-cut as for peptic ulcer disease and gastric carcinoma. The results of different studies often give conflicting interpretations and, in some studies, the number of patients investigated are few, making the results statistically questionable.

Conditions of the small and large intestine

Conditions that have been suggested as being linked with infection by Helicobacter pylori include: colonization of Meckel's diverticulum with subsequent ulceration; inflammatory bowel disease (IBD); and colon cancer.

Meckel's diverticulum is a common congenital abnormality where the vitelline duct does not close off correctly, leaving a diverticulum on the anti-mesenteric border of the small intestine comprising all parts of the bowel cell wall (**3.12**). Frequently, the lining epithelium is heterotropic gastric mucosa, which may become colonized by Helicobacter pylori, possibly leading to ulceration and rectal bleeding. The common symptoms

of Meckel's diverticulum are pain, obstruction and melaena. In a study of 32 cases of Meckel's diverticulum, 12 had heterotropic gastric mucosa and three were colonized by Helicobacter pylori. On the contrary, in a retrospective study of 30 histological sections, 13 had heterotropic gastric mucosa of which 10 presented with acute bleeding. Using PCR, none of the 13 specimens were found to be colonized by Helicobacter pylori. A similar study of 92 patients did not show a relationship between heterotropic gastric mucosa, Helicobacter pylori and bleeding. Overall, colonization of gastric mucosa in Meckel's diverticulum by Helicobacter pylori is uncommon, although individual cases have been identified and its association with clinical presentation is poor.

The importance of the intestinal microflora in relation to IBD has been demonstrated in animal models (**3.13**). Non-pylori Helicobacter spp., such as Helicobacter bilis and Helicobacter hepaticus, can induce a condition resembling IBD in certain types of mice. Recombinase-activating gene-2-deficient knockout mice (Rag2$^{-/-}$) develop IBD following infection with Helicobacter hepaticus, and the same in severe combined immunodeficiency (SCID) mice

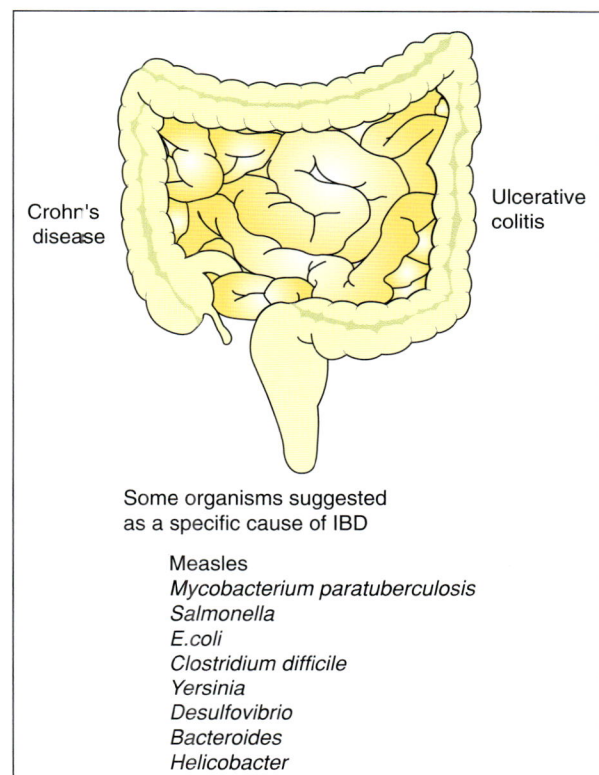

Crohn's disease

Ulcerative colitis

Some organisms suggested as a specific cause of IBD

Measles
Mycobacterium paratuberculosis
Salmonella
E.coli
Clostridium difficile
Yersinia
Desulfovibrio
Bacteroides
Helicobacter

3.13 Association between microbes, including Helicobacter pylori and IBD.

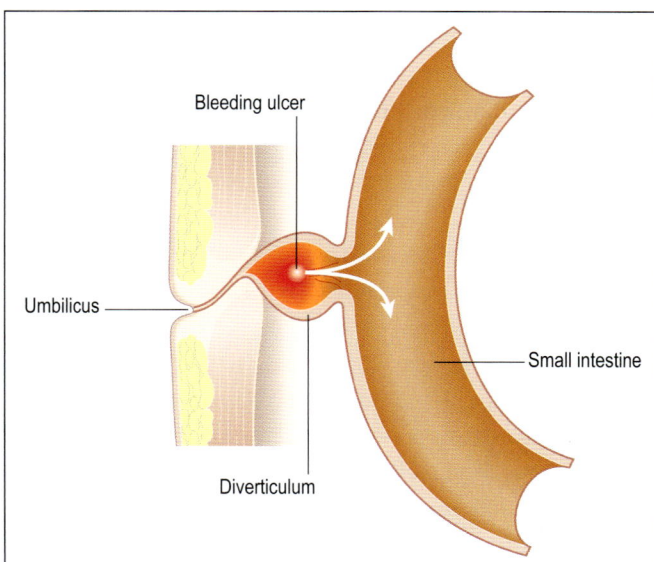

Bleeding ulcer

Umbilicus

Small intestine

Diverticulum

3.12 Meckel's diverticulum and Helicobacter pylori.

infected with *Helicobacter bilis*. A more intensively studied bacterial/host interaction has been with interleukin (IL)-10 knockout mice infected with *Helicobacter hepaticus*, which develops IBD. Additionally, cotton-top tamarinds develop IBD when held in captivity and a *Helicobacter* sp. has been isolated from these animals. This raises the question whether the only known *Helicobacter* sp. to infect humans, *Helicobacter pylori,* is involved in the aetiology of IBD. Seroprevalence studies of *Helicobacter pylori* have shown an inverse correlation between infection and IBD. In one study, involving 100 patients with Crohn's disease (CD), 100 patients with ulcerative colitis and 100 matched controls, the prevalence of *Helicobacter pylori* was 13%, 18% and 43%, respectively. In a larger study of 386 patients with CD compared with controls, the seroprevalence was 12% and 35%, respectively. All seroprevalence studies have shown identical results and studies indicate this low prevalence is not due to taking antibiotics. The results of detecting *Helicobacter pylori* in colonic tissue have been contradictory. A study of 30 patients undergoing colectomy for IBD or other reasons could not detect *Helicobacter pylori* in any specimens. A study of 39 patients undergoing colonoscopy and biopsy detected *Helicobacter pylori* in one patient with IBD and one non-IBD control. In a study of 75 patients using PCR with *Helicobacter* spp. primers, none was detected in 50 patients with IBD and 25 controls. On the other hand, in a study of 60 patients with IBD, *Helicobacter pylori* was detected using PCR in six patients. In a study of 42 patients with IBD compared with 74 non-IBD patients, the organism was cultured from colonic tissue in patients with IBD on three occasions and once in the control population. It was detected by PCR in eight patients and seven controls. The detection of *Helicobacter pylori* in these patients with IBD did not correlate with symptoms. A later study by the same group, however, found a higher prevalence (by culture and PCR) in patients with CD compared with controls, although antibody levels were lower in the patient group.

The lower seroprevalence in patients compared with controls raises the question of whether colonization by *Helicobacter pylori* is protective of developing IBD, or at least modulates the illness. In a study of 296 patients with IBD, the patients who were seropositive had a higher age of onset compared with controls and a bimodal pattern of peak onset, whereas the seronegative patients had a unimodal peak of onset. One case report of a patient with dyspepsia who was given *Helicobacter* eradication therapy developed CD 3 months later. In a second study of 193 patients with CD, those patients who were seropositive for *Helicobacter pylori* and who were non-smokers, had more flare-ups and more surgery than the seronegative group. These results all suggest some form of modulation of the course of the illness by colonization with *Helicobacter pylori*.

Some studies have suggested a link between colon adenocarcinoma and colonization by *Helicobacter pylori* due to the hormonal changes induced by the organism, which could stimulate tumour growth. Gastrin is a mitogen and elevated levels of gastrin can induce cyclo-oxygenase 2. A study of expression of gastrin, gastrin receptor and cyclo-oxygenase 2 in patients with colon cancer colonized by *Helicobacter pylori* demonstrated a higher level of expression in cancer tissue compared with normal tissue. Another study of 29 patients with colon cancer recorded higher gastrin and lower ghrelin (an orexigenic hormone—*see* p.59) levels in patients compared with controls. However, a further study could find no relationship between colonization by *Helicobacter pylori*, gastrin levels and colon cancer, although there was an association between AG and rectal cancer.

Although *Helicobacter pylori* may be isolated from faeces, particularly if diarrhoea is present, it is not an established cause of diarrhoea. However, there are a number of non-pylori *Helicobacter* spp. that are recognized gastrointestinal pathogens linked to diarrhoea (**3.14**) and the low acid associated with chronic *Helicobacter pylori* infection may predispose to other causes of gastroenteritis (e.g. giardia).

Helicobacter pylori has been implicated as a cause of chronic diarrhoea in children in tropical countries. Over 50% of children with chronic diarrhoea in the Gambia were seropositive, although in Peru no association was found. If any association exists it is likely not to be a direct one, but due to hypochlorhydria induced by *Helicobacter pylori*, thereby increasing the chances of other primary gastroenteritis pathogens infecting the child. Some *Helicobacter* spp., however, have been implicated as causing gastroenteritis. *Helicobacter cinaedi* and *Helicobacter fennelliae* have both been isolated from diarrhoeal stools in patients who were HIV positive and who clinically had proctocolitis. They complained of bloody diarrhoea, fever and abdominal cramps, symptoms

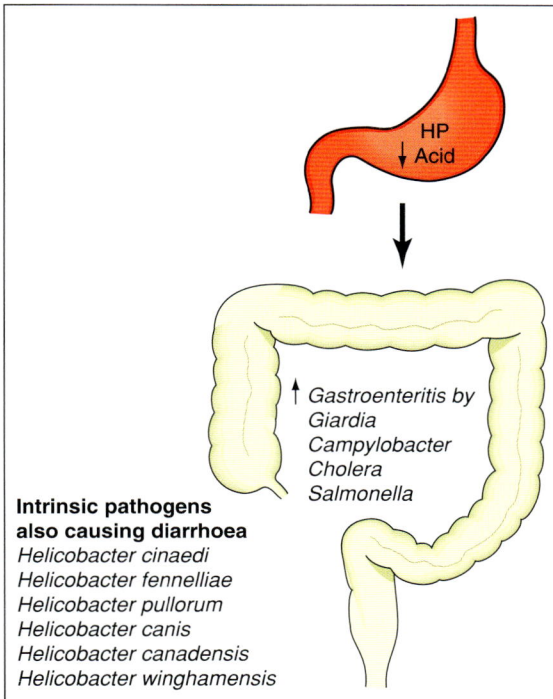

3.14 *Helicobacter pylori*, non-pylori *Helicobacter* spp. and diarrhoea.

very similar to infection with *Campylobacter jejuni*. Although predominantly associated with homosexuals this can occur in other immunocompromised individuals or otherwise healthy persons. Other *Helicobacter* spp. associated with gastroenteritis are *H. pullorum*, *H. canadensis*, *H. canis* and *H. winghamensis*. These latter organisms have only been isolated from a small number of patients and whether they are important causes of gastroenteritis remains an open question.

Conditions of the pancreatohepatobiliary system

Animal *Helicobacter* species (*H. hepaticus*, *H. bilis* and *H. pullorum*) have been shown to be associated with inflammatory and neoplastic lesions of the liver in mice and chickens, raising interest in whether *Helicobacter pylori* and other *Helicobacter* spp. are involved in similar disease in humans. Several studies have demonstrated the presence of *Helicobacter* sp. in pancreatohepatobiliary conditions, although whether there is a causal relationship is uncertain (**3.15**).

Because *Helicobacter* spp. can be found in the liver of animals, *Helicobacter pylori* has been sought and detected in the pancreatohepatobiliary system in humans.

A PCR study of bile detected the organism in 3 of 6 specimens. In a study of 46 Chilean patients, who had the gallbladder resected because of chronic cholecystitis, *Helicobacter* spp. were present in 13 of 23 specimens of bile and 9 of 23 specimens of gallbladder tissue. On sequencing, the organisms were identified as *H. bilis*, *H. pullorum* and *H. rappini*; culture was unsuccessful.

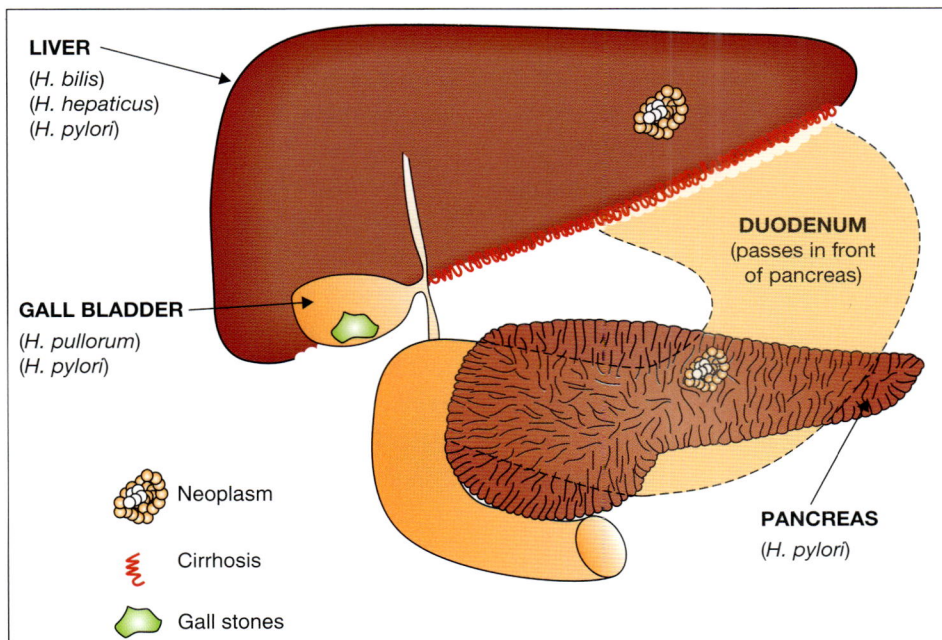

3.15 Suggested associations between *Helicobacter* spp. and inflammatory or neoplastic conditions of the liver, biliary system and pancreas.

In a study of 122 cholecystectomy patients with non-malignant gallbladder disease, *Helicobacter* spp. DNA was present in 50% of samples, principally patients with symptomatic gallstones. A similar study in Brazilian patients demonstrated *Helicobacter* spp. DNA in gallbladder tissue (31%) and bile (42%), and the presence of the DNA in tissue was significantly associated with cholelithiasis, suggesting that *Helicobacter* spp. may be causal for gallstones. Supporting these conclusions are studies in which not only *Helicobacter pylori* DNA but CagA antigen and anti-CagA antibodies were detected in bile. A further study demonstrated that *Helicobacter pylori* antigens were found only is some gallstones (composite and brown) found in the gallbladder but not in ductal stones or single cholesterol stones in the gallbladder, implying that *Helicobacter pylori* may only be associated with the development of some types of gallstones. In a study of 111 patients, *Helicobacter pylori* was detected in 45% of gastric metaplastic tissue in the gallbladder and in 8 of 11 gallstones by PCR. However, not all studies have demonstrated an association between gallstones and colonization by *Helicobacter pylori*. In a study from Mexico, only one specimen of 95 (by immunohistochemistry) and one of 32 (by PCR) was positive for *Helicobacter pylori*. The presence of *Helicobacter* spp. has also been demonstrated in cases of primary sclerosing cholangitis, biliary cirrhosis and carcinoma of the gallbladder.

There have been a number of studies investigating the presence of *Helicobacter* spp. in liver disease. In a seroprevalence study, *Helicobacter pylori* was more common (77%) in patients with hepatitis C virus-associated cirrhosis compared with age-matched non-hepatitis C virus controls (59%), and *Helicobacter* spp. were detected in 90% of liver biopsies by PCR. In a PCR study of hepatocellular carcinoma, *Helicobacter* sp. DNA was detected in all 8 specimens. The organism could not be identified but was neither *Helicobacter pylori* nor *Helicobacter hepaticus*. A seroprevalence study for *H. hepaticus* did not demonstrate any difference between patients with chronic liver disease and controls. The majority of studies have demonstrated an association between liver disease and colonization by unidentified presumptive *Helicobacter* spp., but to date there is no evidence these are causal of any liver illness in humans.

Similarly, the role of *Helicobacter* spp. in pancreatic disease has been investigated. A seroprevalence study of 92 patients with pancreatic cancer compared with controls demonstrated a seroprevalence of 65% and 45%, respectively. Similarly, a population study of 29 133 patients identified 122 with pancreatic cancer—when compared with matched controls, the seroprevalence of *Helicobacter pylori* was 82% and 73%, respectively. A survey of 88 338 patient records in Sweden demonstrated that patients with unoperated gastric ulcer had a 20% increased risk of subsequently developing pancreatic cancer, whereas those with unoperated duodenal ulcer had no increased risk. The authors propose that these results suggest excess nitrosamines as a mechanism for pancreatic carcinogenesis. However, in a study of 104 patients with pancreatic cancer compared with 262 matched controls, there was no association between colonization by *Helicobacter pylori* or the *cagA* status and pancreatic cancer.

As a result of these contradictory findings, further work is needed to identify whether any causal relationship exists between *Helicobacter pylori*, *Helicobacter* spp. and pancreatohepatobiliary disease, and to elucidate biological mechanisms of pathogenesis.

Extra-gastrointestinal conditions

It has been suggested that *Helicobacter pylori* may be related to a wide range of extra-gastrointestinal diseases affecting the oropharynx, respiratory system, heart and vasculature, haemopoietic system, immune system, endocrine system, central nervous system (CNS) and skin. In many of these cases only occasional studies have demonstrated a significant association, while several studies have given conflicting results. This makes it difficult to claim conclusively that *Helicobacter pylori* is associated with any of these conditions, although two conditions—idiopathic thrombocytopenic purpura (ITP) and iron deficiency anaemia (IDA)—have the highest claim.

The association between colonization by *Helicobacter pylori* and a number of diverse conditions affecting several organ systems has been investigated principally by seroepidemiological studies (*Table 3.2*).

Conditions of the oropharynx (3.17)

There have been a number of studies suggesting an association between colonization by *Helicobacter pylori* and various infections (e.g. otitis media), neoplasms (e.g. laryngeal carcinoma) and ulceration (aphthous

Table 3.2 Suggested extra-gastrointestinal associations of *Helicobacter pylori*.

Organ system and/or region	Suggested association
Head and neck	Infections and neoplasms of head and neck, mainly because of detection of *H. pylori* in studies of oropharynx
CNS	Parkinson's disease sufferers have association with peptic ulceration of GI tract; study of 124 patients showed correlation between *H. pylori* seroprevalence and Parkinson's disease
Respiratory system	Small number of studies show association between *H. pylori* seroprevalence and infections, cancer and respiratory disorders (COPD, bronchiectasis, asthma)
Cardiovascular (vascular) system	Association through chronic inflammation caused by *H. pylori*: artheroma, coronary heart disease, cerebrovascular disease, migraine and Raynaud's disease
Haemopoietic system	Association between *H. pylori* eradiction and improvement of idiopathic thrombocytopenic purpura symptoms Some studies link *H. pylori* colonization with iron deficiency anaemia
Immune-mediated allergic disorders	Contrasting results from studies suggest *H. pylori* seroprevalence has both negative and positive correlations with asthma, urticaria, atopy and food allergies Some interaction between *H. pylori* colonization and coeliac disease
Endocrine system	Studies in from small patient groups suggest association between *H. pylori* infection and onset of diabetes or thyroiditis, although some conflicting results Complex interaction between *H. pylori* colonization and leptin and ghrelin signalling
Skin	Small study showed association between eradication of *H. pylori* infection and improvement of rosacea symptoms Possible association between autoimmune disorders such as psoriasis and Henoch-Schönlein purpura

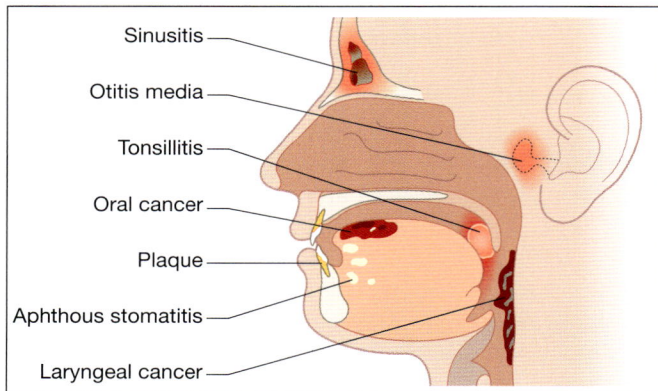

3.17 Suggested associations between *Helicobacter pylori* and oropharyngeal conditions.

stomatitis, or AS) in the oropharynx. An important area that has received much attention is the presence or absence of *Helicobacter pylori* in dental specimens (*see* Chapter 2), not only because of a possible association with dental disease but also because, if present, it may act as a reservoir for reinfection of the stomach.

The detection of *Helicobacter pylori* in dental specimens reported in many studies opens the question whether or not its presence in the oral cavity is related to diseases in this area—particularly neoplasm, as it is a recognized class I carcinogen—but also infections in the oropharynx.

In a study of 134 Indian patients, there was no association between oral colonization with *Helicobacter pylori* and poor oral hygiene and periodontal disease. However, a high rate of colonization by *Helicobacter pylori*, detected by a rapid urease test (RUT), was noted in patients with or without gastric *Helicobacter pylori*. The use of the RUT to detect *Helicobacter pylori* in dental specimens is open to dispute. Additionally, in a Finnish study of 29 104 subjects, which was part of a cancer prevention study, there was no association between tooth loss and colonization by *Helicobacter pylori*. A study of seropositivity to *Helicobacter pylori* and tooth loss in the UK did show an association, but when socio-economic status was taken into account the association did not reach statistical significance.

The role of *Helicobacter pylori* in otitis media has been investigated. In a study of 18 children aged 3–8 from the Lebanon there was no evidence that *Helicobacter pylori* was linked to otitis media. The organism was not detected by culture or PCR from any of the middle ear fluid specimens. However, other studies have detected *Helicobacter pylori* in specimens from these patients. Five studies from Turkey detected *Helicobacter pylori* in 66% (RUT), 33% (RUT), 67% (PCR), 16% (PCR) and 8% (PCR). One study from Turkey detected *Helicobacter pylori* by PCR and culture, and one study from Japan detected *Helicobacter pylori* by immunohistochemistry. A review of these studies, covering 203 patients, indicated that there was little evidence for an association between *Helicobacter pylori* and otitis media in children.

The role of *Helicobacter pylori* in chronic tonsillitis has been investigated. In a study of 52 patients from Turkey who were due for tonsillectomy because of chronic tonsillitis, *Helicobacter pylori* was detected both in the core tonsillar tissue and overlying mucosal tissue, using a RUT. Because there are many unculturable bacteria in the oropharynx and because other bacteria (e.g. *Corynebacterium* spp.) can give a positive RUT, the detection of *Helicobacter pylori* in this study has to be questioned. However, a study using culture and hybridization probes for *Helicobacter pylori* did detect the organism in cases of chronic tonsillitis and cancer.

The role of *Helicobacter pylori* in laryngeal disease has been reported. A study of 35 patients with chronic laryngitis detected 17% apparently colonized by *Helicobacter pylori*, but the study relied on RUT for detection. A study of laryngopharyngeal reflux disease studied 44 adults but did not demonstrate an association between symptoms and presence of gastric *Helicobacter pylori*. Organisms in the larynx were not looked for. Incidentally, this study could not find any association between *Helicobacter pylori* and GORD either.

Because *Helicobacter pylori* is a class I carcinogen and linked to the development of gastric cancer and MALT lymphoma, studies have also investigated the relationship between the organism and head and neck neoplasm. A seroprevalence study of 21 patients with squamous cell carcinoma (SCC) of the head and neck did not show any relationship to colonization by *Helicobacter pylori*. On the other hand, a similar study of 61 patients compared with controls demonstrated a 63% compared with 40% seroprevalance. A seroprevalence study of 26 patients with SCC of the larynx compared with controls demonstrated a prevalence of 73% compared with 40% respectively. In a case-controlled study of 120 patients with SCC of the larynx or pharynx, the seroprevalence of *Helicobacter pylori* was 32% in patients compared with 27% in controls. The difference was greater in the subgroup of laryngeal SCC (39%) compared with pharyngeal SCC (28%). Although no definite causal association was shown, the authors suggest a possible role for *Helicobacter pylori* in SCC of the larynx and further work is required.

Oral cancer is known to be related to betel, areca nut and tobacco chewing and is prevalent in Sri Lanka. A seroprevalence and culture study was undertaken in 30 patients with oral SCC, 30 patients without carcinoma but who chewed betel/areca nut, and 30 healthy controls who did not chew betel. Sixty-seven per cent of patients with oral cancer were chewers of betel/areca nut. Three patients with oral cancer tested positive for *Helicobacter pylori* by serology (two were also culture positive). Three of the non-cancer betel chewers were positive for *Helicobacter pylori* by serology. However, none of the non-betel chewers (non-cancer patients) tested positive for *Helicobacter pylori* by serology demonstrating no significant difference in the presence of *Helicobacter pylori* between patients with oral cancer and control subjects. Colonization by *Helicobacter pylori* in betel chewers occurred in 5 subjects (of 50) compared with non-betel chewers where 1 person was colonized (of 40) suggesting in this preliminary study a potential role for betel chewing in predisposing to colonization by *Helicobacter pylori*.

The role of *Helicobacter pylori* in AS has been investigated. Most studies have detected *Helicobacter pylori* by PCR. A seroprevalence study did not find an association between AS and *Helicobacter pylori*. One study detected *Helicobacter pylori* in 71% of ulcers but six other studies could either find no evidence of *Helicobacter pylori* in the ulcer or did not find a difference between the ulcer and normal mucosa. One study detected *Helicobacter pylori* in 67% of ulcers on mucosa overlying lymphoid tissue, compared with 10% in ulcers on non-lymphoid mucosa and zero in subjects without AS. In two studies in which symptoms of AS were investigated after eradication of *Helicobacter pylori*, one study demonstrated an improvement in symptoms, the other an improvement in the relapse rate.

There has been a small number of studies investigating the relationship between *Helicobacter pylori* and chronic cough, nasal polyps and sinusitis. *Helicobacter pylori* was detected in the faeces using the faecal antigen test more frequently in subjects with chronic cough (86%) compared

with control subjects (45%), and, after eradication of the *Helicobacter pylori*, symptoms improved in 75% of those with chronic cough. A study of patients with nasal polyps, using serology and immunohistochemistry, demonstrated no difference in seroprevalence compared with a control group (87% *vs* 85% respectively), although the organism was detected in polyp tissue but not in normal tissue. Three of 19 specimens from 2 of 11 patients with chronic sinusitis were positive by PCR and immunohistochemistry for *Helicobacter pylori*, suggesting no role for this organism in sinusitis. Overall, these studies indicate that *Helicobacter pylori* plays little if any role in various oropharyngolaryngeal diseases with the possible exception of SCC of the larynx.

Conditions of the respiratory system (3.18)

A small number of studies have shown an association between *Helicobacter pylori* and both chronic obstructive pulmonary disease (COPD) and bronchiectasis. In a study of 126 patients with COPD, the seroprevalence for *Helicobacter pylori* was 77% compared with 54% for a matched control population. Additionally, the seroprevalence for CagA-positive isolates was 54% in the patients compared with 29% in controls and in both cases, the titre of *Helicobacter pylori* antibodies was higher in the patient population than in the control population. A similar association was found in a smaller study of 68 patients where the prevalence was 66% compared with 57%. In a Chinese study of 46 patients

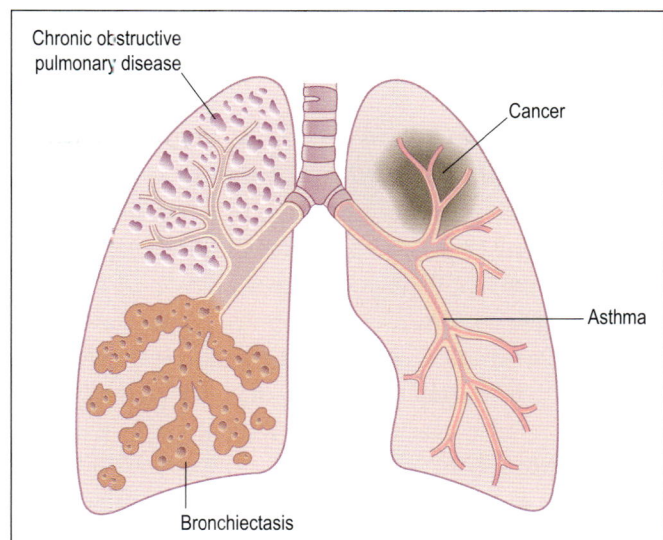

3.18 Suggested associations between *Helicobacter pylori* and respiratory conditions.

with chronic bronchitis, a higher seroprevalence for *Helicobacter pylori* and cagA was found in the patients (86% and 67% respectively) compared with the controls (60% and 20%). In one study, the forced expiratory volume of patients with COPD who were seropositive for *Helicobacter pylori* was lower than in the *Helicobacter pylori* negative COPD group.

In patients with bronchiectasis, the seroprevalence rate for *Helicobacter pylori* was 76% compared with tuberculosis (52%) and controls (54%). In a further study, *Helicobacter pylori* was not detected in any bronchial biopsy from 46 patients, despite 21 being seropositive. Similarly, a study of 26 patients with bronchiectasis did not show any difference in the seroprevalence to *Helicobacter pylori*, nor was *Helicobacter pylori* detected in bronchial lavage or lung biopsy specimens.

A study of 40 patients with lung cancer in Turkey demonstrated a seroprevalence to *Helicobacter pylori* of 93% compared with controls (12%) but studies from Greece and Iran could find no relationship between seroprevalence to *Helicobacter pylori* and lung cancer.

Transmission of *Helicobacter pylori* and *Mycobacterium tuberculosis* share the same demographics, with higher transmission associated with low social class and overcrowding. In addition, *Helicobacter pylori* may induce hypochlorhydria, which may be a risk factor for *M. tuberculosis*. However, two studies investigating the seroprevalence of *Helicobacter pylori* in patients with or without tuberculosis could demonstrate no difference.

Overall, there is enough circumstantial evidence to suggest an association between *Helicobacter pylori* and chronic bronchitis/bronchiectasis to warrant further investigation.

Conditions of the cardiovascular system (3.19)

There have been many studies investigating the relationship between *Helicobacter pylori* and thrombotic cardiovascular disorders (ischaemic heart disease and stroke) and vasospastic disorders (migraine and Raynaud's disease). The studies have involved serological investigations and detection of the organism in affected tissue.

Studies investigating the relationship between atherosclerosis/ischaemic heart disease and *Helicobacter pylori* have given conflicting results. *Helicobacter pylori* has been associated with a number of cardiovascular risk factors. In a study of 1650 Japanese subjects, those that were *Helicobacter pylori* seropositive had significantly

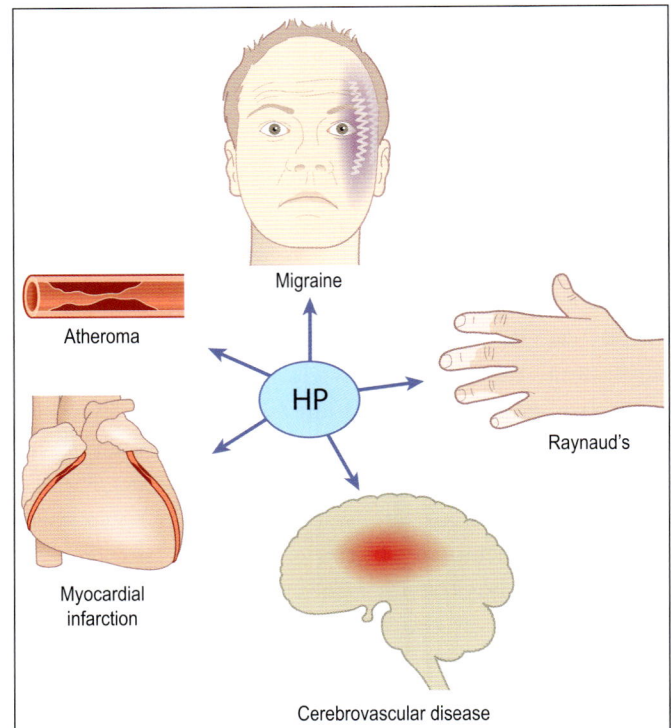

3.19 Suggested associations between *Helicobacter pylori* and cardiovascular illnesses.

lower high-density lipoprotein cholesterol. In a study of 58 981 subjects, seropositive patients had higher triglyceride, low-density lipoprotein cholesterol and apolipoprotein B levels, and lower high-density lipoprotein levels. *Helicobacter* infection also increases insulin resistance, which in turn has an association with atherosclerosis. In a study of 34 patients with AG compared with patients without AG, levels of serum homocysteine were higher (a risk factor for atherosclerosis) in patients with AG. In addition, carotid intima-media thickness was higher in this group, although it did not reach the level of statistical significance.

At variance with the above, many studies that have looked at cardiovascular risk factors have found no association with *Helicobacter pylori*. In a prospective study of 684 subjects, there was no relationship between being *Helicobacter* seropositive and classical cardiovascular risk factors. There was, however, an association between carotid artery intima-media thickness and CagA-seropositive subjects but not for CagA-negative *Helicobacter pylori*-seropositive subjects. In a study of patients with large vessel stroke compared with patients with cardio-embolic stroke and controls, there was no difference in the seroprevalence of *Helicobacter pylori*, despite the seroprevalence of CagA being 42%, 19% and 17%, respectively. A similar study in Japan confirmed an association between seropositivity for *Helicobacter pylori* and ischaemic stroke, principally small vessel disease rather than cardio-embolic disease. The presence of CagA was not reported. Studies have also confirmed an association between *Helicobacter pylori* and coronary atheroma. Clinical correlations with disease presentation have been reported in cases of angina where 81% of patients and 53% of matched controls were colonized by *Helicobacter pylori*. Classical risk factors for ischaemic heart disease were equally present in both seropositive and seronegative individuals. Similar associations have been reported in other studies of coronary heart disease with a seroprevalence of 81% in cases compared with 51% in controls, and, for CagA, 47% compared with 28% in controls. A similar study from Japan confirmed the association of seropositivity of *Helicobacter pylori* with acute coronary syndromes. In one study comparing 80 patients with coronary artery disease (CAD) against 160 controls, although the seroprevalence for *Helicobacter pylori* was similar (78% and 76%, respectively) the seroprevalence for CagA was 71% compared with 52% in the controls. Additionally the antibody titre to bacterial heat shock protein 60 (HpHSP60) was higher in those patients infected with CagA-positive *H. pylori* than in the control group, the implication being that *Helicobacter pylori* CagA strains and anti-HpHSP60 antibodies are both involved in disease.

A study of 90 patients with CAD compared with 90 control subjects demonstrated a seroprevalence of 78% for *Helicobacter pylori* in the patients but only 58% in the controls. However, another study of 175 patients compared with 88 controls was inconclusive: the seroprevalence in both groups was not significantly different and the rate of reintervention after angioplasty was similar in *Helicobacter pylori*-positive and -negative patients. A study of 353 patients with CAD confirmed by angiography, and comprising patients with infarction and unstable or stable angina, compared with patients with angiographically-proven patent coronary arteries, showed that the seroprevalence of *Helicobacter pylori* was similar in the patient and control groups (82–86%); so too was the titre of anti-*Helicobacter pylori* IgG, and

there was no correlation between the level of C-reactive protein and the levels of *Helicobacter pylori* IgG. This study suggests that the levels of anti-*Helicobacter pylori* IgG might be related to the extent of atheroma. A further study of 1754 subjects with ECG-confirmed CAD screened for a number of infectious agents (*Chlamydia pneumoniae*, *Helicobacter pylori*, herpes simplex virus type I and cytomegalovirus) did not demonstrate any correlation between antibodies to *Helicobacter pylori* (nor any of the other agents) and CAD; neither did the study demonstrate any relationship between an elevated C-reactive protein and CAD, unless there was concurrent infection with one of the infectious agents. This study suggests that chronic infection and the subsequent inflammatory response may be related to CAD. A similar study investigating the role of *Helicobacter pylori*-related proinflammatory cytokines and ischaemic heart disease could not demonstrate any significant correlation with circulating cytokines (IL-1, IL-6, tumour necrosis factor [TNF], IL-8), although there was a correlation between gastric mucosal levels of IL-6, TNF and ischaemic heart disease. These results suggest that a gastric inflammatory response induced by *Helicobacter pylori* may have some role in the genesis of ischaemic heart disease.

Two studies have reported on the relationship between *Helicobacter pylori* and atrial fibrillation in patients with CAD. One study demonstrated a marginally higher seroprevalence of *Helicobacter pylori* in patients with atrial fibrillation (65% vs 55%), particularly under 50 years old, and the second study demonstrated a higher prevalence of CagA in the atrial fibrillation group.

Some studies have attempted direct detection of potential pathogens in atheromatous plaques by PCR. *Helicobacter pylori* DNA has been detected in 20 of 38 atherosclerotic plaques in one study and in 4 of 29 coronary endarterectomy plaques in another. However, a second study could not demonstrate any difference in the detection of a range of infectious agents, including *Helicobacter pylori*, in the normal aortic wall compared with the atheromatous wall.

Helicobacter pylori has also been suggested as a cause of vasospastic disorders, including migraine and Raynaud's phenomenon. Again, contradictory results have been reported for both conditions, highlighting the uncertainty of the relationship between colonization by *Helicobacter pylori* and vasospastic vascular problems.

Conditions of the haemopoietic system (3.20)

Initial reports suggested an association between *Helicobacter pylori* and ITP and that eradication of *H. pylori* resulted in an increase in the platelet count. In 18 patients with ITP, 11 were colonized by *H. pylori* and a significant elevation in the platelet count occurred in 8 following eradication. Similarly, in 30 patients with ITP, 43% were colonized and an elevated platelet count occurred in 16% following eradication. In a study of 36 adults with ITP, 20 patients responded with an elevation of the platelet count following eradication of *Helicobacter pylori*, and this response was higher in patients who had the TNF-beta (TNFβ) G/G or G/A genotypes. A similar improvement in the platelet count occurred in 48% of patients in whom *Helicobacter pylori* was successfully eradicated and no improvement in those in whom it was not. In another study of 74 adult patients with ITP, of which 51% were seropositive for *Helicobacter pylori*, a sustained improvement in the platelet count occurred in 68% following eradication. A meta-analysis of 788 patients from 17 studies demonstrated that an increase in the platelet count occurred following eradication compared with untreated (an increase of $40.77 \times 10^9/L$) or *Helicobacter pylori*-negative subjects ($46.35 \times 10^9/L$). Overall, there appears to be a link between *Helicobacter pylori* and a reduced number of platelets, probably immune mediated, and eradication of the organism leads to an elevation of the platelet count. Eradication of *Helicobacter pylori* in patients with ITP is currently a recommendation of the Management Guidelines of the European Helicobacter Study Group—Maastricht III Consensus Report.

A number of small studies have shown an association between colonization by *Helicobacter pylori* and iron deficiency anaemia (IDA), particularly in children. In one study of 52 children, 31 had IDA, of whom 28 were colonized with *Helicobacter pylori*. In those patients with IDA, pan-gastritis was twice as common compared with those without IDA. *Helicobacter pylori* (but not anaemia) was associated with low gastric ascorbic acid levels and was more pronounced if the strain was *cagA* positive. *Helicobacter pylori* was also associated with low serum iron concentrations. In a study of 105 patients with unexplained IDA, *Helicobacter pylori*-associated chronic gastritis was found in 60% of the cases compared with 45% of the controls, particularly if AG was present. In a study of 116 pre-menopausal women who had chronic IDA, 16% had *Helicobacter*-associated gastritis. Eradication of *Helicobacter pylori* can lead to restoration of normal haemoglobin and serum iron. In 30 patients with chronic IDA where the only pathology to be found was chronic gastritis, 91% had normal haemoglobin 12 months after eradication of *Helicobacter pylori*. In contrast, in a study from Alaska where *Helicobacter pylori* colonization is high, 219 children who were colonized by *Helicobacter pylori* and had IDA were all given iron supplements and half were given *Helicobacter* eradication therapy. After 14 months, IDA was present in 65% of

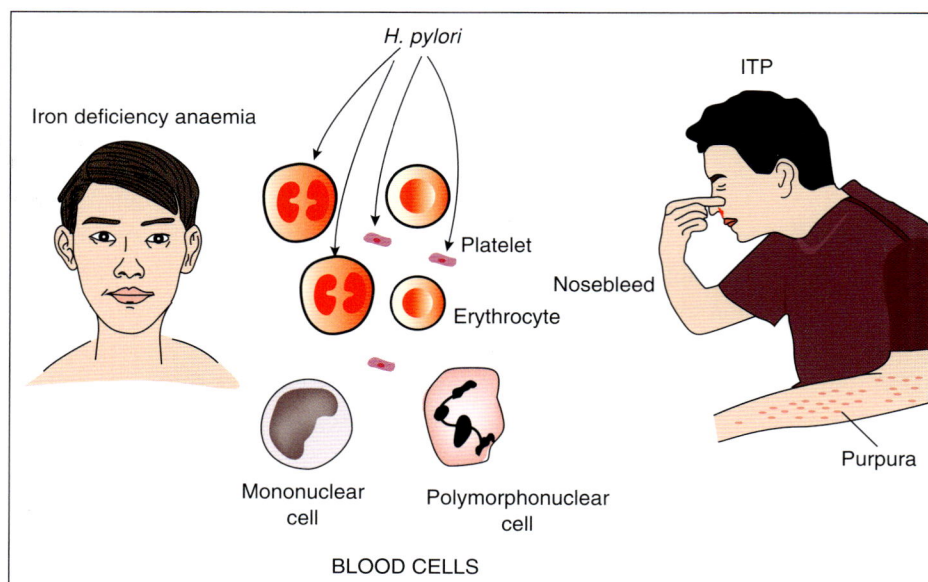

3.20 Suggested associations between *Helicobacter pylori* and haemopoietic diseases.

those given eradication therapy and 72% in the control group—*Helicobacter pylori* was eradicated in 68% of the treatment group and 4% became *Helicobacter* negative in the control group. In a study of 209 children, the difference in frequency of *Helicobacter pylori* in those with anaemia (43%) and those without anaemia (50%) was not statistically significant.

Conditions of the immune system (3.21)

The 'hygiene hypothesis' suggested that repeated immune stimulation by contact with environmental organisms has a beneficial effect by protecting against allergic conditions. Because the prevalence of these allergic conditions (food allergy, atopic dermatitis, urticaria, asthma) has increased while prevalence of a number of infections, including *Helicobacter pylori*, has decreased, the relationship between *Helicobacter pylori* and various allergic conditions has been investigated. In a cross-sectional study of Danish adults, those who were seropositive for markers of poor hygiene (*Helicobacter pylori*, hepatitis A virus, *Toxoplasma gondii*) were less likely to have allergic conditions compared with those who were seropositive for intestinal pathogens (*Campylobacter jejuni*, *Clostridium difficile*, *Yersinia enterocolitica*), who were more likely to have allergic conditions. A similar study comparing 266 children in both Russia and Finland also found a protective effect

from infection by *Helicobacter pylori* on atopic conditions. In addition, in one study of 240 patients with rhinitis and asthma, a lower incidence of *Helicobacter pylori* was detected compared with controls. In another study of the seroprevalence of *Helicobacter pylori* in Finnish children between 1973 and 1994, an inverse relationship between IgE levels and *Helicobacter pylori* was demonstrated, with high IgE levels of 21% in the *Helicobacter pylori*-negative subgroup compared with 5% in the *Helicobacter pylori*-positive group in 1994. Similarly, a negative association was demonstrated between skin hypersensitivity (as a marker for atopy), and seroprevalence to *Helicobacter pylori* in a group of asthmatics compared with controls. In this study, it was noted that certain polymorphisms of IL-4 (–590T/T) were related to a decreased risk of being seropositive for *Helicobacter pylori*. In patients with chronic idiopathic urticaria, eradication of *Helicobacter pylori* improved the condition in 72%. However, a study of 16 patients with chronic urticaria compared with controls could not demonstrate a significant difference between colonization by *Helicobacter pylori* in the two groups.

Furthermore, in a study of 97 patients, colonization by *Helicobacter pylori* had no effect on the expression of allergy and, in a study of 90 middle-aged asthmatics, there was no difference in the seroprevalence of *Helicobacter pylori* when compared with a control

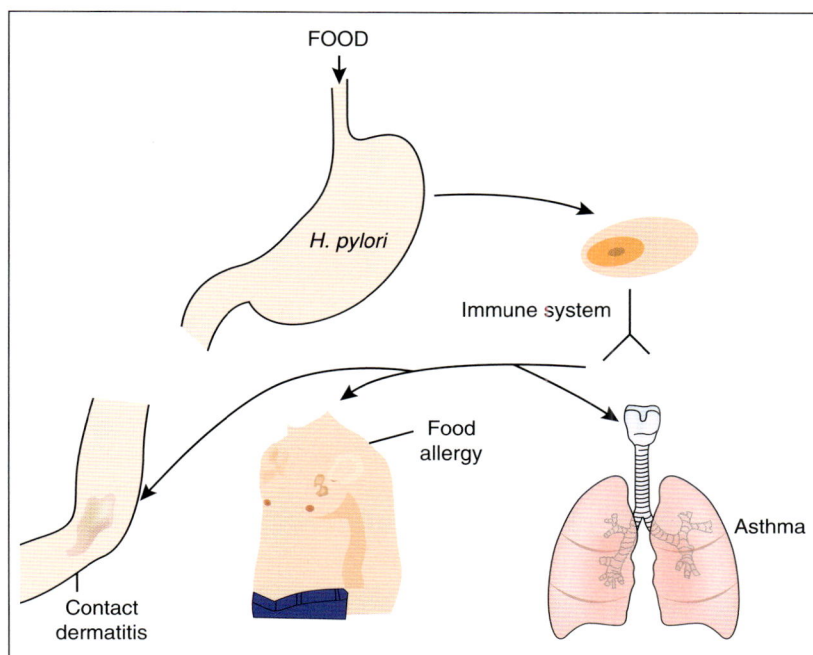

3.21 Suggested associations between *Helicobacter pylori* and atopic disease and asthma.

population. However, a study of 90 patients with either atopic dermatitis, food allergy or asthma showed an increased titre of anti-*Helicobacter pylori* antibodies in the atopic dermatitis and food allergy groups compared with the asthmatic group. In a study of urticaria in children, recent infection, including with *Helicobacter pylori*, was more likely to be linked to presentation.

A number of studies have investigated the relationship between *Helicobacter pylori* and food allergy. A seroprevalence study of 38 patients with food allergy compared with matched controls demonstrated that although the seroprevalence of *Helicobacter pylori* was similar (42% vs 48%) the seroprevalence of anti-CagA antibodies was significantly higher in those patients with food allergy (62%) compared with controls (28%), and the serum level of IgE to food allergens was also higher in CagA-positive patients (3.2 U/ml vs 1.9 U/ml). In a different study in children, when patients with food allergy were compared with patients with asthma or IBD, the titre of anti-*Helicobacter pylori* IgG was higher in patients with food allergy but there was no difference in the titre of anti-CagA antibodies. A further study showed that the degree of inflammation was higher in patients who had food allergy and were colonized by *Helicobacter pylori* compared with patients who were not colonized but had food allergy. On the other hand, a study of food-specific IgE demonstrated no significant difference in the prevalence between those infected with *Helicobacter pylori* (33%) compared with those who were not infected (26%).

Histopathologically, subjects with food allergy have a similar appearance to those with coeliac disease (i.e. an increased permeability of the mucosa to food antigens is common to both). The clinical presentation of both is unrelated, although villous atrophy appears milder in patients with coeliac disease that are also infected with *Helicobacter pylori*. Additionally, follicular gastritis was more common in patients with infected coeliac disease but AG was less. These findings demonstrate a complex immunological interaction between coeliac disease and *Helicobacter pylori* colonization.

Conditions of the endocrine system (3.22)

Studies on the relationship between *Helicobacter pylori* and endocrine abnormalities (thyroiditis, diabetes) have given conflicting results. In a group of 80 patients with insulin-dependent diabetes mellitus (type 1 diabetes),

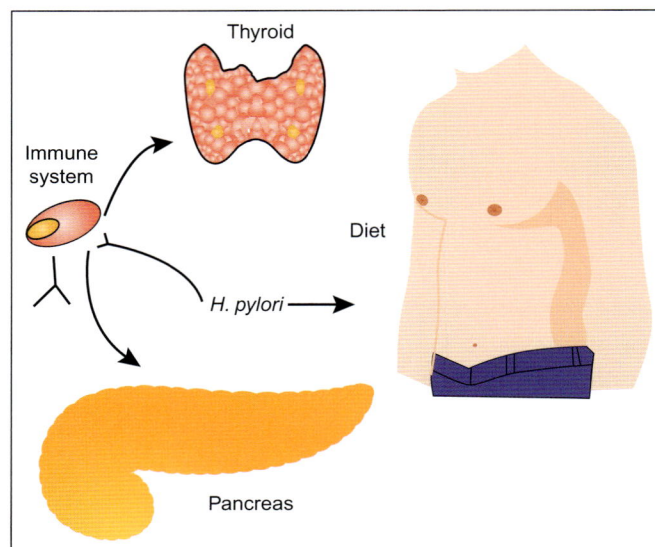

3.22 Suggested associations between *Helicobacter pylori* and endocrine disease.

the seroprevalence to *Helicobacter pylori* was higher than in the control group if <24 y, but over 24 y was similar. The titres of antibodies to parietal and islet cells were higher in the *Helicobacter pylori*-positive group compared with *Helicobacter pylori*-negative diabetics. A similar association has been demonstrated for adult-onset (or type 2) diabetes in 210 patients compared with matched controls where the seroprevalence was 76% and 64% respectively. A study of type 2 diabetics from Turkey, however, could not detect any significant difference in 141 diabetics compared with 142 non-diabetics (61% and 58%), nor was there any correlation with complications of diabetes, except for neuropathy, where patients who were colonized were more likely to have neuropathy.

A seroprevalence study of 59 patients with autoimmune thyroiditis demonstrated a seroprevalence for *Helicobacter pylori* of 85% compared with 40% in non-toxic nodular goitre and 45% in Addison's disease. A second seroprevalence study of 90 patients with autoimmune thyroiditis compared with controls demonstrated a seroprevalence of 26% compared with 12%. The authors further demonstrated that a significant association was present between infection with *Helicobacter pylori* and HLA-DRB1*0301. A second study has demonstrated higher numbers of seroreactive individuals with anti-*Helicobacter pylori* IgA in patients compared with controls, and higher numbers of seroreactive individuals with anti-VacA IgG in addition to both a 17 kDa and 30 kDa antigen.

The effect of colonization by *Helicobacter pylori* on orexigenic hormones (leptin, ghrelin) and on body mass index (BMI) has also been investigated. A complex hormonal interaction exists to control appetite, metabolism and growth. Ghrelin, a recently discovered hormone produced principally by epithelial cells in the fundus of the stomach, has two major biological activities: first, regulation of energy balance (i.e. by increasing hunger through its action upon the hypothalamus and suppression of fat utilization in adipose tissue); and, secondly, stimulation of growth hormone (GH) secretion from the anterior pituitary. The release of growth hormone is also regulated by growth hormone-releasing hormone secreted from the hypothalamus, and somatostatin (an inhibitory factor) synthesized by many tissues, including D cells in the stomach. GH has a direct effect upon adipose tissue, increasing triglyceride breakdown, and a direct effect upon the liver by stimulating production of insulin-like growth factor-1 (IGF-1). It is this increase in IGF-1 that is responsible, in part, for growth-enhancing effects by: stimulating the proliferation of chondrocytes and myloblasts; stimulating protein synthesis in many tissues; increasing fat utilization; plus IGF-1 is, in part, responsible for the control of blood glucose levels. The plasma concentration of GH is highest during deep sleep. For ghrelin, plasma levels increase before a meal and are lowest postprandially; plasma ghrelin levels also reduced in obesity. Acylated ghrelin is the active form, although de-acylated ghrelin may also have biological relevance. Leptin is an important factor in regulating body weight and metabolism as well. It is found predominantly in adipose tissue but also in the stomach and placenta. As triglycerides accumulate in the adipocytes, the level of leptin also increases, and there is a correlation between body fat and blood leptin levels. Leptin acts upon the hypothalamus to decrease hunger and food consumption and to increase energy metabolism. Leptin also has effects upon reproduction.

Leptin and ghrelin are key regulators of the release of GH and metabolic control, and disturbances in these pathways may represent a plausible biological explanation for short stature and the evolution of atherosclerosis. Both hormones are affected by *Helicobacter pylori* colonization.

Ghrelin levels in a *Helicobacter pylori*-positive group of patients were significantly lower compared with a *Helicobacter pylori*-negative group. Similarly, serum ghrelin and leptin concentrations were significantly lower in *Helicobacter pylori*-infected than non-infected children. Histologically, ghrelin-immunoreactive cells were significantly reduced in *Helicobacter pylori*-positive individuals. The degree of gastric atrophy associated with *Helicobacter pylori* colonization also appears to be linked to the plasma ghrelin levels. Eradication of *Helicobacter pylori* leads to an increase in plasma ghrelin levels. As ghrelin stimulates the release of GH, ghrelin deficiency may provide an explanation for the reduced height in children colonized by *Helicobacter pylori*. In addition, the high incidence of *Helicobacter pylori* infection in children in some countries seems to contribute to decreased serum levels of ghrelin and to decreased appetite and dyspeptic symptoms in children. On the other hand, some studies have found no relationship between colonization by *Helicobacter pylori* and ghrelin or leptin levels. These (few) studies confirm that these hormones have not been thoroughly investigated in *Helicobacter pylori* infection, particularly in relation to virulence characteristics of *Helicobacter pylori*.

Little is known about the role of ghrelin in the body or the physiological circumstances controlling its release from the stomach. Neither is much known about the relationship between *Helicobacter pylori* virulence factors (e.g. CagA/VacA) and appetite hormones, and there are few published data available on the effect of different gastric pathologies and these factors, especially in children. The issue regarding the differences in plasma ghrelin between *Helicobacter pylori*-positive and -negative patients is still under debate. In addition, other important questions remain to be answered, such as whether colonization by *Helicobacter pylori* affects ghrelin dynamics and its relation to obesity and its associated diseases over the long term. Thus, in developed countries, *Helicobacter pylori*-negative children may have relatively high concentrations of ghrelin, may reach their full growth potential and may grow into overweight adults with obesity and associated problems. In developing countries, however, where *Helicobacter pylori* prevalence is high, children may not achieve full stature, and some will develop peptic ulcer disease or adenocarcinoma of the stomach.

Special interest has been focused on the relationship between body weight regulation, stature and BMI after it was reported that the eradication of *Helicobacter pylori* was associated with a significant increase in body weight and BMI, and a report linked colonization by *Helicobacter pylori* with short stature. Indeed, it has also been suggested that decreasing prevalence of *Helicobacter pylori* in the population may be causally related to increasing obesity and, therefore, GORD and an increasing incidence of oesophageal adenocarcinoma.

A study of 4742 subjects in Northern Ireland demonstrated that colonization by *Helicobacter pylori* was related to low stature in females. Studies on 24 children in Turkey with constitutional delay of growth and puberty had a seroprevalence to *Helicobacter pylori* of 66%, compared with a matched control population of 37%. This suggests that colonization by *Helicobacter pylori* could be a risk factor for short stature or delayed puberty. In a further study of 3315 healthy children in Germany, those who were colonized by *Helicobacter pylori* were shorter than the *Helicobacter*-negative cohort. In boys, the weight of those who were colonized was less than that of the non-infected control. A study of 41 Japanese children with growth hormone deficiency ($n = 27$) or idiopathic short stature ($n = 14$) were assessed for seroprevalence to *Helicobacter pylori*. The highest prevalence was in the idiopathic group (28% compared with the control or GH deficiency group [6.4% and 7.4%, respectively]). In a prospective study of 347 Colombian children, those colonized with *Helicobacter pylori* showed a reduced growth velocity and short stature. A further study from Turkey in 40 children with growth retardation showed a 78% seroprevalence of *Helicobacter pylori*, and an 85% seroprevalence of CagA compared with a control population (10% and 15%, respectively).

On the other hand, some studies have not found any association between colonization by *Helicobacter pylori* and growth retardation or BMI. A study of native Alaskan children failed to demonstrate any relationship between colonization by *Helicobacter pylori* and growth retardation. Two studies in the USA could not demonstrate any relationship between *Helicobacter pylori* colonization and BMI. In one study, 6724 subjects were screened for seroprevalence to *Helicobacter pylori* and CagA and, in a second study, 7003 subjects were similarly screened for seroprevalence, resulting in an overall OR 1.17–1.20 for being colonized by *Helicobacter pylori* and developing obesity. A study from Taiwan has demonstrated an inverse relationship between colonization by *Helicobacter pylori* and morbid obesity, and has suggested that lack of colonization by *Helicobacter pylori* in childhood might be a risk factor for the development of morbid obesity. Similarly, in Japan, a study of 932 subjects showed that eradication of *Helicobacter pylori* led to an increase in BMI.

Conditions of the central nervous system

Patients with the neurodegenerative disorder Parkinson's disease have inflammation in the brain and an association with peptic ulceration of the gastrointestinal tract; consequently, the role of *Helicobacter pylori* has been investigated. A serological study of patients with Parkinson's disease has demonstrated a higher seroprevalence compared with controls. Using IgG antibodies against *H. pylori* antigens, a study of 124 subjects with Parkinson's disease demonstrated that presence of CagA seroreactivity was a predictive marker for the illness.

Conditions of the skin (3.23)

Helicobacter pylori colonization and skin conditions have also been investigated. Higher seroprevalence has been found in patients who have rosacea, and improvement occurred following eradication of the organism in 29 patients, with 35% having a complete improvement and 31% a good improvement, with only five patients showing no improvement. A possible association between *Helicobacter pylori* and both psoriasis and Henoch–Schönlein purpura has also been documented.

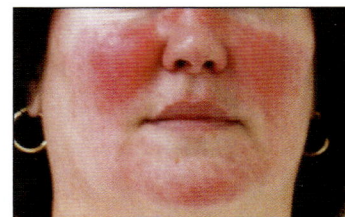

3.23 A patient with rosacea.

Further reading

Anon. Schistosomes, liver flukes and *Helicobacter pylori*. IARC Working Group on the Evaluation of Carcinogenic Risks to Humans. *IARC Monogr Eval Carcinog Risks Hum* 1994; 61: 1–241.

Bohr UR, Annibale B, Franceschi F, Roccarina D, Gasbarrini A. Extragastric manifestations of *Helicobacter pylori*-other helicobacters. *Helicobacter* 2007; 12(Suppl): 43–53.

Corley DA, Kubo A, Levin TR, *et al*. *Helicobacter pylori* infection and the risk of Barrett's oesophagus: a community-based study. *Gut* 2008; 57: 727–33.

Halder SL, Talley NJ. Functional dyspepsia: a new Rome III Paradigm. *Curr Treat Options Gastroenterol* 2007; 10: 259–72.

Hellmig S, Hampe J, Schreiber S. *Helicobacter pylori* infection in Africa and Europe: enigma of host genetics. *Gut* 2003; 52: 1799.

Holcombe C. *Helicobacter pylori*: the African enigma. *Gut* 1992; 33: 429–31.

Leong RWL, Sung JJY. *Helicobacter pylori* and hepatobiliary disease. *Aliment Pharmacol Ther* 2002; 16: 1037–45.

Nordenstedt H, Nilsson M, Johnsen R, Lagergren J, Hveem K. *Helicobacter pylori* infection and gastroesophogeal reflux in a population based study (the HUNT Study). *Helicobacter* 2007; 12: 16–22.

O'Morain C. Role of *Helicobacter pylori* in functional dyspepsia. *World J Gastroenterol* 2006; 12: 2677–80.

Quigley EM, Keohane J. Dyspepsia. *Curr Opin Gastroenterol* 2008; 24: 692–7.

Santacroce L, Cagiano R, Del Prete R, *et al*. *Helicobacter pylori* infection and gastric MALToma: an up to date and therapeutic highlight. *Clin Ther* 2008; 159: 457–62.

Singh K, Ghoshal UC. Causal role of *Helicobacter pylori* infection in gastric cancer: an Asian enigma. *World J Gastroenterol* 2006; 12: 1346–51.

Tsuji S. The 'Costa Rica enigma' of *Helicobacter pylori* CagA and gastric cancer. *J Gastroenterol* 2006; 41: 716–17.

Chapter 4

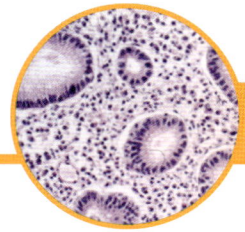

Pathogenesis

Virulence

Virulence factors encompass all determinants that enable pathogens to invade the host and survive. The study of *Helicobacter pylori* determinants of pathogenicity is complicated by the fact that everything concerning *Helicobacter pylori* infection is unusual, for example:

- The bacterial habitat (restricted to the stomach, an environment in which no other bacteria are able to survive).
- The genomic variability (strains from different patients have different genomic patrimonies).
- The infection itself (which lasts for the entire patient's life if it is not treated).

In addition, the methods for investigating the virulence characteristics of bacteria have been established mostly for fast-growing, non-fastidious organisms, which develop well in broth and nearly always cause acute infections: moreover, they were laid down before the existence of *Helicobacter pylori* infection was discovered. On the contrary, *Helicobacter pylori* is a peculiar, fastidious, slow-growing organism, which does not develop in broth if the inoculum is not dense.

Once it became apparent that *Helicobacter pylori* infection was a *sine qua non* in ulcerogenesis, and a risk factor for the development of gastric cancer, the search for putative virulence factors of *Helicobacter pylori* received a vigorous boost. Perhaps the most striking aspect of *Helicobacter pylori* infection is that the majority of subjects who harbour this organism remain asymptomatic throughout their entire lives and never develop ulcers or cancer. Possible explanations for this are variations in the virulence of *Helicobacter pylori* or polymorphisms in the host. However, *Helicobacter pylori* is a primary pathogen, as gastric epithelial colonization with these bacteria is practically always associated with mucosal inflammatory lesions. A certain proportion of isolates (from about 20% to 80% according to where patients live) possess factors of increased pathogenicity.

The first steps in pathogenesis are the ability to penetrate the mucus and adherence to the gastric epithelial cells. Motility, spiral shape and the ability to survive acid conditions for a short period of time are, thus, important initial virulence characteristics and, in this, the urease activity of *Helicobacter pylori* is important for modulation of the bacterial intracellular pH while transiently in an acid environment. The organism adheres by a number of different adhesins, the most important of which is BabA, whose ligand is the Lewis blood group antigens (*see* Chapter 2). Other loci that have been reported to be important virulence markers are *sabA* (*see* Chapter 2), *cagA*, *vacA*, *iceA*, *oipA*, *dupA* and *napA*, although there is increasing recognition that none of these markers can robustly predict clinical outcome. It has been suggested that only the presence of the *cag*PAI (and its association with an inflammatory response), and *cag*PAI-independent *oipA*, *dupA* and *babA* are the only markers that could be considered related to virulence. More crucially, the host response to the presence of *Helicobacter pylori* may be more important than the strain in determining clinical outcome.

Once adherent, the organism begins to initiate inflammation and, in a proportion of patients, symptoms of disease. There are four general pathophysiological mechanisms whereby *Helicobacter pylori* causes gastroduodenal disease: the production of surface-damaging agents; interference with normal physiological mechanisms; interference with cell signalling and cell dynamics; and inflammatory and immunopathological mechanisms.

Surface-damaging factors

Helicobacter pylori produces a number of extracellular products important in the pathogenesis of cell damage: urease; phospholipase; alcohol dehydrogenase (ADH); and, importantly, the VacA cytotoxin. Certain enzymes produced protect the organism against damaging free radicals or acid—these include urease, carbonic anhydrase, superoxide dismutase (SOD) and catalase. Additional extracellular products, such as neuroaminidase, indirectly damage the mucosa; yet others appear to have little relationship to pathogenicity, e.g., isocitrate dehydrogenase and fucosidase.

Urease

Urease is one of the most abundant proteins produced by *Helicobacter pylori*, comprising about 10–15% of the total protein content, testifying to its importance to the organism. Urease is composed of two major subunits and, although synthesized in the cytoplasm, it is found on the surface of the organism due to a process of 'altruistic autolysis' whereby spontaneous lysis of *H. pylori* cells releases urease (among other cellular proteins), which then adheres to the surface of intact bacteria. The 26 kDa (UreA) and 62 kDa (UreB) subunits of *H. pylori* urease form a trimeric assembly of UreA–UreB dimers, (AB)$_3$. Nickel is transported into the cell by NixA and bound into the active site on the UreB subunits (making 12 Ni atoms per enzyme) with the aid of UreG, one of four urease accessory proteins (UreE–H) involved in nickel binding to the active site. UreI is a proton-gated pore controlling access of urea to the bacterium on which the UreA–UreB complex is bound. *In vivo* colonization by *Helicobacter pylori* and modulation of urease activity is dependent upon a metal efflux pump CznA-C.

The urease protein has four main effects:

1. Catabolic function, by incorporating nitrogen into the organism

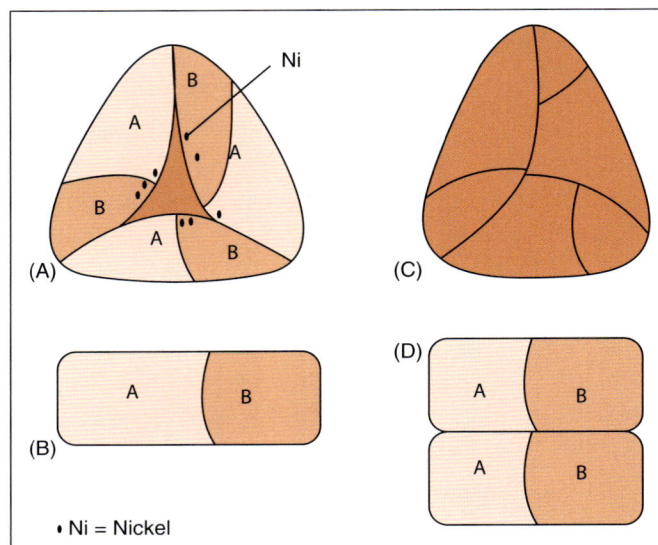

4.1 Idealized diagram showing the subunit structure of *Helicobacter* urease: (A) top view and (B) side view. Two of these subunits associate to form the holoenzyme that has a central empty spherical cavity: (C) top view and (D) side view.

2. Mucinolysis
3. Direct cell-damaging and proinflammatory effect
4. Allowing bacterial survival in an acid environment

Urease-negative mutants are unable to colonize, although adherence is unaffected.

The urease enzyme (pH optimum of 7.0–8.0) splits urea according to the following general equation:

$$(NH_2)_2CO + H_2O \rightarrow 2NH_3 + CO_2$$

One of the functions of the urease enzyme is to provide nitrogen in the form of ammonia/ammonium that can be incorporated into cell anabolism according to the following equation:

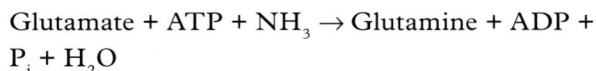

$$\text{Glutamate} + ATP + NH_3 \rightarrow \text{Glutamine} + ADP + P_i + H_2O$$

The ammonia produced by the urease enzyme can have a direct toxic action upon epithelial cells and on the tight junctions affecting paracellular permeability. This effect of NH_3/NH_4^+ is through the endocytosis and accumulation of an altered occludin protein. Also, the activity of myosin regulatory light chain kinase is increased, mediated by UreB protein, which in turn leads to increased phosphorylation of myosin regulatory

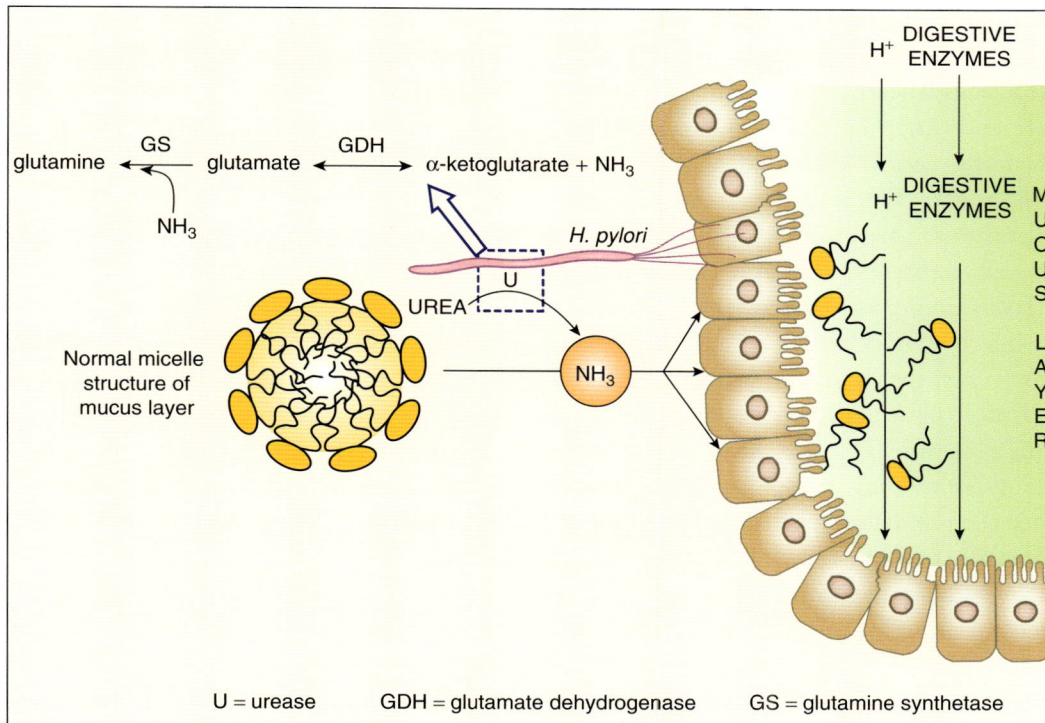

U = urease   GDH = glutamate dehydrogenase   GS = glutamine synthetase

4.2 The local effects of *Helicobacter pylori* through the action of urease.

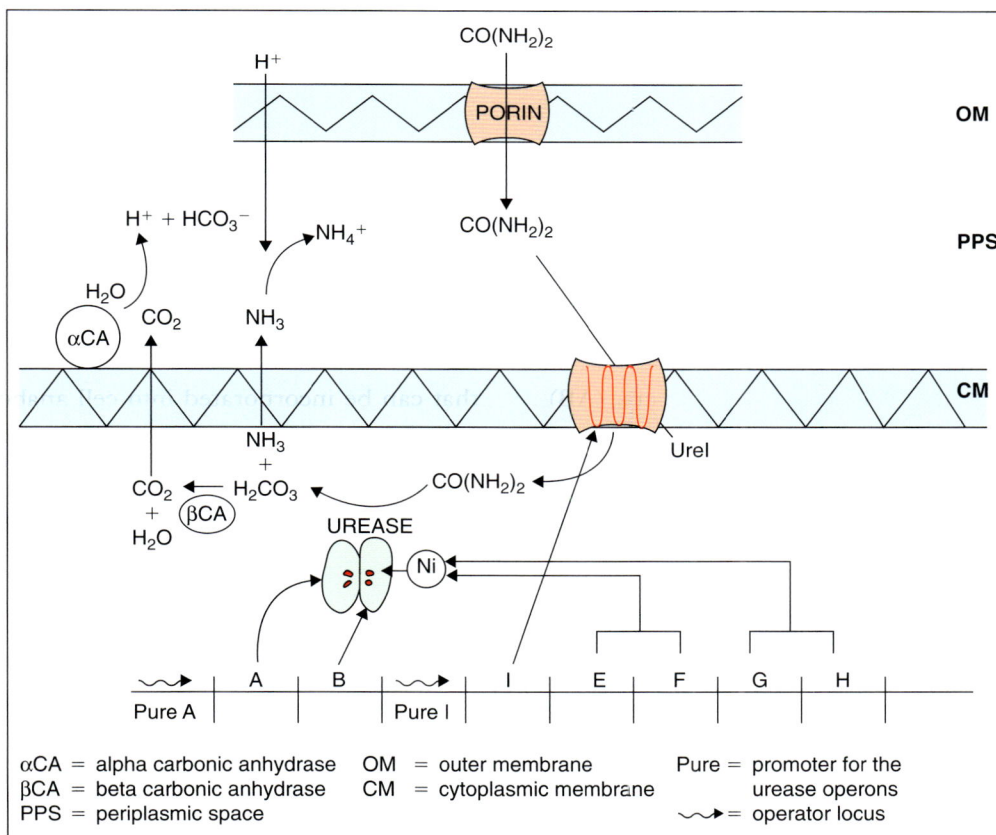

αCA = alpha carbonic anhydrase   OM = outer membrane   Pure = promoter for the
βCA = beta carbonic anhydrase   CM = cytoplasmic membrane   urease operons
PPS = periplasmic space   ⤳ = operator locus

4.3 Chemical protection of *Helicobacter pylori* in an acid environment.

light chain and, hence, functional regulation of tight junctions. Additionally, NH_3/NH_4^+ disrupt the micellar structure of the mucus, thereby making the mucus thin and watery and allowing stomach enzymes and acid to directly affect the gastric epithelial cells (**4.2**; the so-called 'leaking roof'). The micellar structure is also affected by the phospholipase enzymes.

The fourth, and perhaps most important, function of *Helicobacter pylori* urease is to protect it while in the acid milieu of the stomach, producing a cytoplasmic buffering capacity for the acid and maintaining the microbe periplasm at neutral. This is achieved by the proton-gated urea channel, UreI, which is a 21 kDa transmembrane protein lying across the cytoplasmic membrane. Once the pH decreases in the environment, UreI becomes protonated and the gate opens allowing ingress of the urea from the periplasmic space. The assembled dodecameric urease apoenzyme (UreAUreB)$_6$ moves from the cytoplasm to lay adjacent to the UreI pore on the inner leaflet of the cytoplasmic membrane and acquires nickel with the aid of the accessory proteins UreE–H. The functioning enzyme then hydrolyses the urea to ammonia and carbonic acid. The carbonic acid is converted to carbon dioxide by cytoplasmic β-carbonic anhydrase according to the following equation:

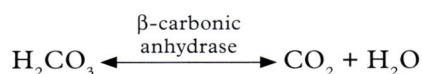

$$H_2CO_3 \xleftarrow{\substack{\beta\text{-carbonic} \\ \text{anhydrase}}} CO_2 + H_2O$$

The volatile ammonia and carbon dioxide diffuse into the periplasmic space where the following reactions occur spontaneously and by periplasmic α-carbonic anhydrase, the ammonia thus buffering hydrogen ions in the periplasmic space (**4.3**):

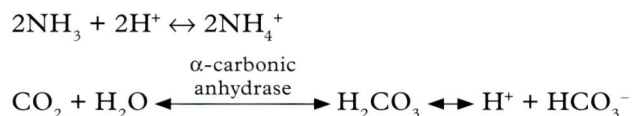

$$2NH_3 + 2H^+ \leftrightarrow 2NH_4^+$$

$$CO_2 + H_2O \xleftrightarrow{\substack{\alpha\text{-carbonic} \\ \text{anhydrase}}} H_2CO_3 \leftrightarrow H^+ + HCO_3^-$$

Phospholipase

Phospholipases are an important and diverse group of enzymes that are virulence factors for several micro-organisms and important modulators of cell signalling in host cells. There are four main groups of phospholipases: A_1, A_2, C and D. Each major group has several subgroups. One of the groups, PLA_2, can be subdivided into five

main subgroups: secreted phospholipase ($sPLA_2$), cytosolic phospholipase ($cPLA_2$), calcium-independent phospholipase ($iPLA_2$), platelet-activating factor (PAF) acetylhydrolases, and lysosomal phospholipase (L-PLA_2). $sPLA_2$ is secreted from the pancreas and is found in other body fluids (e.g. synovial fluid). $cPLA_2$ hydrolyses arachidonic acid and is important in cell signalling. Phospholipase C (PLC) also comprises a large family of enzymes that are phosphoinositide specific and are involved in cell signalling.

The putative targets of these enzymes are the phospholipid-rich zone of gastric epithelial cells and the phospholipid components of the gastric mucus. Phospholipases attack phospholipids and generate amphipathic lysolecithin and fatty acids (**4.4**). Lysolecithin is an ulcerogen and is also a precursor for PAF, which is also an ulcerogen. Colonization by *Helicobacter pylori* activates host $cPLA_2$ via its lipopolysaccharide, which, in addition, results in decreased mucus secretion. Increased levels of bacterial PLA enzyme by strains isolated from patients with gastric carcinoma have been noted and it has been suggested that infection by hypersecretory strains may have a role in gastric carcinogenesis.

The effect of bacterial PLA_2 is to modify the cell membrane of *Helicobacter pylori*, increasing the lysophospholipid content but also decreasing membrane stability. However, membrane stability is maintained by cholesterol pyranosides content. This PLA_2 activity appears to be pH regulated and mechanistically is due to phase variation of the PLA_2 gene. *Helicobacter pylori* with higher lysophospholipid content in the cell membrane are more acid resistant and bind to gastric epithelial cells more strongly. In summary, *Helicobacter pylori* produces clinically relevant concentrations of PLA_2 and PLC that may affect the quality of the mucus barrier as well as the integrity of the gastric epithelial cell, and leads to the production of an ulcerogenic cascade of inflammatory mediators.

Alcohol dehydrogenase

There are several families of ADH that have either zinc or iron at the catalytic site and require nicotinamide adenine dinucleotide (NAD^+) or NAD phosphate ($NADP^+$) as cofactors, although some require quinoids as cofactors. The ADH from *Helicobacter pylori* is a protein of 38 kDa that uses NAD^+ as a cofactor and preferentially

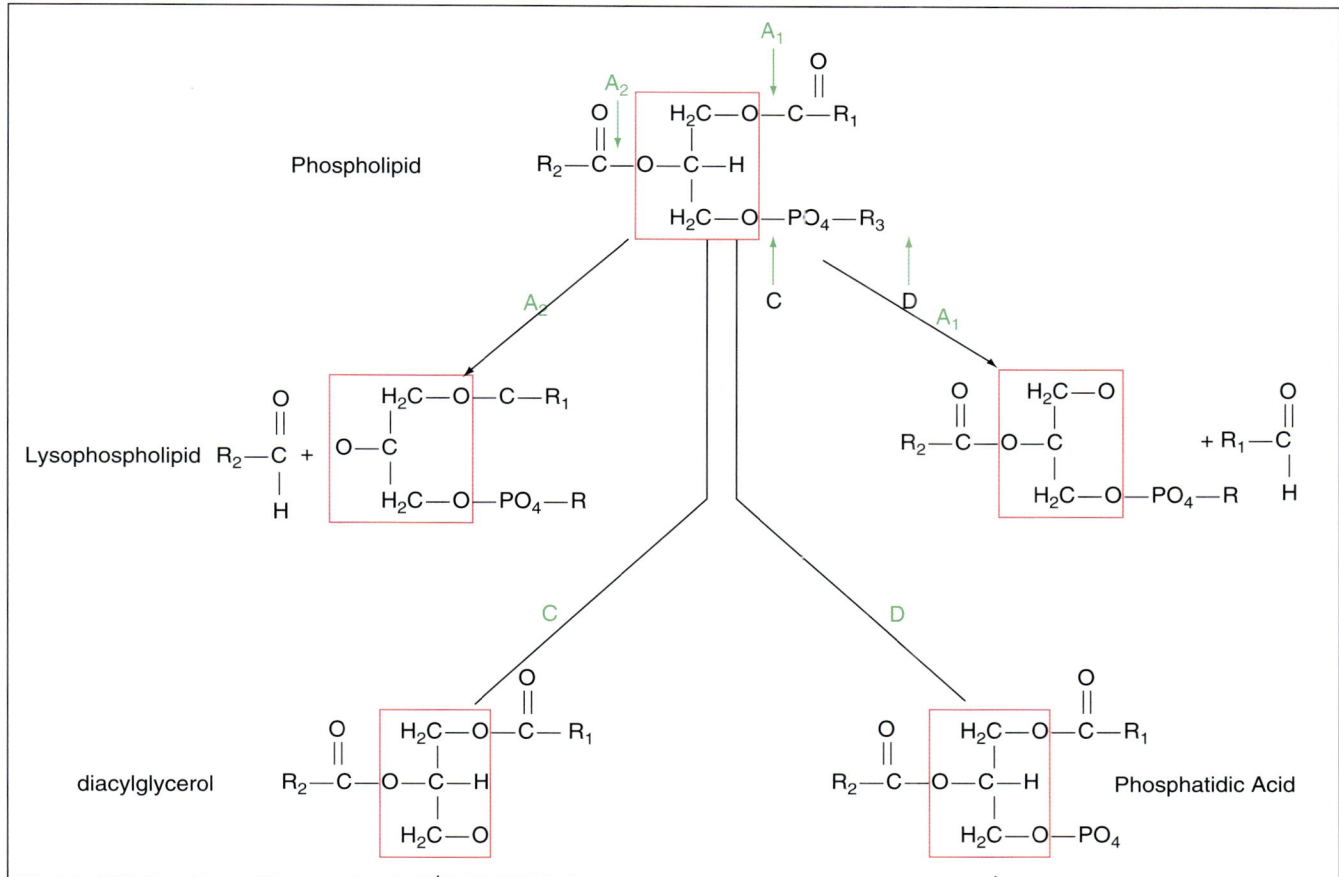

4.4 The action of various phospholipases.

hydrolyses primary alcohols. The ADH monomer consists of two catalytic domains and a binding domain. Two monomers combine to give the holoenzyme and the alcohol fits into a cleft with NAD^+ next to the catalytic site. ADH acts upon ethanol to produce acetaldehyde according to the following equation:

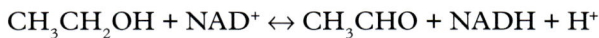

$$CH_3CH_2OH + NAD^+ \leftrightarrow CH_3CHO + NADH + H^+$$

As the organism lacks acetaldehyde dehydrogenase activity, acetaldehyde can accumulate in the gastric tissues, possibly causing damage by promoting tissue erosion and ulceration. The acetaldehyde produced inhibits proliferation of gastric cells and this may be involved in the development of disease. In addition, acetaldehyde *in vitro* reacts with phospholipids and proteins to form adducts. Acetaldehyde can also bind various proteins *in vivo* and may induce lipid peroxidation, which may have a direct toxic effect on gastric mucosa (**4.5**).

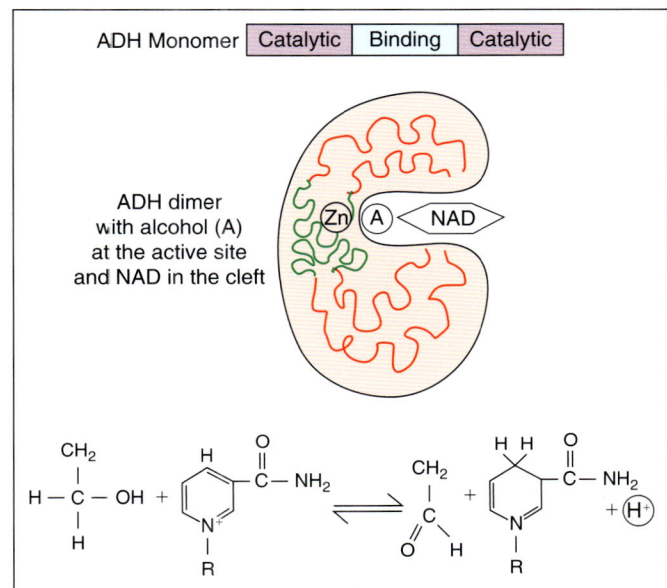

4.5 The action of ADH.

Helicobacter pylori also produces a cinnamyl-ADH (45 kDa), which can react on both cinnamyl alcohols and cinnamaldehydes, and an aldoketose reductase (39 kDa), which can reduce a wide range of aromatic aldehydes and is an important enzyme that allows growth of the organism under acidic conditions.

Humans have five isoenzymes of ADH distributed in different tissues. In the stomach, class I, III and IV are found. Colonization with *Helicobacter pylori* leads to a decrease in classes III and IV (in males) in the stomach but an increase in serum levels. Class I ADH levels are unaffected.

Vacuolating cytotoxin

The *vacA* gene encodes for a protoxin of 1296 amino acids with a mass of 140 kDa, initially secreted into the environment as monomers after cleavage of the N-terminal leader sequence (*see* p.13), which then aggregate to form a high molecular weight (700–1000 kDa) toxin having the shape of a flowerhead (**4.6**). The soluble VacA monomers released by the bacteria form oligomers with the appearance of a hexameric rosette resembling the head of a flower. The rosette has a size of ≈30 nm, with a central ring of ≈15 nm encircled by six or seven ≈6 nm 'petals'. A larger complex is made of two of such flower-like overlapped structures. The 95 kDa monomers are structured in two distinct fragments joined by an exposed loop. *In vitro*, monomers undergo proteolytic cleaving at the level of the loop (without disrupting the oligomeric structure of the toxin), to yield an N-terminal fragment of 37 kDa (p37) and a C-terminal fragment of 58 kDa (p58). Following activation (see below) the 58 kDa fragment appears to form the base and lobes, while the 37 kDa fragment forms the centrally raised area of the toxin in the host cell membrane (**4.6**). The amino-terminal fragment contains three GXXXG tandem repeats, forming a hydrophobic segment which is important for oligomerization.

This type of cleavage is characteristic of the A/B family of bacterial toxins that exploit one subunit (the B, or binding subunit) to adhere to and penetrate into the target cell, while the other subunit (the A, or active subunit) exhibits the toxic activity. VacA constitutes the prototype of a new family of toxins with a characteristic mode of action and characteristic morphological effect on cells. Moreover, the fact that the effect can be reversed is peculiar for this toxin.

The VacA toxin is mainly released from *Helicobacter pylori* as a free soluble toxin but it is believed that some is released within outer membrane vesicles. Many Gram-negative bacteria release surface blebs from the cell wall and something similar occurs with *Helicobacter pylori*. Although free soluble toxin accounts for about 75% of the released VacA protein, roughly 25% is detected in outer membrane vesicles. The release of these outer membrane vesicles by *Helicobacter pylori* may represent a mechanism for the delivery of bacterial virulence factors and antigens into the gastric mucosa that is additional to the secretory pathway (**4.7**).

The toxin is activated by exposure to acid, presumably inducing a conformational change that makes it resistant to pepsin and facilitates oligomerization in the host cell membrane. VacA affects different host cells leading to various pathophysiological effects. It can target several cell types, e.g., gastric epithelial cells, macrophages, neutrophils, mast cells, T cells and goblet cells. It can interact with several cellular compartments, such as the cytoplasmic membrane, the late endosomal and lysosomal compartments and the mitochondria. Cells affected by the toxin will die either by apoptosis or necrosis, with the pathophysiological effects depending upon the cell type affected (**4.8**).

Endo-lysosomal trafficking

The most obvious direct effect causing damage to the gastric epithelial cells is on normal endosome vesicle trafficking, resulting in vacuolation of cells. Endocytic pathways include: intracytoplasmic vesicles carrying recycled molecules from the cytoplasmic membrane; the major histocompatability complex class II protein; and ingested bacteria, food or secreted products. Material can be taken into cells: (a) by binding to specific receptors (receptor-mediated endocytosis), which occurs at specific pits coated with a protein called clatherin; (b) in a non-specific manner, which can occur at any point of the cytoplasmic membrane (pinocytosis) and is a mechanism for taking up solutes; or (c) by enveloping particulate matter, such as a bacterium in which the particulate matter is enclosed in pseudopodia (phagocytosis). This latter type of endocytosis is mainly employed by specific immune cells and is a mechanism of host defence.

Once the material has been taken up by one of these mechanisms the pathways of the vesicles within the cell

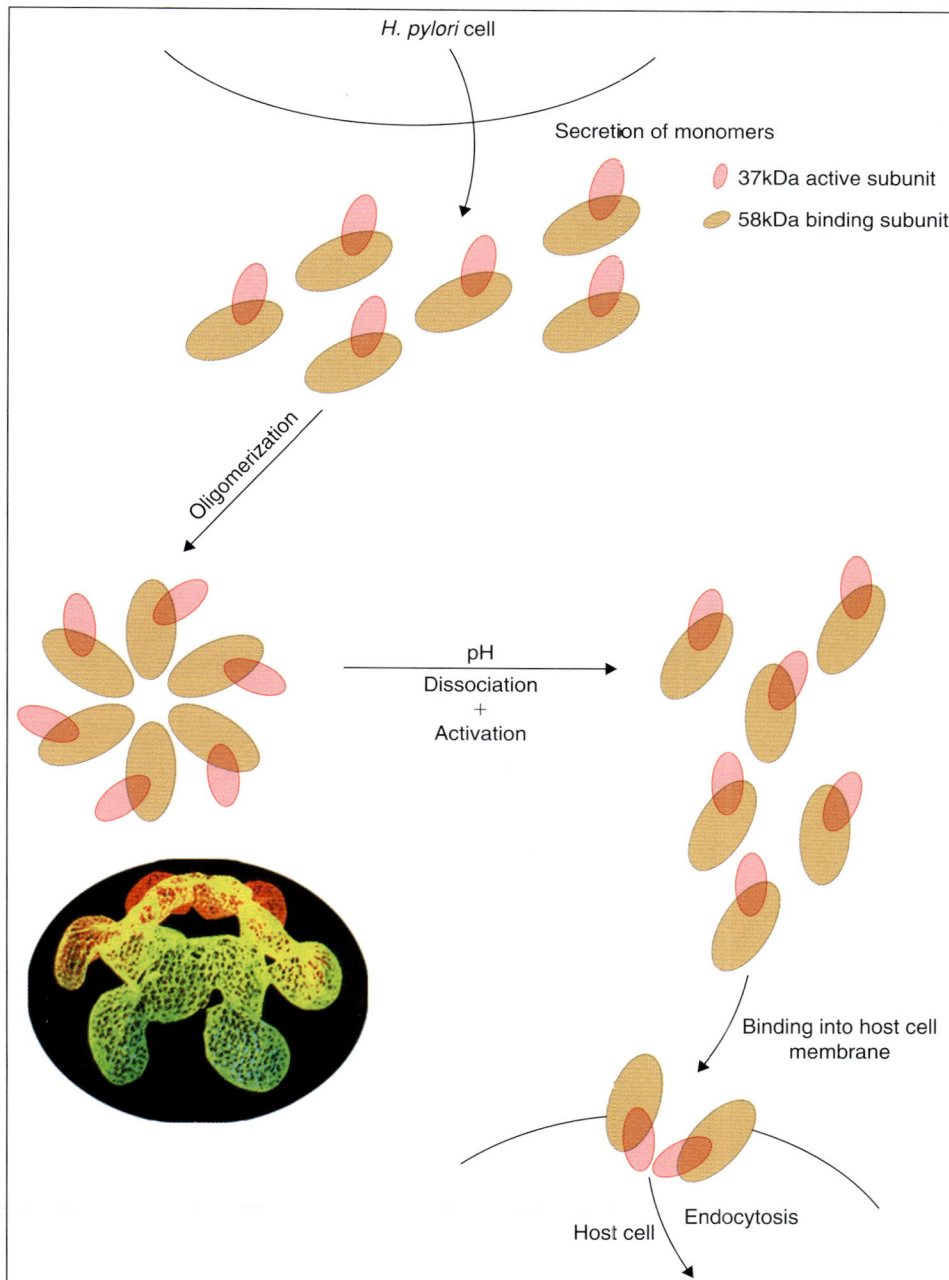

4.6 Structure, oligomerization of VacA toxin and binding to host cell membrane.

may differ (**4.9**). One main route is to traffic material between intracytoplasmic compartments (e.g., to recycle the material back to the cytoplasmic membrane or to transfer the material to the trans-Golgi apparatus). The second major pathway is to deliver the vesicle (in this case called a phagosome) to the lysosome, which is responsible for digesting the material.

After uptake of material, the vesicle with a single compartment is called an early (sorting) endosome—as it is routed along a specific pathway it 'matures' into a multivesicular body by invagination of the vesicle membrane and eventually becomes a late endosome. Each stage in the process is associated with specific marker proteins (small GTPases called Rab), although there is some overlap. Vesicles that are destined to be recycled have a protein, Rab11, in the vesicle membrane. Early endosomes are identified by Rab5, and late endosomes by Rab7, Rab9 and LAMP1. If the contents

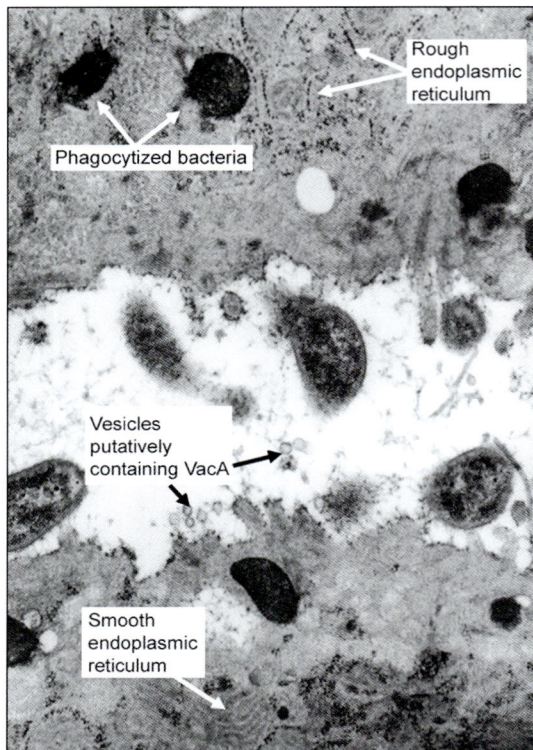

4.7 Electron micrograph showing outer membrane vesicles.

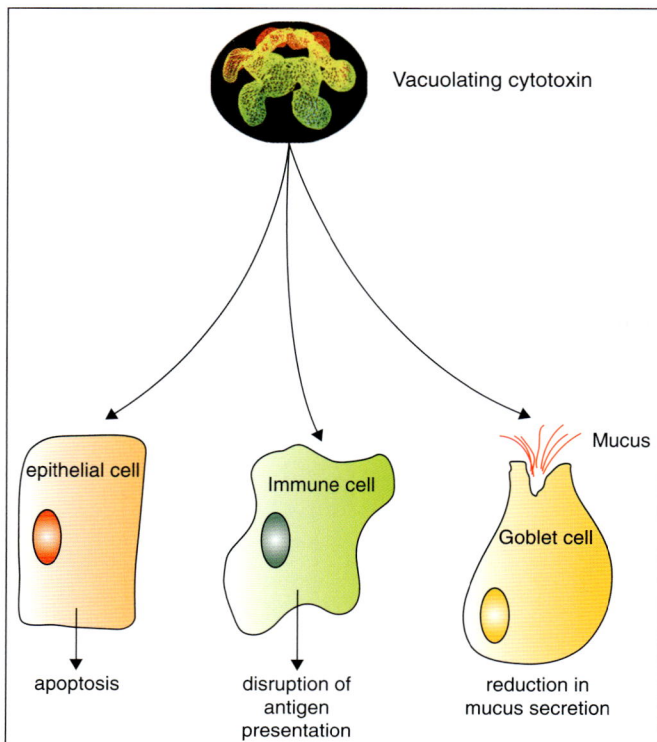

4.8 Host cells affected by vacuolating cytotoxin.

of the vesicle are to be digested, the late endosome will fuse with a lysosome that contains digestive enzymes or cationic proteins. Progressive acidification of the vesicles occurs during the development to late endosomes, which is due to a vacuolar-type H^+-ATPase (V-type ATPase). This process aids digestion or release of the ligand from its receptor.

The endosomes are transported through the cytoplasm by the actin cytoskeleton or microtubules.

VacA internalization and vacuolization in cells

VacA associates with lipid rafts on the surface of epithelial cells and cholesterol is required for strong membrane binding. Studies have indicated that VacA can bind glycosphingolipids, in particular galactosylceramide, galabiosylceramide and glucosylceramide. VacA also binds to receptor-like protein tyrosine phosphatase α and β. The interaction with glycoconjugate receptors leads to a membrane-close attachment, which may facilitate the internalization of the toxin by a clatherin-independent pathway.

The A/B-type toxins usually gain access to the cytoplasm by endocytosis of the complete toxin following binding to host cell-surface receptors. In this case, both the A and B moieties are required for binding and internalization of the toxin, as well as for the vacuolating effect. However, the VacA p58 subunit (i.e., the B moiety) is not internalized. There is evidence that p58 may form pores in the plasma membranes, creating hexameric anion-selective channels of low conductance through which bicarbonate and organic anions are released from the cell cytosol to support bacterial growth.

The VacA toxin may also alter the tight junctions by an as yet unidentified mechanism and increase the paracellular route of permeability from the underlying mucosa, providing iron, nickel and other nutrients essential for *Helicobacter pylori* growth. Some observations suggest that the adhesion of bacteria to the epithelial cells (or even their phagocytosis) facilitates the entrance of VacA into the cytoplasm. Although both duodenal and gastric epithelia can undergo vacuolization, *in vivo* vacuoles are a rare finding; in the infrequent instances in which vacuole formation can be observed in gastric biopsies by transmission electron microscope, one can perceive *Helicobacter pylori* organisms in close proximity to them.

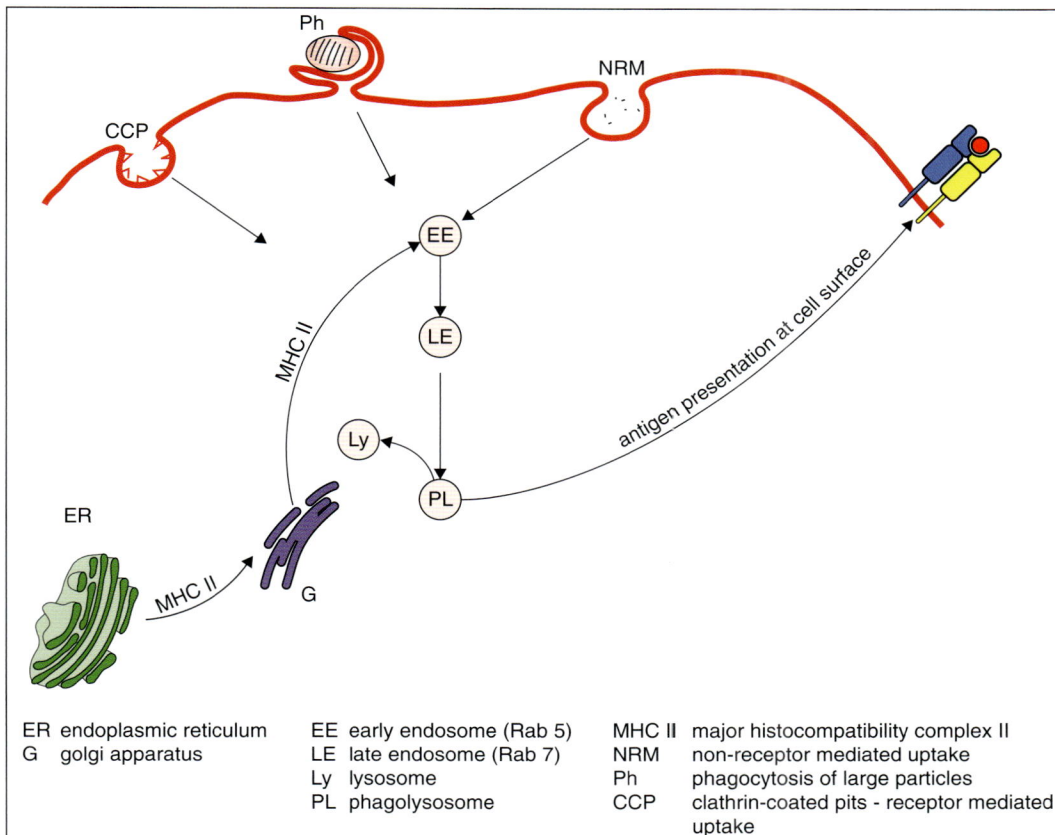

ER endoplasmic reticulum
G   golgi apparatus

EE early endosome (Rab 5)
LE late endosome (Rab 7)
Ly lysosome
PL phagolysosome

MHC II major histocompatibility complex II
NRM non-receptor mediated uptake
Ph phagocytosis of large particles
CCP clathrin-coated pits - receptor mediated uptake

4.9 Various types of endocytosis.

Once inside the cell the VacA toxin finds its final target, the V-type ATPase, which is normally present on vesicles formed via invagination of the cell membrane. These vesicles undergo a process of maturation and serve to enrich the Golgi apparatus and other intracellular compartments. The toxin binds to the late endosomal compartments that express Rab7, making them no longer available to the Golgi apparatus, lysosomes and other cytoplasmic complexes. At this point, vesicles fuse with each other. The activity of the V-type ATPase (which is a proton pump that regulates the flux of H^+) causes hydrogen ions to accumulate inside the fused vesicles, forming an acidic pH gradient across cell membranes. Basic substances such as ammonia (produced by urease activity from *H. pylori*) diffuse passively into the vacuoles being formed, and are protonated because they find an acidic environment (**4.10**). Protonated substances cannot cross back out from the vacuoles because the endocellular membranes are semipermeable; they are bound to remain inside the vacuoles where they accumulate and attract water osmotically, thereby causing enlargement of the vacuole and eventual cell lysis (**4.11**).

Endosomal vesicle fusion requires complex formation between Q- and R-SNARE family proteins. The SNARE proteins Syntaxin 7 and VAMP-7 appear to be important for the induction of vacuoles by the *H. pylori* VacA toxin.

Additional actions of VacA

VacA reduces the prostaglandin E_2-stimulated secretion of bicarbonate by about 50% through increasing the release of histamine. This reduction in bicarbonate levels is likely to have a detrimental effect upon the capacity of the mucosal defence against damaging agents.

The *vacA* gene is also harboured by non-cytotoxic strains, which secrete a biologically truncated VacA protein. Various mutations account for the non-cytotoxic proteins, which include deletions, duplications, insertions and non-sense mutations. As bacteria tend to lose their genomic material, if the gene product has no advantageous function, this suggests that the non-cytotoxic *vacA* product may have more targets and another activity. If the purpose of the secretion of VacA were only to induce vacuolation and, consequently, to

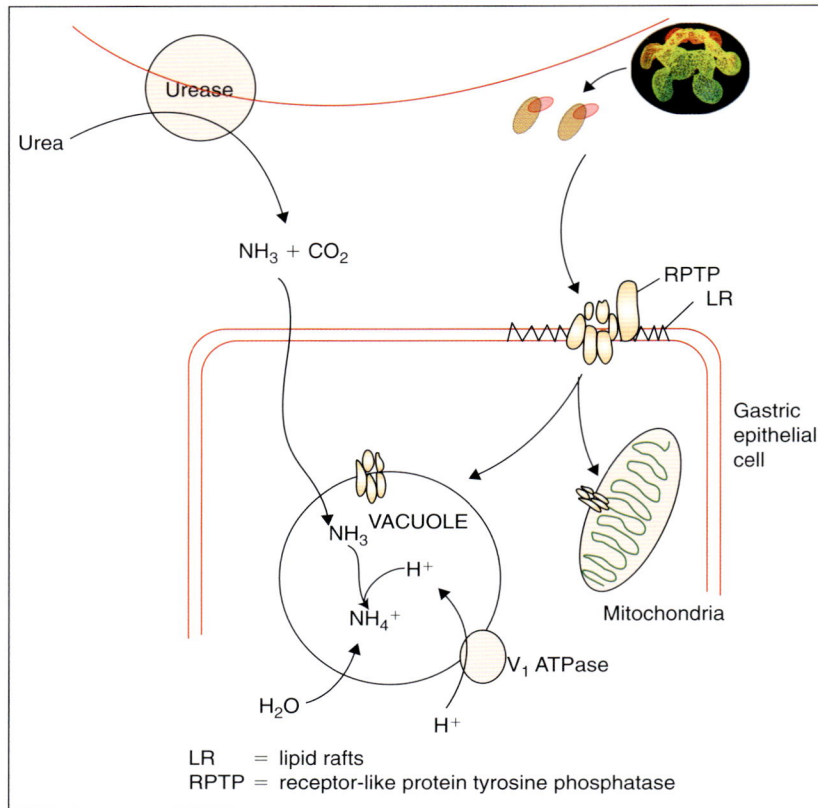

4.10 Disruption of endosome cycling: vacuolation.

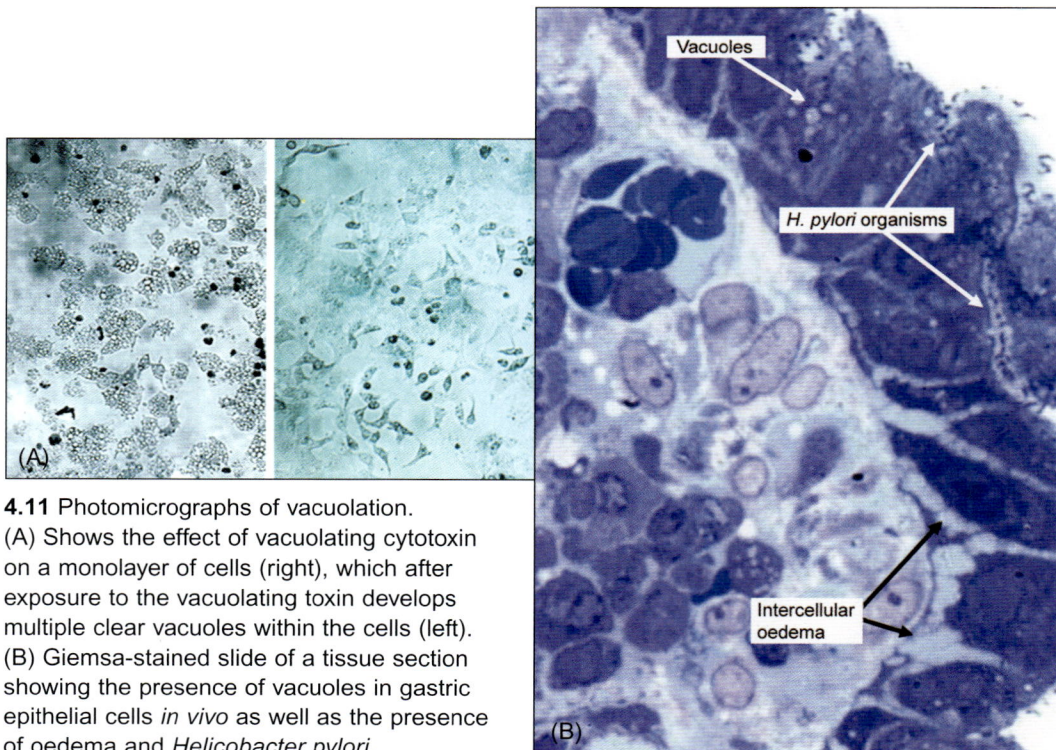

4.11 Photomicrographs of vacuolation.
(A) Shows the effect of vacuolating cytotoxin on a monolayer of cells (right), which after exposure to the vacuolating toxin develops multiple clear vacuoles within the cells (left). (B) Giemsa-stained slide of a tissue section showing the presence of vacuoles in gastric epithelial cells *in vivo* as well as the presence of oedema and *Helicobacter pylori*.

increase the mucosal damage, there would be no reason for non-cytotoxic *Helicobacter* to maintain replication of the non-cytotoxic *vacA* product.

Other enzymes

Isocitrate dehydrogenase

Helicobacter pylori produces isocitrate dehydrogenase but, although this stimulates a strong host immune response, it does not appear to stimulate proinflammatory cytokine production.

Carbonic anhydrase

Carbonic anhydrase catalyses the following reaction:

$$CO_2 + H_2O \longleftrightarrow HCO_3 + H^+$$

Carbonic anhydrase is found in two forms (α and β) in *Helicobacter pylori*. The α-carbonic acid anhydrase is found in the periplasm and is involved in acid resistance (**4.3**). The β class is found in the cytoplasm. There is significant homology between the α-carbonic anhydrase and human class II carbonic anhydrase, suggesting a possible relationship to autoimmune pancreatitis.

Superoxide dismutase and catalase

SOD is an almost ubiquitous enzyme among living things that either has the metal cation cofactor Cu, Fe, Mn, Ni or Zn (Fe in *H. pylori*) at the active site and the valence alternates during the reaction. The enzyme catalyses the reduction of superoxide radicals (produced during inflammation or respiration) to hydrogen peroxide according to the following scheme:

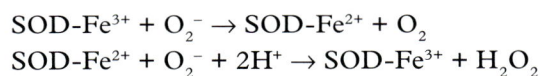

$$SOD\text{-}Fe^{3+} + O_2^- \rightarrow SOD\text{-}Fe^{2+} + O_2$$
$$SOD\text{-}Fe^{2+} + O_2^- + 2H^+ \rightarrow SOD\text{-}Fe^{3+} + H_2O_2$$

Catalase then converts the peroxide to water and oxygen according to the following scheme:

$$2H_2O_2 \leftrightarrow 2H_2O + O_2$$

Platelet-activating factor

Platelet-activating factor (PAF) is produced by numerous host cells and is a potent ulcerogen in the gastrointestinal tract. *Helicobacter pylori* can be stimulated to produce PAF by exposure to acetyl coenzyme A or lyso-PAF (both of which are found in the host), and thus may be involved

in the direct damage to gastric epithelial cells caused by *Helicobacter pylori*. The mechanism of this damage may be by platelet aggregation in microcirculation leading to ischaemia or an effect upon mucin synthesis. An additional pathway induced by *Helicobacter pylori* that decreases mucin production may be stimulation of endogenous cytosolic PLA_2 by lipopolysaccharide, which in turn leads to increasing PAF synthesis.

Neuraminidase

Neuraminidase is produced by all *Helicobacter pylori* strains tested. Its putative target is neuraminic acid, a component of the gastric mucin which is believed to have a protective function. Thus, neuraminidase may undermine the mucus gel and enable *Helicobacter pylori* to better penetrate the mucus layer.

Fucosidase

The role of fucosidase in damaging the gastric mucosa is only speculative. The production of this glycosidase by *Helicobacter pylori* may convert the fucosylated gastric mucin to non-fucosylated. As a result, the functional properties of gastric mucus could be impaired. However, no correlation between fucosidase production and pathogenic potential has yet been found.

Effects on gastric physiology

Acid secretion

Acid in the stomach is an important biocide and failure of acid secretion may be associated with an increase in gastrointestinal infections. Acid is also important as part of the digestive process, and its control is a balance between initiation of secretion with positive and negative feedback loops that control the level of stomach acid.

Mechanisms of stimulating secretion of acid

Gastric acid secretion occurs following the thought or sensory perception of food and is mediated via: (a) cholinergic fibres of the vagus nerve; (b) a paracrine route mediated by histamine release; and (c) a hormonal route mediated by gastrin release (**4.12**).

Acid is released directly from parietal cells (which are found mainly in the fundus of the stomach) by cholinergic

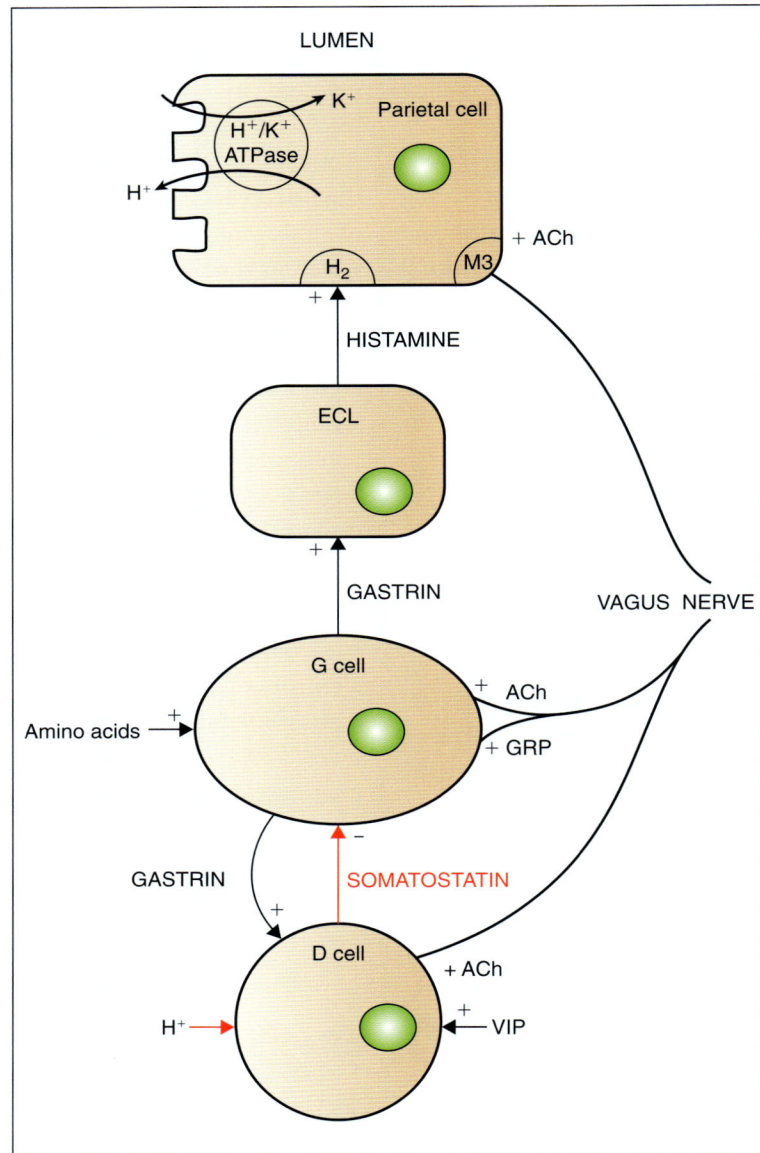

4.12 Normal control of acid secretion. ACh = acetylcholine; ECL = enterochromaffin-like cell; GRP = gastrin related peptide; H$_2$ = histamine-2 receptor; M3 = muscarinic-3 receptor.

fibres of the vagus nerve innervating muscarinic-3 receptors. A further, indirect, route of release of acid involves gastrin and histamine.

Gastrin is synthesized by G cells found mainly in the antrum of the stomach. The hormone is synthesized initially as a larger peptide, which is then cleaved, amidated and cleaved again to produce gastrin-17 and gastrin-34, which are secreted from the cell. In addition to stimulating histamine release, gastrin affects cell dynamics by stimulating cell growth and migration,

inhibiting apoptosis and increasing angiogenesis; therefore, it has carcinogenic potential.

G cells are stimulated to release gastrin by cholinergic and peptinergic innervation, and by luminal amino acids. Gastrin stimulates the release of histamine from enterochromaffin-like cells by binding to cholecystokinin-2 receptors.

Histamine is synthesized from arginine by arginine decarboxylase and is released from enterochromaffin-like cells after stimulation by the binding of gastrin. In turn, histamine binds to histamine-2 (H_2) receptors on parietal cells, activating a cAMP signalling cascade that recruits the proton pump to the apical membrane and activates it to release acid.

The direct and indirect route of stimulation activates the H^+/K^+ ATPase antiporter (proton pump) to release H^+. The proton pump carries out the electroneutral exchange of intracellular H^+ for extracellular K^+ and is the target for proton pump inhibitors used as part of the standard *Helicobacter pylori* eradication regimen.

The acid is released from the parietal cell with some force, penetrating the overlying mucus by viscous fingering to emerge in the lumen of the stomach with a pH of ≈ 2.0.

Mechanisms of inhibiting secretion of acid

The main negative regulator of acid release is somatostatin (SST). SST is a family of peptides produced by D cells in the stomach with SST-14 and SST-28 being the active products. SST inhibits the release of gastrin, histamine and acid from the appropriate cell.

Antral D cells have luminal-facing apical membranes and may sense the pH and, thus, can release SST when acid increases. SST is also directly released in response to: histamine binding to H_3 receptors; gastrin; and vasoactive intestinal peptide secretion from postganglionic peptinergic innervation. Indirectly, the release of SST is also under the positive control of atrial natriuretic peptide, which is secreted from enterochromaffin cells by postganglionic peptinergic fibres releasing pituitary adenylate cyclase-activating polypeptide. Cholinergic innervation of D cells and enterochromaffin cells inhibits the release of SST.

This acid regulatory network can be disturbed by the presence of *Helicobacter pylori* leading to an increase in gastrin (hypergastrinaemia) and, eventually, basal acid levels. Initial colonization by *Helicobacter pylori* leads to hypochlorhydria, which may be mediated by reducing parietal cell numbers due to the action of vacuolating cytotoxin or the production of water-soluble factors that directly inhibit acid secretion. Cytokines produced as part of the inflammatory process, particularly interleukin (IL)-1β and tumour necrosis factor (TNF)-α, also inhibit acid secretion. *Helicobacter pylori* inhibits the expression of histidine decarboxylase, which leads to a reduction in histamine secretion and the gene expression of the α-subunit of the ATPase proton pump, thereby also reducing acid production.

Patients who develop duodenal ulcers have many more G cells compared with people who do not; thus, they have both a higher meal-stimulated and maximal output of acid. Following colonization by *Helicobacter pylori* the lipopolysaccharide inhibits SST, leading to hypergastrinaemia and hyperchlorhydria. The mechanism of this effect is not clear but may involve the production of an H_3 receptor agonist or be due to the proinflammatory cytokines. Additionally, gastrin secretion is directly stimulated by IL-8 and PAF, and PAF also stimulates acid secretion directly from parietal cells. In these circumstances, inflammation is predominantly antral, and the high acid may manifest itself with symptoms of duodenal ulcer, possibly accompanied by a type III or type II gastric ulcer, which can also be found in high acid conditions.

More commonly, with time, there is pan-gastritis associated with hypochlohydria, which may be accompanied by a type I or type IV gastric ulcer. The reduction in acid is due to the pronounced inflammation in the main acid-producing area of the stomach—the fundus—caused by loss of parietal cells due to the inflammatory process or an immune-mediated process (**4.13**).

Leptin, grehlin, appetite and obesity

Humans have a drive to eat just as they have a drive to breathe. A complex neuronal and hormonal interaction exists to control appetite, metabolism and growth. The feeling of hunger is controlled in part by the levels of leptin and ghrelin (**4.14**). Ghrelin, a hormone produced principally by epithelial cells in the fundus of the stomach, has two major biological activities. These are: first, regulation of energy balance by (a) increasing hunger through its action upon the hypothalamus, and (b) suppression of fat utilization in adipose tissue; and second, to stimulate secretion of growth hormone (GH) from the anterior pituitary.

Leptin is also an important factor in regulating body weight and metabolism. It is found predominantly in adipose tissue but also in the stomach and placenta. As triglycerides accumulate in the adipocytes the level of leptin also increases and there is a correlation between body fat and blood leptin levels. Leptin acts upon the hypothalamus to decrease hunger and food consumption and increase energy metabolism. Both leptin and ghrelin hormones are key regulators of the

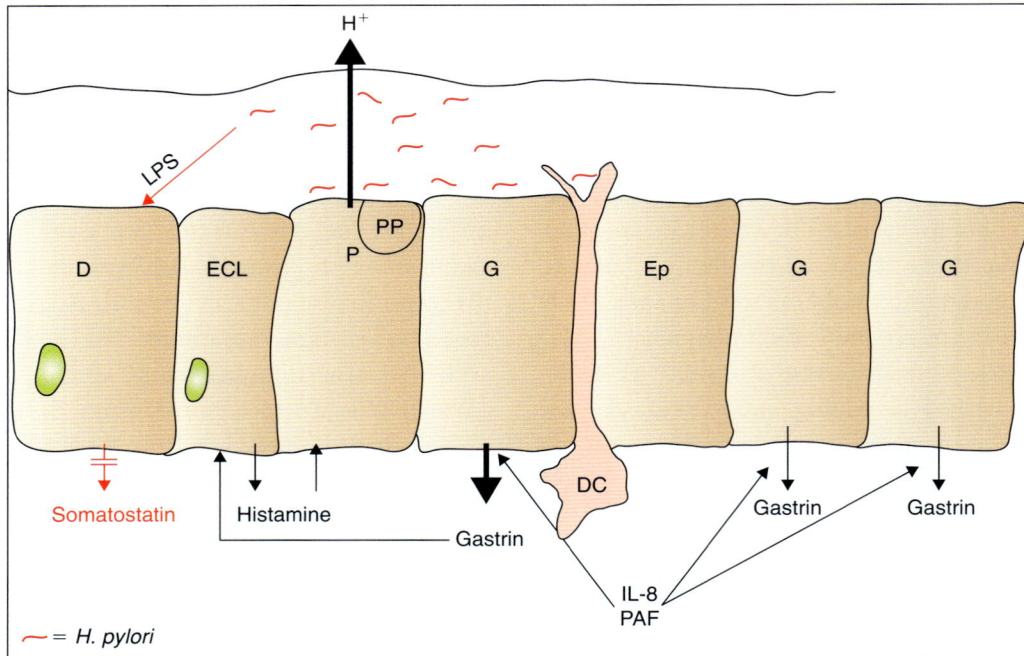

4.13 The effect of *Helicobacter pylori* on gastric acid secretion illustrating the inhibition of somatostatin by the LPS of the organism and the subsequent increase in gastrin and H⁺.

release of GH and metabolic control and their levels are affected by *Helicobacter pylori*.

Leptin also negatively affects the activation of PLA_2 and therefore PAF synthesis by *Helicobacter pylori* lipopolysaccharide, which in turn suppresses the increase in apoptosis and reduction in mucus secretion induced by PAF. Leptin also has effects upon reproduction.

Both ghrelin and leptin act upon the arcuate nucleus, the former stimulating the orexigenic neurons, and the latter stimulating anti-orexigenic neurons while inhibiting the orexigenic neurons (**4.14**). Signals pass from the arcuate nucleus to the paraventricular nucleus thence to the limbic system (controlling emotive states) and ultimately to the motor cortex. Signals also pass to the brain stem and, depending upon the relative effects of leptin and ghrelin, the person decreases or increases their food uptake.

The levels of these hormones can be disturbed in patients colonized by *Helicobacter pylori* (**4.15**). *Helicobacter pylori* and obesity are both major socio-economic health problems. Colonization with *Helicobacter pylori* may be associated with anaemia, short stature and insulin resistance on the one hand, but eradication of *Helicobacter pylori* may be linked to obesity, and GORD, the latter increasing predisposition to adenocarcinoma of the oesophagus. With obesity also

comes an increased risk of diabetes and cardiovascular problems (diabetes is also an independent risk factor for cardiovascular disease). Obesity, growth retardation, insulin resistance and consequent cardiovascular problems (such as atheroma, stroke, ischaemic heart disease and thromboembolism) can all be linked through the control of appetite and energy metabolism. This metabolic balance can be disrupted by *Helicobacter pylori* colonization. Whether this affects ghrelin/leptin dynamics over the long term, and the potential sequelae of obesity and associated comorbidities, is an important question that is still under debate. Clinical findings regarding the relationship between metabolic/endocrine disease and *H. pylori* colonization are discussed in Chapter 3 (pp. 58–60).

Helicobacter pylori type IV secretion system (T4SS) and intracellular signalling

Most vacuolating cytotoxic *Helicobacter pylori* strains also express a high molecular weight protein called CagA, which is injected into host cells by the type IV secretion system (*see* Chapter 1), which is highly immunogenic in humans. The *cagA* gene is part of the PAIs present in

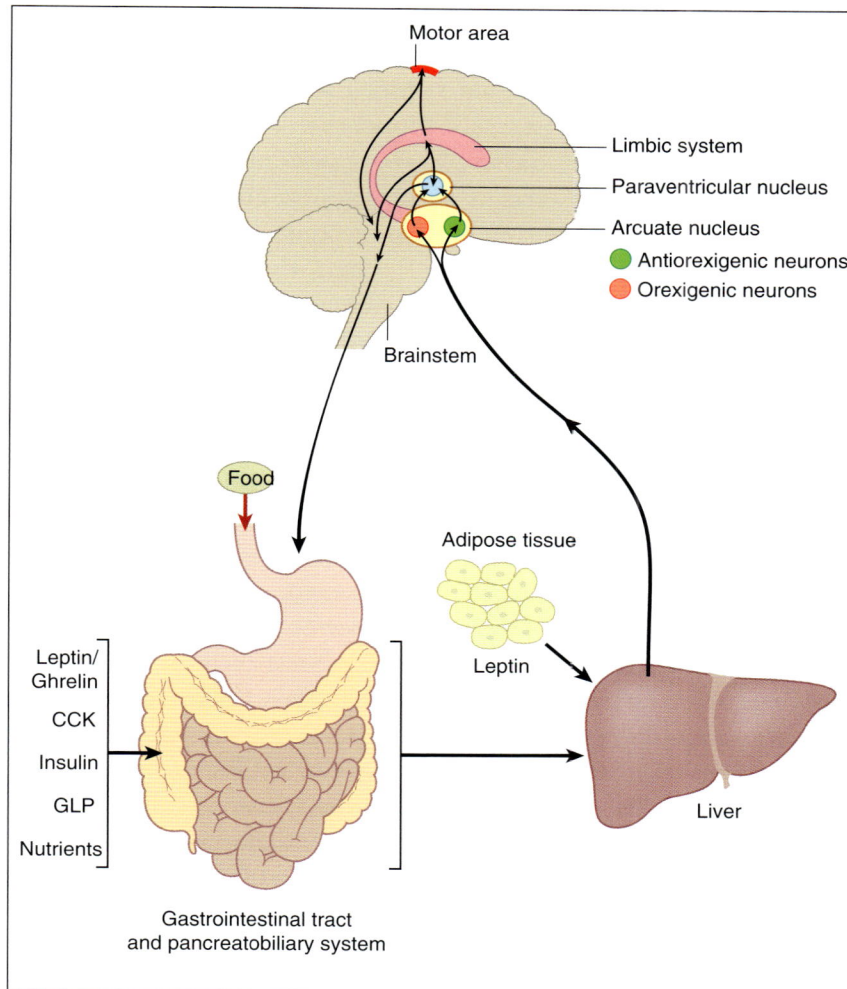

4.14 Control of appetite by leptin and ghrelin. CCK = cholecystokinin; GLP = glucagon-like peptide.

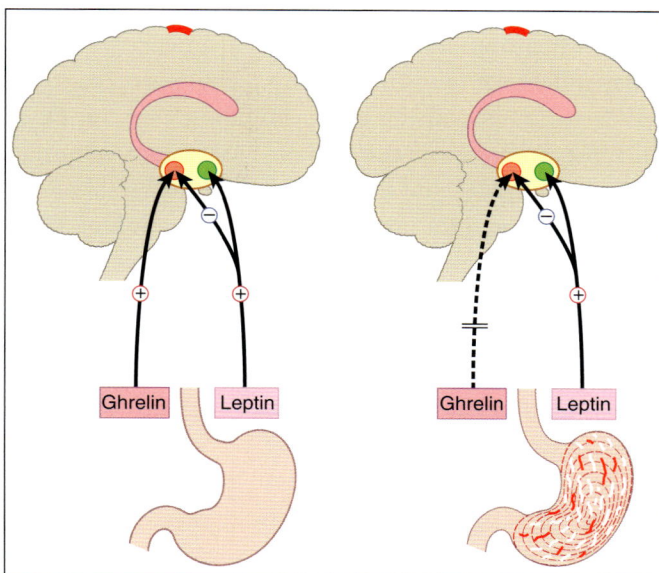

4.15 The effects of *Helicobacter pylori* on leptin and ghrelin.

some bacterial pathogens. The *cag*PAI residing in type I strains (*see* p. 14) can be considered as the 'command centre' for the strategy executed by virulent strains of *H. pylori*. Most genes in the *cag*PAI encode for proteins involved in modifying host cell regulatory pathways that depend on contact with bacteria. It has been suggested that in natural infections CagA-positive strains are 10–1000-fold more numerous in the gastroduodenal tract than strains that do not express CagA, although current evidence suggests that there is no difference between density of colonization and CagA status. Non-cytotoxic CagA-negative bacteria have little tendency to gather at the junctional complexes between adjacent mucous cells, whereas CagA-positive bacteria are often found at cell margins and damage the junctional apparatus.

Injection of CagA into host cells by type I *Helicobacter pylori* leads to multiple effects on intracellular signalling.

The CagL protein, coded for on the *cag*PAI and located at the tip of the pilus, binds to integrin $\alpha_5\beta_1$ on the surface of the host cell. This interaction stimulates the injection of CagA across the pilus and into the host cell, activating the Src kinases and focal adhesion kinases (FAKs). Another product of the *cag*PAI, CagF, acts as a chaperone protein by binding to the C-terminal end of CagA to facilitate its transfer. A further product of the *cag*PAI required for effective translocation of CagA is CagD. The precise function of CagD is unknown, although it is present at both inner membrane of the bacterium and extracellularly and may be involved in pilus assembly; it is also required for secretion of IL-8.

CagA injection into host cells induces the following: cytoskeletal rearrangement; membrane dynamics and motility; plus various mitogenic, proinflammatory, cell-to-cell adhesion and apoptotic effects, either in its phosphorylated or non-phosphorylated form. CagA is tyrosine phosphorylated at EPIYA sites by Src and Abl kinases (*see* p. 15). The phosphorylated CagA binds SHP-2 phosphatase and activates it, which in turn activates extracellular-signal-regulated kinase (Erk). The degree of CagA phosphorylation depends on the number of tyrosine residues phosphorylated, which varies with the number of specific EPIYA motif repeats. There is also a variation in the sequence at the phosphorylation sites between Western and East Asian strains. Both these variations lead to differential binding and activation of the SHP-2 phosphatase. Phosphorylated CagA specifically binds SHP-2 via the EPIYA-C motif (Western) or EPIYA-D motif (east Asian). Activation of the SHP-2 phosphatase and the Erk pathway induces the 'hummingbird' (an extremely elongated cell shape) morphological change and eventual apoptosis. This morphological change is modulated by phosphorylated CagA also binding to another kinase, Csk (C-terminal Src kinase) via the EPIYA-A or EPIYA-B site and activating it. The activated Csk in turn inactivates Src kinases, thereby reducing the availability of phosphorylated CagA that can bind to SHP-2. In both cases, the greater the degree of binding, which depends upon the number of repeats of the EPIYA motifs, the greater the resultant effect.

Phosphorylated CagA binds Crk adaptor proteins, which leads to mitogenic effects and actin reorganization. It also induces dephosphorylation of the Pak-interacting exchange factor (αPix), which affects cytoskeletal changes via activation of PAX (p21 activated tyrosine kinase). In addition, Src and FAK are tyrosine phosphorylated, which in turn activates Erk, causing actin stress fibre formation and morphological changes the cell. The *Helicobacter pylori* product OipA is necessary for these changes, as mutations in *oipA* reduce phosphorylation, stress fibre formation and morphological changes.

CagA, the T4SS and peptidoglycan all contribute to activating the PI3K/AKT pathway via Src and epidermal growth factor receptor (EGFR) activation, which in turn has an anti-apoptotic effect. AKT activation is also involved in nuclear factor κ B (NFκB) induction.

CagA also has phosphorylation-independent effects on cell signalling, including stimulation of nuclear factor of activated T cell (NFAT) transcription, which is abrogated by VacA activity. A conserved motif called 'conserved repeat responsible for phosphorylation independent activity' (CRPIA) interacts with the hepatocyte growth factor receptor (MET) and activates the PI3K/AKT pathway: the end result of this is activation of NFκB, leading to a proinflammatory response, and β-catenin activation, leading to a mitogenic response. Non-phosphorylated CagA also activates cAbl kinase, which phosphorylates EGFR blocking endocytosis and degradation of the receptor.

CagA has effects upon cell adhesions due to its inactivation of Src kinases. Src inactivation leads to dephosphorylation of vinculin, which means vinculin is unable to bind to the actin-related protein 2/3 (Arp2/3) complex, thus reducing cell matrix adhesion. Also, CagA induces dissociation of β-catenin and E-cadherin, thus disrupting adherens junction integrity. CagA, independent of phosphorylation, also perturbs tight junctions by recruiting the scaffolding protein ZO-1 and the transmembrane protein junctional adhesion molecule (JAM-1) to sites where *H. pylori* is attached adjacent to the tight junctions. Mislocalization of ZO-1 at junctions thus lead to a scattering phenotype with cell disaggregation. In addition, translocation of CagA dysregulates MET signalling, initiating cellular motility.

Helicobacter pylori recruits MARK2/PAR1b (a serine/threonine kinase involved in the regulation of cell polarity) to the adhesion site where it binds to CagA. This prevents PAR1b phosphorylation by atypical protein kinase C (aPKC), thereby dissociating PAR1b from the membrane and inducing effects on cell polarity, cell-to-cell junctions and differentiation. PAR1b stabilizes

CagA-SHP2 binding, promoting morphological changes (hummingbird morphology) as well as cell polarity effects; induction of these effects seemingly requires the simultaneous inhibition of PAR1b. The diversity of the CagA multimerization sequence that mediates PAR1b binding is important for the induction of hummingbird phenotype and junctional effects. The sequence from the East Asian strains bind PAR1b more strongly compared with Western strains. CagA also activates signal transducers and activators of transcription (STAT-3), which are involved in carcinogenesis.

VacA, secreted by type I strains, can mitigate the morphological effects of CagA by inactivating the EGFR and Erk mitogen-activated protein kinase, which are necessary for morphological changes. Additionally, VacA counteracts upregulation of NFAT induced by CagA. Similarly, CagA reduces the vacuolating effects of VacA. Teleologically, these counterbalancing effects of CagA–VacA on each other moderate the degree of pathological damage the host suffers.

Helicobacter pylori heat shock protein (Hsp60) also activates intracellular signalling pathways mediated by Toll-like receptor 2. These pathways involve cross-talk with mitogen-activated protein kinase (MAPK), p38 and Erk signalling downstream to increase NFκB transcription, leading to release of the chemokine IL-8. *Helicobacter pylori* also upregulates decay accelerating factor (DAF) in a CagA-dependent manner. DAF normally acts to protect epithelial cells from complement-mediated lysis, but, as with many microbial pathogens, *Helicobacter pylori* uses it as receptor for binding to cells.

The net result of these effects on cell signalling is to induce the hummingbird phenotype, characterized by spreading and elongation of the cell shape, and a deregulation of cell growth. This last event probably plays a critical role in the development of gastric cancer, as CagA increases the expression of cyclin D3, phosphorylation of the tumour suppressor Rb (a substrate of the cdk-cyclin D complexes) and expression of transcription factor c-jun; this leads to an increase in cell proliferation, probably caused by deregulation of the G_1/S checkpoint of the cell cycle. CagA also alters cell barrier function and affects cell-to-cell and cell matrix adhesion, all of which might contribute to cell migration and invasiveness (**4.16**, **4.17**).

Additionally, peptidoglycan is also passed into the host cell, which is recognized by NOD-1 and eventually leads to upregulation of NFκB, as does binding of the B-subunit of urease to CD74 on gastric epithelial cells.

NOD family proteins are intracellular pattern recognition molecules that have nucleotide oligomerization domains (NOD) and are part of the innate immune system. They have an N-terminal domain that binds effectors (for NOD-1 and -2 this is a caspase recruitment domains, or CARD), a central NOD and a C-terminal ligand recognition domain.

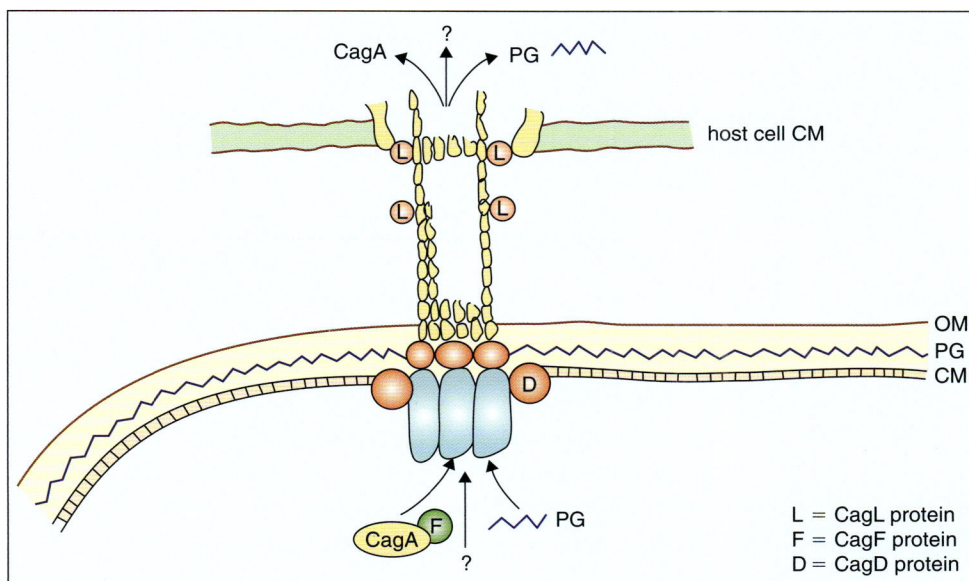

4.16 Entry of cagA and other bacterial products into host cells by the type IV secretion system.

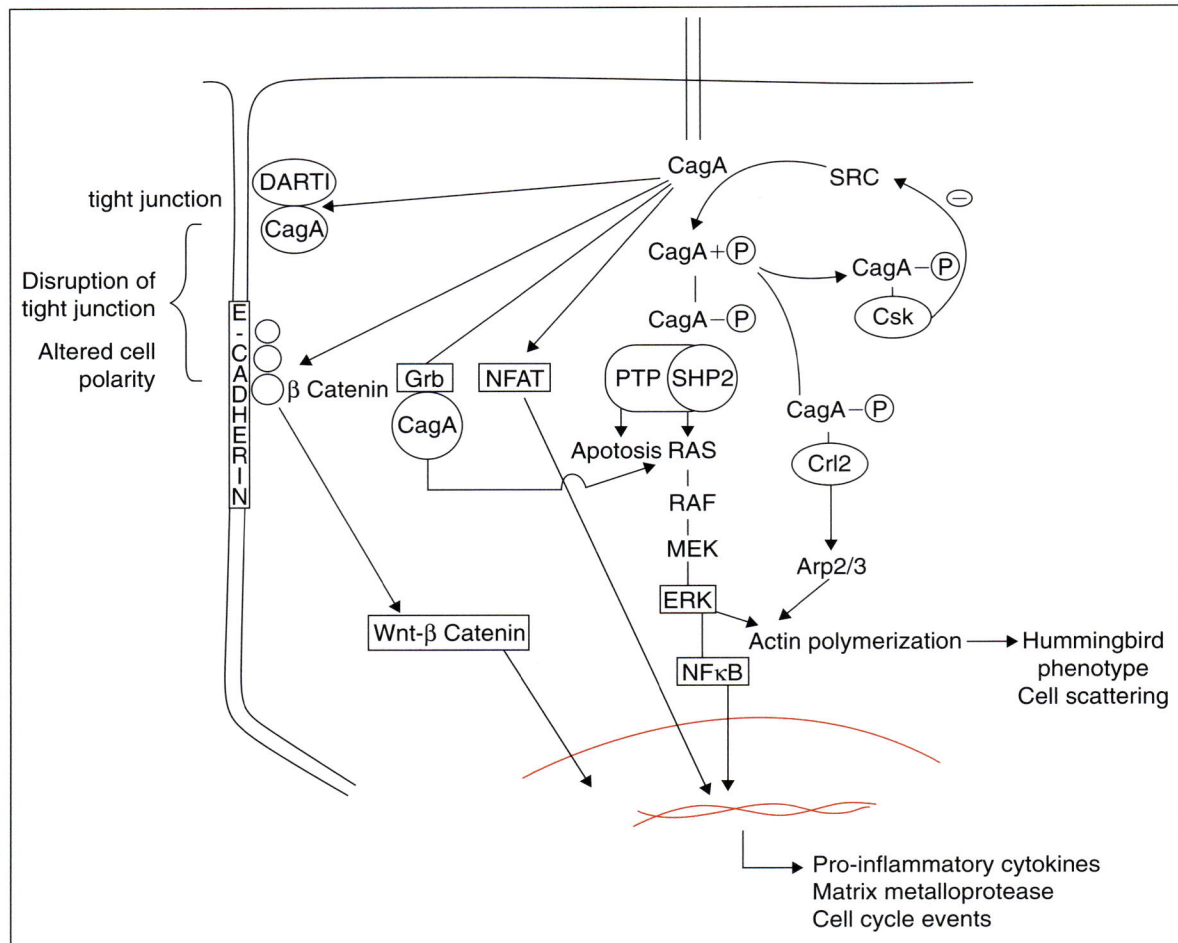

4.17 The effects of CagA on intracellular signalling.

The CARD mediates homophilic protein interactions. Other effector binding domains are: pyrin domain (PYD), found in NOD-6, NOD-8 and NALP1; baculovirus inhibitor of apoptosis repeats (BIR), such as neuronal apoptosis inhibitory protein (NAIP); or the NOD protein may lack an effector binding domain (and is thus a non-DNA-binding protein), e.g., the MHC II transactivator (CIITA), which is involved in MHC II expression (**4.18**).

NOD-1 and NOD-2 effector domains (CARD4 and CARD15, respectively) recognize cell wall components of bacteria: NOD-1 recognizes a dipeptide incorporating diaminopimelic acid, and NOD-2 recognizes a muramyl dipeptide (*see* also **1.3** in Chapter 1). Recognition and binding induces activation of the NFκB transcriptional activator. Polymorphisms in NOD proteins may result in clinical conditions, e.g., Crohn's disease in the case of a NOD-2 R702W polymorphism.

As well as activation of NFκB, downstream signalling of peptidoglycan components binding to NOD proteins include: production of proinflammatory cytokines such as TNFα and IL-1β; activation of caspases; and activation of c-Jun N-terminal kinase pathways, which may lead to further production of proinflammatory cytokines. The activation of caspases by binding to NOD may be related to cytokine processing rather than induction of apoptosis, as activation of NFκB is anti-apoptotic. Alternatively, this may be a way of regulating apoptosis by *Helicobacter pylori* so that it does not induce serious effects that may harm its host (**4.19**).

It is possible that the correlation between infection by the *cagA*-positive strain and severe mucosal damage cannot be always applied. In certain countries, for instance, the prevalence of infection by *cagA*-positive *Helicobacter pylori* strains is close to 100%. Therefore,

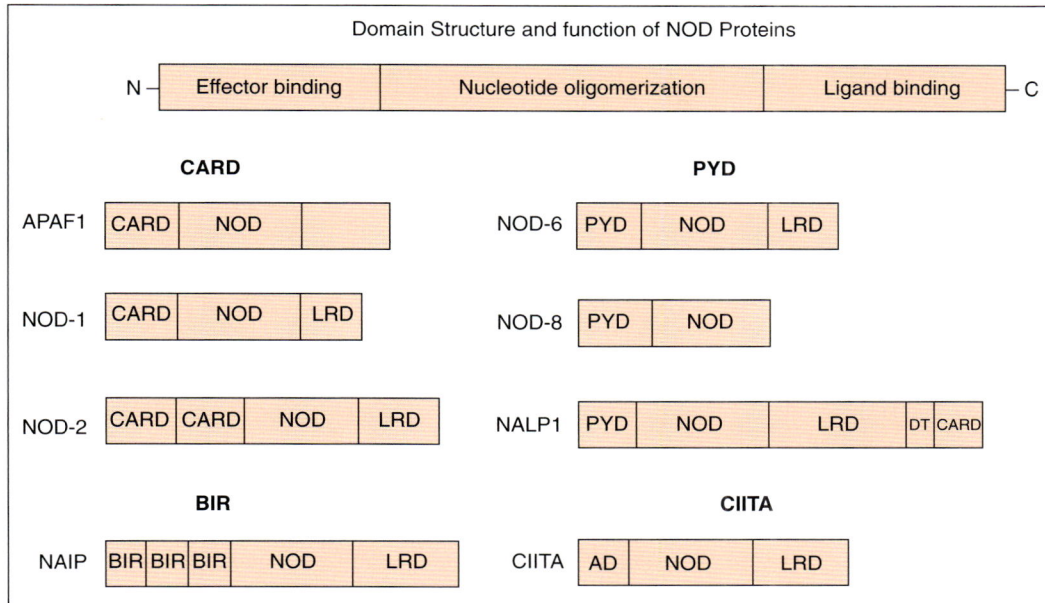

4.18 Domain structure of the NOD proteins. CARD = caspase recruitment domain; LRD = ligand recognition domain; NOD = nuclear oligomerization domain; PYD = pyrin domain.

the detection of *cagA* is not reliable as a single marker to discriminate for the risk of developing serious gastroduodenal diseases because the second term of comparison (the frequency of pathologies associated with infection of *cagA*-negative strains) is lacking. However, in countries where the frequency of infection with *cagA*-positive *Helicobacter pylori* strains is particularly elevated, a high prevalence of both peptic ulcer and gastric cancer commonly occurs, lending some credence to the theory that infections with *cagA*-positive strains may contribute to the high prevalence of severe gastroduodenal pathologies. An observation on Alaska natives, however, contradicts this conclusion: despite the high prevalence of *Helicobacter pylori* infection and the high incidence of gastric cancer observed in that area, a relatively low frequency of *cagA* positivity was found.

Inflammation and immunopathology

Colonization by *Helicobacter pylori* is largely asymptomatic. Histologically, it is evident the stomach is infiltrated with inflammatory cells, which, rather than eradicating the organism, induce bystander damage to the gastric epithelium. Similarly, there is a pronounced systemic and local immune response involving IgG and IgA but, again, this does not lead to eradication of the organism—instead some of the antibodies produced cross-react with host proteins and lead to host damage.

After infection, there is an increase in the mucosa CD4[+] T-cell population, and some studies have also shown an increase in γδT cells. The infection produces a T helper (Th)-1 cell cytokine profile.

Inflammation

Activation of NFκB in gastric and immune cells by *Helicobacter pylori* increases transcription of genes for a number of proinflammatory cytokines and chemokines (**4.20**), which leads to an inflammatory response with large numbers of neutrophils infiltrating the lamina propria of the stomach. Following NFκB activation, IL-8, IL-1α, IL-1β, CXCL1 (chemokine [C-X-C motif] ligand 1), TNF-α, IL-12 and IL-23 are secreted and CCL20 expressed. IL-8 is an inflammatory cytokine constitutively expressed by inflammatory cells, as well as by epithelial cells such as gastric mucocytes. IL-8 is induced by CagE, -F and -D of the T4SS rather than CagA. IL-8 attracts and activates granulocytes and therefore has a pivotal role in the neutrophil infiltration of *Helicobacter pylori*-colonized gastric mucosa. CXCL1

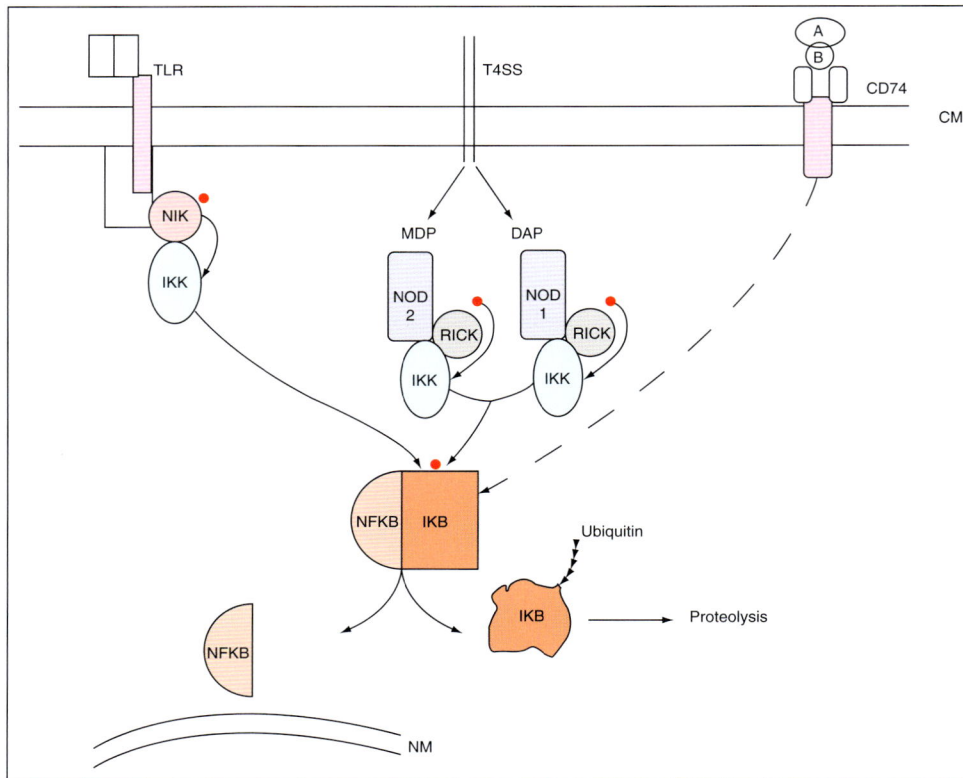

4.19 Activation cascade for NOD.

is a member of the CXC chemokine subfamily, which is involved in leucocyte recruitment and is increased in *cagA*-positive *Helicobacter pylori* infection. The other major subfamily of chemokines consists of the C-C type cytokines, which include CCL2, -3, -4, and -5; these chemokines recruit immune cells and induce the release of proinflammatory cytokines, such as IL-1. Cytokine IL-1, in addition to being proinflammatory,

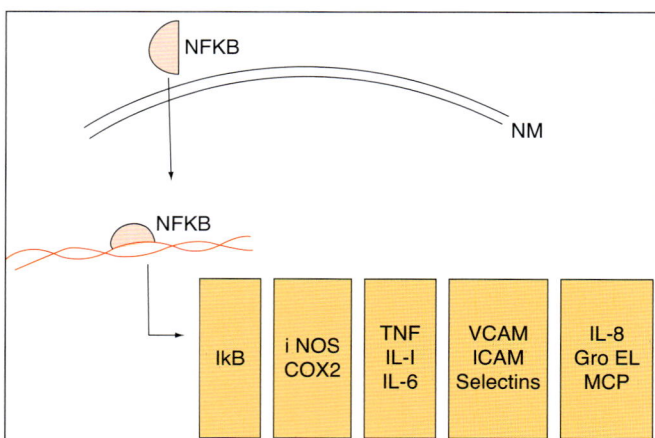

4.20 Secretion of gene products after NFκB binds to the DNA and stimulates a range of proinflammatory proteins.

is also a potent inhibitor of acid secretion from parietal cells. CCL20, another C-C type cytokine, attracts naïve dendritic cells.

In addition to the cytokines produced, NFκB controls the transcription of matrix metalloproteinase 9 (MMP-9), which is involved in both ulcer and cancer development.

Neuraminidase can also have a pathophysiological implication in inflammation. Neutrophils exposed to neuraminidase adhere to endothelial cells with an increased efficacy and can therefore enhance bystander damage to the gastric epithelial cells. In addition, this same effect is further induced by another product secreted by *H. pylori*, called neutrophil-activating protein (HP-NapA). This cytosolic protein is expressed by virtually all *H. pylori* strains examined.

HP-NapA has a dodecameric structure with a mass of 150 kDa and is able to bind iron via its N-terminus (the sequence of which is similar to other bacterial iron-binding proteins). HP-NapA is released into the extracellular medium by autolysis, whence it binds to the bacterial surface and acts as an adhesin. The presence of HP-NapA increases trans-endothelial migration of neutrophils, stimulating their adhesion to endothelial cells and inducing neutrophilic release of reactive oxygen species. HP-NapA is able to stimulate neutrophils and monocytes to increase their expression of IL-12, a key cytokine for the differentiation of naïve Th cells into the Th1 phenotype. HP-NapA also induces monocytes to produce IL-23. Finally, HP-NapA might favour fibrin deposition, by inducing the coordinate expression of cell pro-coagulant and antifibrinolytic activities, which contributes to the inflammatory reaction of gastric mucosa provoked by *Helicobacter pylori* (**4.21**).

Immunopathology

Gastric epithelial cells are also subject to damage by an autoantibody and cellular response following *H. pylori* colonization. Gastritis is associated with an increase in $\gamma\delta$ T cells and CD4$^+$ T cells in the mucosa. The number of $\gamma\delta$ T cells is directly related to the severity of gastritis when associated with high levels of antibodies to *Helicobacter* urease. The presence of the $\gamma\delta$ T cells also is associated with expression of the GroEL heat shock protein expression in gastric epithelial cells. Autoantibodies directed against gastric tissue have been detected in about 50% of patients infected by *Helicobacter pylori*, mostly directed at the surface antigens of the gastric cells and the H$^+$/K$^+$ ATPase in secretory canaliculi of parietal cells. However, autoantibodies to extra-gastric antigens have also been demonstrated, leading

to suggestions that *Helicobacter pylori* may be causally linked to some extra-gastric diseases. Additionally, the disruption of the epithelial barrier has been implicated in the precipitation of abnormal immune responses leading to food allergies and inflammatory bowel disease (**4.22**).

Autoantibodies directed against Le^b epitopes on the H$^+$/K$^+$ ATPase of parietal cells cause cell damage, leading to eventual atrophy, fibrosis and loss of parietal cells. This loss of acid-producing capacity leads to achlorhydria. The level of autoantibodies correlates with the degree of gastric atrophy. Achlorhydria is associated with pan-gastritis, and is a risk factor for intestinal metaplasia, dysplasia and adenocarcinoma of the stomach.

A role for *Helicobacter pylori* in food allergy and chronic urticaria has been proposed, with suggestions that raised levels of gastric mucosal IgE and an increase in the leakiness of the gastric mucosa (particularly if colonized by *cagA*-positive strains) leads to sensitization to food allergens and disease. However, studies have demonstrated that the prevalence or eradication of *Helicobacter pylori* has no effect on the course of chronic urticaria and that the presence of *Helicobacter pylori* may even have a protective affect on food allergy (*see also* p. 58). Similarly, studies have not been able to demonstrate an association between *Helicobacter pylori* and atopic disease.

However, it has been suggested that the Th1 response stimulated by *Helicobacter pylori* may counteract the Th2

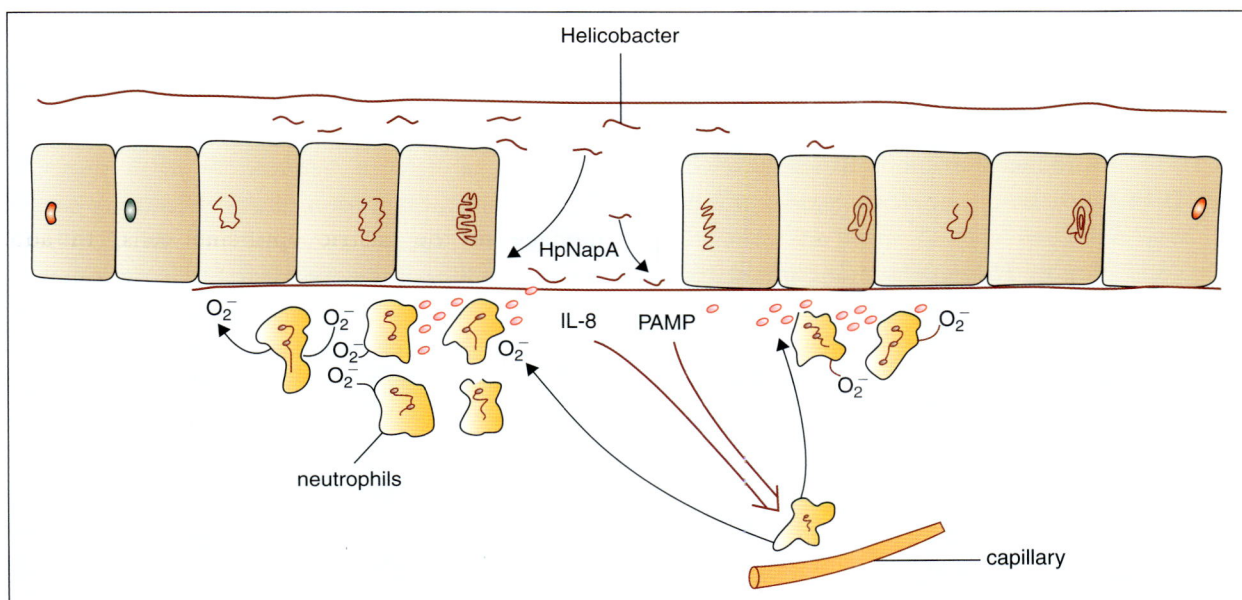

4.21 Action of HP-NapA protein and reactive oxygen species by polymorphonuclear leucocytes.

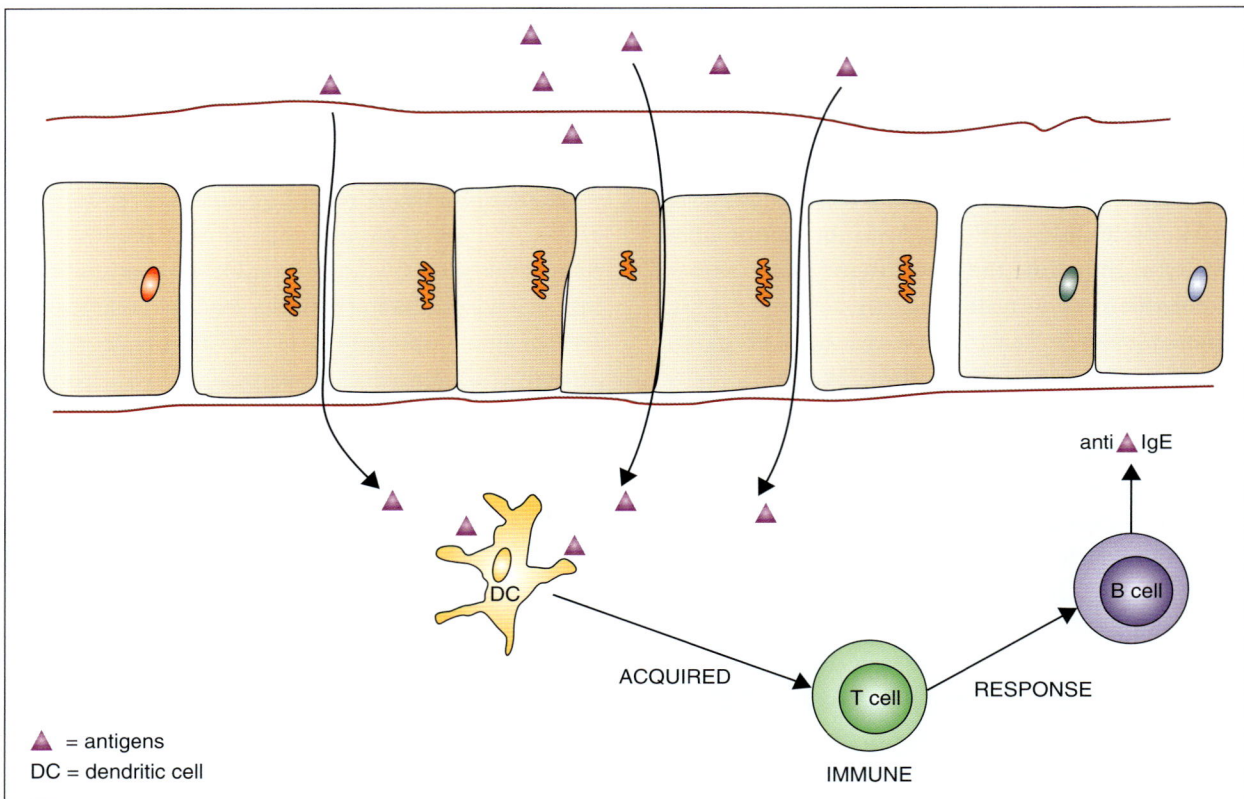

4.22 Potential immune effects of *Helicobater pylori*.

response found in asthma, and that colonization by *Helicobacter pylori* should therefore reduce the severity of asthma. It has been shown that a potential HP-NpaA mediated mechanism exists to reduce the Th2 immune response. HP-NapA stimulates IL-12 and IL-23 via an interaction with Toll-like receptor 2, inducing a Th1 polarization of the immune system, which thus could ameliorate asthma. In an animal model of asthma, systemic HP-NapA reduced eosinophilia and bronchial levels of IL-4 and IL-5. Epidemiological studies, however, have not been able to show an association between colonization by *Helicobacter pylori* and asthma. In fact, colonization by *Helicobacter pylori* has been linked to protection from asthma.

Autoantibodies against extra-gastric tissue have been demonstrated and some evidence supports autoantibodies directed against platelets are involved in idiothrombocytopenic purpura. In contrast, there is currently no convincing evidence that *Helicobacter pylori* is related to inflammatory bowel disease.

The urease of *Helicobacter pylori* can also activate monocytes, inducing IL-1β, IL-2 R, IL-6, TNFα,

IL-8 and HLA-DR expression. The effect on gastric epithelial cells is production of IL-6 and TNFα, but not IL-8. These results suggest that human gastric epithelial cells contribute to the induction of proinflammatory cytokines.

Additional immune effects of *Helicobacter pylori* are directed at the host immune system, thereby protecting the organism from the host's immune defence. As a first line of defence, *Helicobacter pylori* protects itself from complement lysis *in vivo* by becoming coated with complement control proteins such as CD59, thereby preventing lysis of the organism. Similarly, it may express Le^x and Le^y antigens, both of which may be found in the host and thus the organism may remain hidden to the host immune system. The lipopolysaccharide of *Helicobacter pylori* is poorly endotoxic and thus does not induce a strong immune response. Many of the outer membrane proteins of *Helicobacter pylori* are susceptible to phase variation (e.g. BabA) and, thus, during an infection the target for the immune system may alter slightly, hence diminishing the effect of an immune response. Additionally, the organism escapes killing by professional phagocytes through inhibiting its uptake by human neutrophils and monocytes. The mechanism of this is unclear, but once the *H. pylori* are taken up the phagosomes fuse to form megasomes in which the bacteria can survive. *Helicobacter pylori* strains expressing VacA arrest megasome maturation in association with the retention of tryptophan aspartate-containing coat protein (TACO), which is a marker of the early phagosome. This function of VacA is independent of its vacuolating activity. The organism also produces both catalase and SOD, thus nullifying the effect of reactive oxygen species produced by granulocytes.

The second major way in which *Helicobacter pylori* defeats the immune defences is by inducing apoptosis of macrophages. Apoptosis is caused by activation of pro-apoptotic proteins Bax and Bak, which stimulate caspase 8 and cytochrome release from the mitochondria, ultimately resulting in cell death. *Helicobacter pylori* also increases expression of ornithine decarboxylase and arginase II in macrophages, which is linked to polyamine synthesis, activation of c-Myc and apoptosis. Further, the polyamines may become oxidized to H_2O_2, which can also lead to apoptosis through mitochondrial membrane depolarization, cytochrome *c* release and subsequent caspase 3 activation. The arginase also inhibits inducible nitric oxide synthetase and thus the toxic nitric oxide.

A third method of mitigating the effects of the immune system is to inactivate metabolism and oxygen consumption, which induces apoptosis of immune cells and inhibits antigen presentation by B cells and T-cell activation. *In vitro*, VacA inhibits the proliferation of activated Jurkat T cells and fresh human peripheral blood lymphocytes. In Jurkat T cells, inhibition of proliferation is due in part to the inhibition of the nuclear translocation of NFAT, resulting in reduction of IL-2 secretion and IL-2 receptor expression. In fresh human peripheral blood lymphocytes there is a G_1/S cell-cycle arrest. The finding in Jurkat T cells has been confirmed by another study showing that inhibition of NFAT translocation is due to the capacity of VacA to form ion channels in the cell membrane of T cells. Additionally, VacA activates p38 stress kinase and induced Rac-1-dependent cytoskeleton rearrangement; these two mechanisms are also ion channel-independent. A more recent study has demonstrated that the inhibition of the proliferation of activated primary human CD4$^+$ T cells by VacA is neither dependent on inhibition of IL-2 secretion or activation of NFAT, rather the cells become anergic due to an arrest in the cell cycle. Several of these studies underline the complexity of T-cell inhibition by VacA, which seems to depend particularly upon the type and state of T cells used.

Helicobacter pylori is also associated with an increase in CD4$^-$-CD25$^+$-Foxp3 T$_{reg}$ cells, which dampen the proinflammatory response. Finally, there is some evidence that a proportion of the organisms may be intracellular (**4.23**).

Pathological effects of colonization by *Helicobacter pylori*

As already described in Chapter 3, the normal gastric mucosa contains:

- The gastric pits and surface epithelium
- The gastric glands supported by the lamina propria

The gastric gland consists of three regions: (1) gastric pit; (2) neck region containing stem cells that replenish cells in both directions—towards the gastric pit and towards the base of the gland; and (3) the base of the gland.

The gastric glands vary in composition depending on the region of the stomach. In the cardia there are principally mucus-secreting glands, containing goblet cells found in the gastric pit region. In the body of the stomach parietal cells, found mainly in the middle part of the gland, secrete acid and gastric instrinsic factor (to aid absorption of vitamin B$_{12}$); and chief cells, found mainly in the base of the gland, produce digestive enzymes. In the antrum of the stomach the gland produces mucus from goblet cells, gastrin from G cells, and SST from D cells.

A balance between cell loss and renewal maintains the integrity and architecture of gastric mucosa. The surface epithelial cells are renewed every 3–5 days (for other glandular cells it is >3 months), being replaced by cells that migrate from the proliferative zone in the neck of the foveolar glands. Increased gastric epithelial cell proliferation, and movement superficially of the gland's proliferative compartment, have been observed in stomachs colonized by *Helicobacter pylori*. These

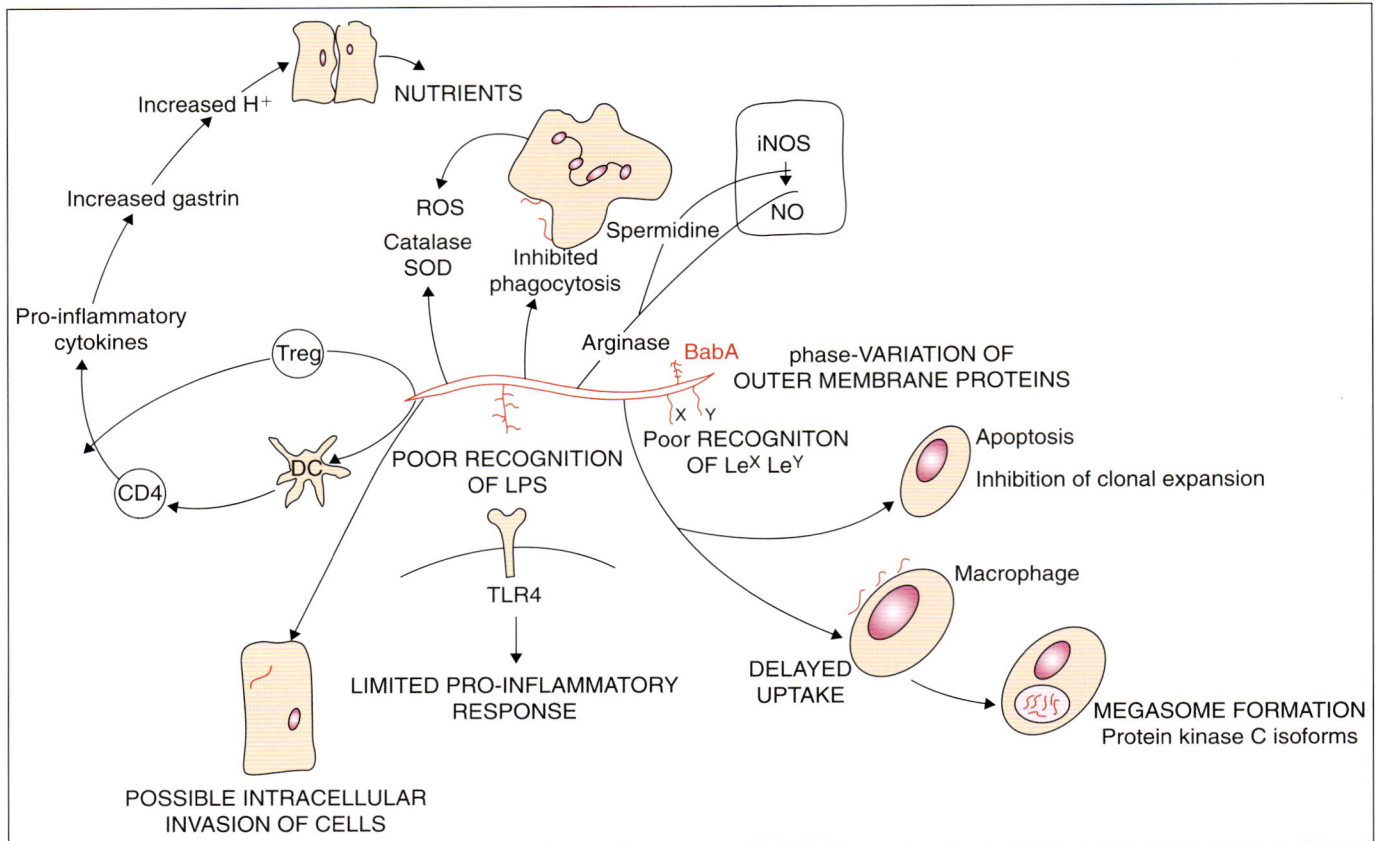

4.23 Effects of *Helicobacter pylori* on the host immune defence mechanisms.

phenomena could increase the probability of polyploid abnormalities with an enhanced risk of gastric cancer development. The key mechanism regulating gastric cell proliferation is still unknown. One of the most important factors that control the turnover of gastric epithelial cells is apoptosis. At present, little information is available on the role of apoptosis in gastric mucosa cell renewal. It is highly regulated at the genomic level: it is repressed by the *bcl*-2 oncogene, and induced by counterbalancing genes.

From a morphological point of view, apoptotic cell death begins with clumping of nuclear chromatin and cell shrinkage; then the nuclei break up (karyorhexis), and cells begin to bleb and undergo necrotic changes (i.e., break up into a cluster of apoptotic bodies). The apoptotic process can be started by a sort of built-in clock or by extracellular agents, including infectious agents. It is therefore conceivable that apoptosis can be involved in the series of events that characterize *Helicobacter pylori* infection, such as cancer and ulcer.

When *Helicobacter pylori* infects humans, it begins as an acute gastritis characterized by a polymorphonuclear infiltrate in the neck of the gastric pits. The acute gastritis evolves into chronic gastritis and may develop lymphoid follicles.

Acute inflammation

Acute inflammation is a defence mechanism comprising cells and soluble factors. The majority of these components are in the blood in an inactive form and must be transferred to the tissues in an active form to combat the invading pathogen. The body recognizes both the presence of tissue injury and *Helicobacter pylori* on the gastric epithelial cells, and responds by producing endogenous mediators (such as histamine and prostaglandins), as well as responding to the presence of exogenous mediators produced by the invading pathogen (such as peptidoglycan and lipopolysaccharide). This response involves activating tissue macrophages, which release additional mediators. The net result of this is dilatation and increased permeability of the local blood vessels, thereby increasing blood flow and allowing plasma containing defensive factors to leak into the tissue. Released into the tissues are such factors as complement, mannose-binding protein, and coagulation proteins. Also activated is the kallikrein cascade, which produces bradykinin. One of the effects of this is to stimulate local sensory nerve endings, thus causing pain. The endothelium of the capillaries respond by upregulating adhesive molecules that trap circulating neutrophils, which pass out of the vessel towards the presence of organisms and injury, guided by a concentration gradient of chemotactic mediators, such as C5a and C3a. IL-8, another chemotactic factor attracting neutrophils, is also produced by epithelial surfaces. The neutrophils then attempt to engulf and kill the invading pathogen, although *Helicobacter pylori* can avoid this, as discussed earlier.

Meanwhile, antigenic material from the organism is being taken up by macrophages, and antigen is also draining into the lymph and being transported to the regional lymph nodes. Macrophages release proinflammatory cytokines such as IL-1, IL-6 and TNF, and present the antigenic material to T cells. Upon activation, the T cells release further cytokines, all of which acts as a positive feedback for the process. IL-1 stimulates the acute-phase reaction, upregulating a collection of proteins produced by the liver; these proteins include C-reactive protein, complement, coagulation proteins and protease inhibitors.

In the regional lymph nodes, the T cells activate B cells, which divide and expand in number. The function of B cells is to produce antibodies, which in turn enhance the phagocytosis of bacteria by neutrophils and memory cells are produced.

On initial infection of the gastric tissue, the host responds strongly to the presence of *Helicobacter pylori* by both the innate and acquired immune responses. Even though the organism does not normally penetrate the gastric epithelium, damage caused by immune factors results in acute inflammation followed by chronic inflammation. Initially, there is a strong recruitment of granulocytes to the area, but phagocytosis by both granulocytes and macrophages of *Helicobacter pylori* is inhibited in some way not yet clearly understood. The acquired immune system is also activated with the production of both local (stomach) and systemic antibodies of the IgM, IgG and IgA classes. It appears that IgA secreted into the stomach is unable to penetrate the mucus and fails to block successfully the adhesins expressed by the bacteria. *Helicobacter pylori* is susceptible to complement lysis *in vitro*, yet *in vivo* it is protected by coating itself in complement control proteins, such as CD59. The induction of anti-*Helicobacter pylori* antibodies of IgM and IgG class suggests that at least parts of the organism are taken up by dendritic cells to generate a systemic adaptive immune response. However, despite a humoral and cellular immune response, the organism is able to evade the immune system. An initial intense acute inflammatory response is invoked with infiltration of the lamina propria by granulocytes and, as the inflammation becomes chronic, a mononuclear cell infiltrate occurs and chronic infection of the stomach ensues. The photomicrograph (**4.24**) demonstrates infiltration of the gastric epithelium by inflammatory cells.

Chronic inflammation

The initial acute inflammatory response may be all that is required to eradicate an organism but, as the antigenic stimulus from *Helicobacter pylori* persists, the acute response subsides and a chronic response develops, with the number of neutrophils declining to be replaced by mononuclear cells. Macrophages engulf remaining bacteria, dead neutrophils and parenchymal cells. The connective tissue of the inflamed area produces fibroblasts that deposit collagen, leading to fibrosis. The new tissue—comprising mononuclear cells, fibroblasts and stroma—is called granulation

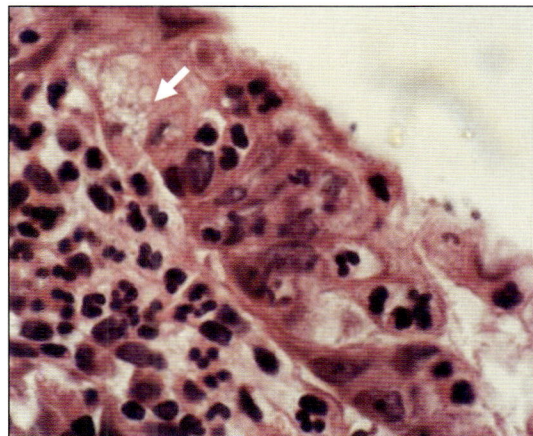

4.24 Acute gastritis micrograph: arrow indicates *in vivo* vacuolation.

tissue and is permeated by new blood vessels. Over time this gradually resolves, with tissue integrity restored and residual damage indicated by scar formation. However, although mononuclear cells are mobilized, *Helicobacter pylori* is able to persist and the chronic inflammatory response lasts a lifetime. This is the basis for atrophy, metaplasia, dysplasia and neoplasia, i.e., the Correa pathway to gastric and mucosal-associated lymphoid tissue (MALT) tumours. The photomicrograph (**4.25**) illustrates that mononuclear cells largely replace the granulocytes.

The mucosa is infiltrated by lymphocytes, plasma cells, eosinophils, monocytes, macrophages and mast cells; sometimes, the lymphocytes organize into lymphoid follicles (follicular gastritis). Chronic gastritis is defined as 'active' when neutrophils persist in the lamina propria and gastric gland epithelium. In the beginning, the inflammatory infiltrate is confined in the superficial mucosa; thereafter, it involves the entire mucosa thickness. The photomicrograph (**4.26**) illustrates a large lymphoid follicle at the lower right of the picture.

Ulcer

The pathophysiological sequence of events leading to ulceration is not known with any certainty, although plausible biological mechanisms can be constructed into a reasonable hypothesis. *Helicobacter pylori* is linked to two types of ulcer: duodenal ulcer and gastric ulcer. In duodenal ulcer, the organism is found principally in the antrum of the stomach, with a high acid load in the stomach induced by the presence of the organism. In gastric ulcer, the converse is true—the organism is not confined to the antrum but can be found throughout the stomach (antrum and fundus), and the amount of acid in the stomach is low. This latter finding is due to death of the acid-producing cells found mainly in the fundus of the stomach, caused by presence of the organism. Several virulence characteristics may combine to lead to ulceration: for duodenal ulcer a diminution of the local host defences, particularly the mucus barrier, and the production of directly-acting toxins combined with an enhanced physiological acid response led to the suggestion of the 'leaking roof' hypothesis for the development of ulceration (*see* also **4.2**).

The helical shape of the organism facilitates its penetration of the mucus layer covering the gastric epithelium. This is followed by binding to the gastric epithelium. Once bound, *Helicobacter pylori* produces ammonia by virtue of its urease enzyme and PLA_2, both enzymes that affect the quality of the mucus barrier and directly damage the host cell. The loss of this protective barrier can allow stomach acid and digestive enzymes to have direct access to the gastric epithelium. In addition, type I strains will secrete VacA and also inject CagA into host cells, inducing further damage to the host epithelium, and ultimately causing release of chemotactic cytokines, which recruit inflammatory immune cells to the area. The release of reactive oxygen species induced by *Helicobacter pylori* activity and cytotoxic proteins from the immune cells leads to additional damage to the host epithelium. Additionally, the levels of stomach acid are increased, causing yet more damage to the gastric epithelium and eventually leading to ulcer formation.

VacA provokes an increased extracellular secretion of acidic hydrolases and a reduction of the degradative

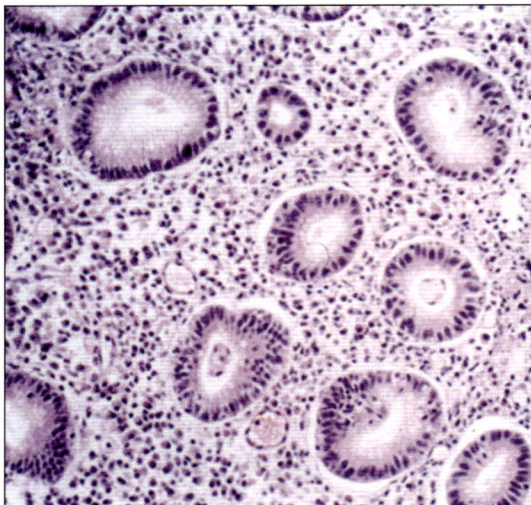

4.25 Chronic gastritis micrograph.

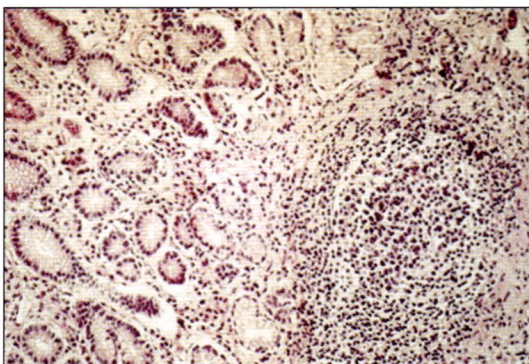

4.26 Lymphoid follicle.

potential of late endosomes and lysosomes. These findings may account for the enhanced gastric mucosa injury associated with cytotoxic *Helicobacter pylori* colonization, consisting of a partial disruption of the extracellular matrix, reduction of mucus viscosity, and weakening of the junctional apparatus between adjacent mucous cells, the spaces of which can therefore be easily invaded by the bacteria. It is conceivable that *Helicobacter pylori* has set up a strategy to modulate mucosal damage through a multiplicity of VacA-mediated functions.

In addition to vacuole formation, VacA may cause cytoskeletal alterations and actin rearrangement, which could hinder ulcer healing. Mucosal restoration is promoted by various growth factors, such as EGF, a potent mitogenic that stimulates epithelial cell proliferation, migration and ulcer healing. Extracts of cytotoxic *Helicobacter pylori* were found to induce expression of EGF-related growth factors in human-derived gastric adenocarcinoma cells in culture; however, stimulatory effects on cell growth were counteracted by prevention of *in vitro* binding of EGF to its receptor, and by reduction of the EGF-activated signal transduction cascade. A negative influence of VacA on cell proliferation was also observed using fibroblast and platelet-derived growth factors to stimulate fibroblasts *in vitro*, and hepatocyte growth factor (HGF) to stimulate isolated rabbit gastric epithelial cells. In any case, HGF did not prevent or revert to *in vitro* vacuolization. There is a significant reduction of *in vitro* cell proliferation under the effect of a vacuolating cytotoxic broth culture filtrate. Experimental infection of mice with cytotoxic and non-cytotoxic *Helicobacter pylori* strains confirmed these *in vitro* findings, as it was found that infection with VacA-positive strains delayed healing of chronic ulcer.

It is not known whether *Helicobacter pylori* determinants or inflammation *per se* (or both) are involved in inducing apoptosis. Most probably, both *Helicobacter pylori* determinants and inflammation are involved in apoptosis, as apoptosis of gastric epithelial cells is increased *in vitro* by inflammatory cytokines such as interferon-γ and TNF-α, which are known to be involved in natural *Helicobacter pylori* infection. As levels of cytokines in the gastroduodenal mucosa are increased in the presence of peptic ulceration, it is conceivable this acts as a positive feedback loop, such that apoptosis is further increased in the presence of gastroduodenal ulcer. Contradictory evidence against this suggestion does exist, however.

In the case of gastric ulcer, the extent of inflammation is throughout the stomach and the acid-producing capacity of the stomach is decreased. As the host mounts an acquired immune response to the presence of the organism, cross-reacting antibodies directed against the proton pump are produced and these can induce antibody-mediated cell death. Although there is atrophic gastritis, the other virulence mechanisms of *Helicobacter pylori* are still produced and this can ultimately lead to gastric ulcer (**4.27**).

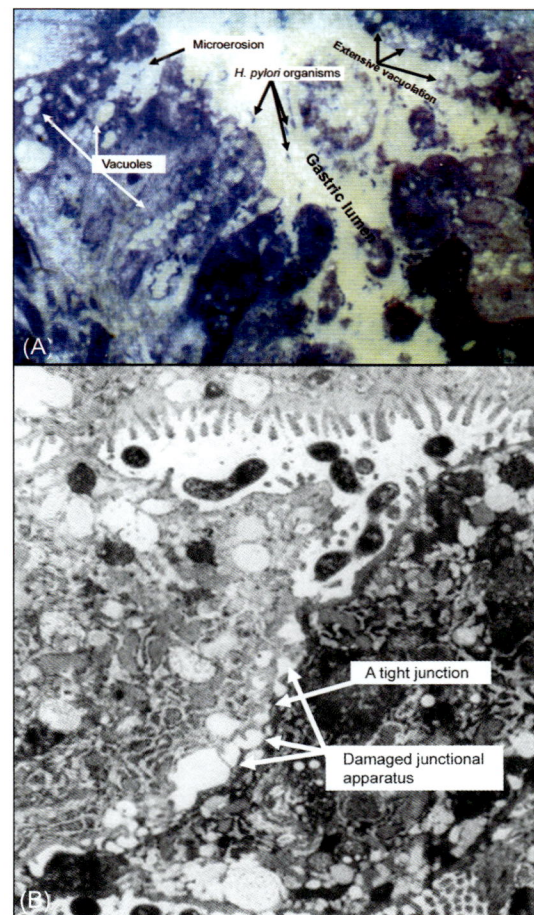

4.27 Photomicrograph and electron micrograph of early stages in ulcer formation. The micrograph (A) of a Giemsa-stained section shows the presence of *Helicobacter pylori*, vacuoles within cells, and drop-out of cells leading to microerosions, whereas the electron micrograph (B) shows damage to intercellular junctions. This initial damage may then lead on to ulcer formation due to disturbed cell dynamics and exposure to cell-damaging substances leading to necrosis.

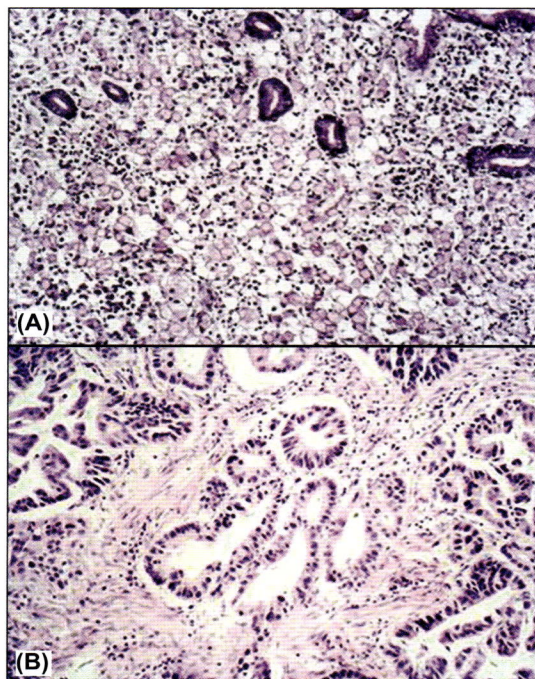

4.28 Intestinal/diffuse carcinoma. The diffuse type gastric carcinoma arises from gastric mucous cells and is characterized by poorly cohesive cells infiltrating the gastric wall without gland formation. It is usually a poorly differentiated adenocarcinoma, often with signet-ring cells (A). The intestinal adenocarcinoma is characterized by recognizable glandular structures that range from well differentiated to moderately and sometimes poorly differentiated tumours (B).

Cancer

According to the Lauren classification, gastric carcinoma is subdivided into two histological types, intestinal and diffuse (**4.28**): *Helicobacter pylori* infection is associated with both.

In long-standing chronic gastritis, gastric atrophy may develop (which is believed to be a precancerous condition) with partial loss of gastric glands, which become shorter, and/or replacement of gastric glands with intestinal glands (intestinal metaplasia). This occurs in association with pan-gastritis and a low acid level. Under these circumstances, the stomach can become colonized with other enteric Gram-negative organisms. After long-term colonization, there may be a sequence of atrophy → metaplasia → dysplasia, followed by eventual carcinoma.

Based on a study of morphology and mucin secretion, three types of intestinal metaplasia have been identified.

Type I, or complete intestinal metaplasia, resembles normal small intestinal mucosa: crypts are straight and regular, and the epithelium consists of mature absorptive cells with a well-developed brush border, goblet cells and often Paneth cells at the base of the pits. The goblet cells secrete sialomucins and the absorptive cells are non-secretory. In incomplete intestinal metaplasia, the crypts are elongated and tortuous (**4.29A**); the epithelium is characterized by few or absent absorptive cells and goblet cells and by columnar mucous cells in various stages of differentiation; Paneth cells disappear.

On the basis of the mucin content of the columnar cells, incomplete intestinal metaplasia has been subdivided into type II and type III. In the incomplete type II form, the columnar mucous cells secrete neutral mucin and sialomucin, and goblet cells secrete sialomucins and, occasionally, sulphomucins (**4.29B**). In the incomplete type III form, columnar cells secrete predominantly sulphomucin, and goblet cells secrete sialomucins and/ or sulphomucins (**4.29C**). Various studies have shown that type III intestinal metaplasia exposes patients to an increased risk of gastric cancer. In a few cases, the chronic atrophic gastritis and intestinal metaplasia are followed by glandular dysplasia.

Gastric dysplasia is considered an important marker for cancer risk and a morphological precursor of intestinal-type gastric carcinoma. The World Health Organization has redefined dysplasia as an unequivocal neoplastic epithelial alteration without invasion and it is characterized by architectural alteration of gastric mucosa, abnormal epithelial differentiation and atypical morphology of cells. It is graded, according to the degree of histological alterations, as low grade and high grade (**4.30**). Dysplasia may then progress to carcinoma (**4.28**), the pathophysiology of which involves disturbance of gastric epithelial cell dynamics.

Helicobacter pylori infection disturbs the gastric epithelial cell cycle and alters the balance between apoptosis and proliferation. Apoptosis may also be controlled in part by a *Helicobacter pylori* gene product that has 3′–5′ exoribonuclease activity, which is involved in post-translational modification of apoptosis-inducing genes. As with the immune cells, VacA also has a similar effect on gastric epithelial cells, impairing mitochondrial metabolism, causing a reduction in ATP, oxygen consumption and mitochondrial membrane potential, leading to an altered cell cycle.

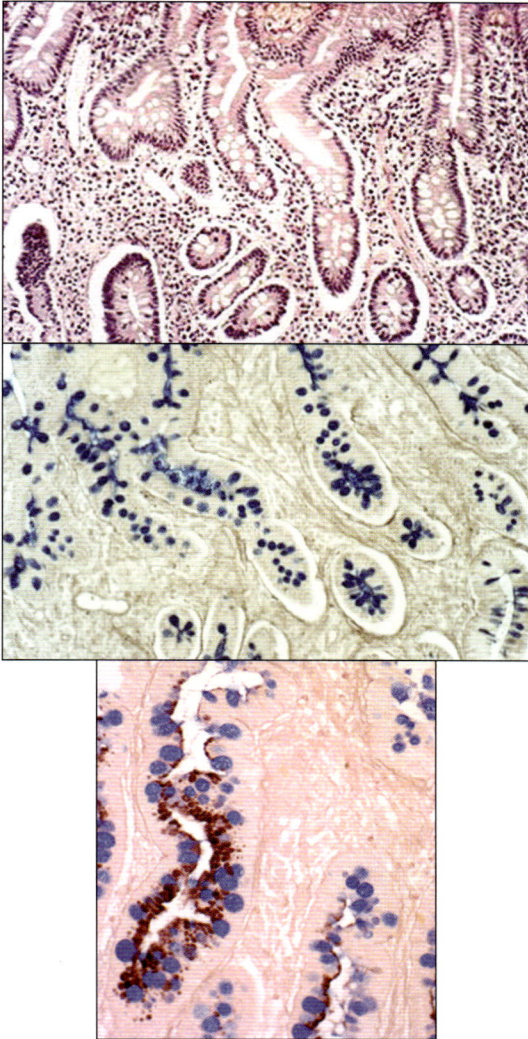

4.29 Metaplasia.

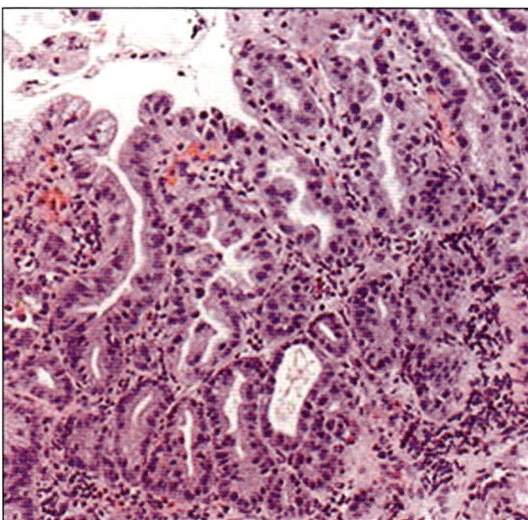

4.30 Dysplasia and carcinoma.

Colonization by *Helicobacter pylori* leads to activation of EGFR (through the release of EGFR ligands via and matrix metalloprotease-17 activity), which is anti-apoptotic. In a study of patients with ulcer or cancer, the effect of *Helicobacter pylori* on upregulation of Bax (pro-apoptotic) is stronger than induction of Bcl-2 (anti-apoptotic) in ulcer patient group; however, in patients with gastric cancer, the upregulation of Bcl-2 was such that the effect of Bax was inhibited and cell proliferation enhanced, which may be relevant to the development of gastric adenocarcinoma.

Gastric carcinogenesis appears to be a multistep and multifactorial process. It is possibly an interaction with environmental and hereditary factors related to gastric carcinogenesis, resulting in the sequence of atrophy, intestinal metaplasia, dysplasia and intestinal type gastric cancer. The carcinogenic process involves genes that control cell proliferation and differentiation. Conversely, genes involved in the control of cell adhesion are affected in the pathogenesis of diffuse-type gastric carcinoma. Alterations of basal membrane proteins and of zonula adherence proteins, such as cadherins and catenins, may lead to diffuse-type gastric carcinoma directly from glandular neck cells.

An increase in apoptosis occurs in a stomach colonized by *Helicobacter pylori*, which falls to normal after the infection is cured. It is not known whether *Helicobacter pylori* determinants or inflammation *per se* (or both) are involved in inducing apoptosis. *Helicobacter pylori* urease was found to be involved indirectly in triggering or stimulating apoptosis of rat gastric cells *in vitro* through the production of monochloramine, which originates from the interaction of urease-generated ammonia, and hypochlorous acid generated by innate immune defence cells.

Development of gastric carcinoma can be explained on the basis of inflammation induced by the colonizing type I *Helicobacter pylori* strains. Granulocytes and other cells stimulated by cytokines exhibit oxidative burst, producing reactive oxygen species (O_2^-, H_2O_2, NO) potentially capable of damaging the DNA of surrounding cells which could, thus, undergo polyploidy abnormalities. IL-8 mRNA is overexpressed in neoplastic gastric tissues and the genomic message levels are related to the degree of tumour vascularization. In addition, IL-8 is able to stimulate the proliferation of endothelial-derived cell lines *in vitro*, thus behaving as an autocrine angiogenic factor potentially capable of promoting the development of gastric carcinoma.

Mutations in the oncosuppressor *p53* gene are a fundamental step in the carcinogenic processes. In normal conditions, when a genotoxic substance damages the DNA of epithelial cells, *p53* is stimulated to express high amounts of p53 protein, which is able to stop the cell replicative cycle, so that the cell endonucleases can repair the injury. If *p53* is mutated, the protein produced does not function properly; hence, the cell cycle is not arrested, damaged DNA is inherited, other mutations may accumulate and, in the end, cancer may develop.

The increased cell proliferation and the diminished apoptotic score found in gastric mucosa colonized by type I *Helicobacter pylori* organisms could account, at least in part, for the observation that infection by type I *Helicobacter pylori* strains increases the risk of gastric cancer development. Exposure of AGS cells (a human gastric adenocarinoma cell line) to a *cagA*-negative *Helicobacter pylori* strain was shown to enhance cell apoptosis in a process that could be reversed by *bcl*-2 expression, while a *cagA*-positive strain upregulated *bcl*-2, thus reducing apoptosis.

However, apoptotic effects mediated by *Helicobacter pylori* still remain to be clarified. The induction of *Helicobacter pylori*-mediated apoptosis would presumably take place through increased expression of the Bak protein by epithelial cells, especially of the luminal portion of the gastric gland. *Helicobacter pylori* binds to MHC II molecules on gastric epithelial cells, and can induce apoptosis through cross-linking of this complex. If colonization by CagA-positive strains induced an increased expression of MHC II molecules, which are used by *Helicobacter pylori* to adhere to epithelial cells, infection with type I organisms should augment, not decrease, apoptosis. This field is in continuous evolution.

The pathways that lead cells to die by apoptosis are numerous. Cytotoxic T lymphocytes, for instance, can induce apoptosis to target cells through a Fas-Fas ligand pathway (also known as CD95 receptor/ligand system). Fas (or CD95) is a receptor present on the surface of T lymphocytes, epithelial cells, including gastric mucosa cells. A Fas-ligand protein, such as the ones secreted by T lymphocytes and epithelial cells, binds to its receptor and induces apoptosis. Cytokines induce apoptosis

because they increase the expression of Fas by cells. Some researchers have recently explored the mechanisms of Fas-mediated apoptosis during *Helicobacter pylori* infection, and have shown that *H. pylori* increases expression of Fas receptors, as well as apoptosis, in cells *in vitro*. While Fas was hardly detectable on gastric epithelial cells from uninfected subjects, almost all epithelial cells from *Helicobacter pylori*-positive patients expressed this receptor. However, the prevention of Fas-mediated killing by a monoclonal antibody to the Fas receptor, did not diminish the induction of apoptosis by *Helicobacter pylori*.

MALT lymphomas (**4.31**) are antigen-driven extranodal marginal B-cell lymphomas. They account for about 10% of all non-Hodgkin lymphomas, of which 50% occur in the stomach. Gastric MALT lymphomas are associated with chronic inflammation caused by *Helicobacter pylori* and are morphologically similar to Peyer's patches in the lower gastrointestinal tract. There are several links between *Helicobacter pylori* and MALT lymphoma: a strong epidemiological association (the organism is found in over 90% of cases); molecular evidence whereby patient and allele-specific PCR of *Helicobacter pylori* chronic gastritis demonstrates that the B cell giving rise to the lymphoma is present before the development of lymphoma; and the regression of low-grade lymphoma following *H. pylori* eradication. *Helicobacter pylori*-associated virulence markers that may be linked to the development of MALT lymphoma are *iceA1*, expression of *sabA*, non-expression of *hopZ*, and presence of the JHP950 open reading frame found in the plasticity zone. Host markers associated with the development of MALT lymphoma vary according to ethnic background but have been variously identified as: *IL-1 RN*2/2* (gene coding for IL-1ra, the allele corresponds to two 86bp variable number

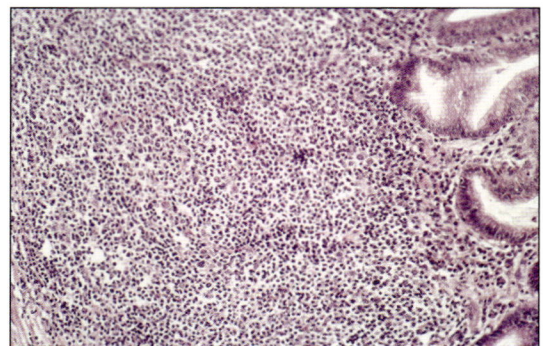

4.31 MALT lymphoma.

tandem repeats); *GST T1* null genotype (a glutathione S-transferase polymorphism); and a *TNF* C-857T functional polymorphism.

Further reading

Andersen LP. Colonization and infection by *Helicobacter pylori* in humans. *Helicobacter* 2007; 12(Suppl 2): 12–15.

Backert S, Selbach M. Role of type IV secretion in *Helicobacter pylori* pathogenesis. *Cellular Microbiology* 2008; 10: 1573–81.

Ferreri AJM, Ernberg I, Copie-Bergman C. Infectious agents and lymphoma development: molecular and clinical aspects. *J Int Med* 2009; 265: 421–38.

Hatakeyama M. Linking epithelial polarity and carcinogenesis by multitasking *Helicobacter pylori* virulence factor cagA. *Oncogene* 2008; 27: 7047–54.

Hatakeyama M. SagA of CagA in *Helicobacter pylori* pathogenesis. *Curr Op Microbiol* 2008; 11: 30–7.

Kaneko H, Konagaya T, Kusugami K. *Helicobacter pylori* and gut hormones. *J Gastroenterol* 2002; 37: 77–86.

Kufer TA, Sansonetti PJ. Sensing of bacteria: NOD a lonely job. *Curr Op Microbiol* 2007; 10: 62–9.

Lupetti P, Heuser JE, Manetti R, *et al.* Oligomeric and subunit structure of the *Helicobacter pylori* vacuolating cytotoxin. *J Cell Biol* 1996; 133: 801–7.

Nardone G, Holicky EL, Uhl JR, *et al. In vivo* and *in vitro* studies of phospholipase A2 expression in *Helicobacter pylori* infection. *Infect Immun* 2001; 69: 5857–63.

Sachs G, Kraut JA, Wen Y, Feng J, Scott DR. Urea transport in bacteria: acid acclimation by gastric *Helicobacter pylori* spp. *J Membrane Biol* 2006; 212: 71–82.

Schubert ML. Gastric secretion. *Curr Opin Gastroenterol* 2008; 24: 659–64.

Schubert ML, Peura DA. Control of gastric acid secretion in health and disease. *Gastroenterology* 2008; 134: 1842–60.

Slomiany BL, Slomiany A. Platelet-activating factor mediates *Helicobacter pylori* lipopolysaccharide interference with gastric mucin synthesis. *IUBMB Life* 2004; 56: 41–6.

Wada A, Yamasaki E, Hirayama T. *Helicobacter pylori* vacuolating cytotoxin, vacA, is responsible for gastric ulceration. *J Biochem* 2004; 136: 741–6.

Wessler S, Backert S. Molecular mechanisms of epithelial barrier disruption by *Helicobacter pylori*. *Trends Microbiol* 2008; 16: 397–405.

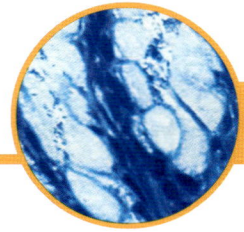

Chapter 5

Diagnosis

Test parameters

The incidental discovery in 1983 of a gastric bacterium led to a dramatic change in the field of gastroenterology and the development of specific diagnostic tests for the organism. *Helicobacter pylori* infects more than half the world's population, causing peptic ulcer disease and chronic gastritis, and is strongly associated with gastric malignancies. It is an important global pathogen with significant morbidity and mortality. Accurate diagnostic tests are thus important for targeted antibiotic therapy. *Helicobacter pylori* infection can be diagnosed by: (1) invasive techniques, which means endoscopy with biopsies for histology, culture and a rapid urease test; and (2) non-invasive techniques, such as serology, ^{13}C-urea breath test, and the stool antigen test.

All the main tests used for the diagnosis of *Helicobacter pylori* have differing sensitivity and specificity and a single test is insufficient to make an accurate diagnosis of active infection, except for a positive culture test. For this reason, according to European guidelines, the gold standard is generally represented by at least two different tests. Nevertheless, in daily clinical practice, just one test is used for diagnosis of infection, making the choice of the 'right test' the most important step.

Any diagnostic test can be characterized by its sensitivity, specificity, and positive and negative predictive values, and these latter parameters vary with the prevalence of the disease in the community. The prevalence of a condition is the proportion of individuals in a population that have the condition. A perfect test will correctly identify all those who have the disease by recording a positive test (sensitivity 100%). Numerically,

this is the number of true positive (TP) divided by the number of TP plus the false negative tests (*see* **Box 5.1A** below [p. 98]). A perfect test will also identify all those who do not have the disease by recording a negative test (specificity 100%). For example, if the prevalence of a condition is 40% (i.e. 400/1000 have the disease) and the test identifies 340/400 persons with the disease correctly, the test sensitivity is 85%; if the test identifies 480/600 persons without the disease correctly, the specificity is 80%. If the prevalence of disease were only 10% the sensitivity and specificity would be unchanged and would detect 85/100 as positive and 720/900 as negative.

There is generally a compromise between sensitivity and specificity in the test characteristics. For diseases amenable to treatment, a test with high sensitivity is preferable, whereas for those conditions that are untreatable or have implications for the population at large, a test with a high specificity is required.

An alternative way of defining sensitivity and specificity is the probability of persons with the disease having a positive test (sensitivity) and the probability of persons without the disease having a negative test (specificity). Such a calculation is possible using a Bayesian approach, which requires a pre-test probability (in this case prevalence) to be converted into a post-test probability. In Bayes' theorem the post-test probability is proportional to the pre-test probability multiplied by the likelihood of the test being positive. This value is the positive predictive value related to the prevalence of disease in the community (*see* Box **5.1B**). Thus, in populations with a low prevalence of disease, the positive predictive value will be low even if the sensitivity and specificity are high and there will be many false-positive results. The converse is true of negative predictive value (*see* **Box 5.1C**).

The likelihood ratio (the ratio of the probability of a positive result in a person with the disease compared with the probability of positive results in a person who does not have the disease) can indicate the value of a test or sequence of tests. The likelihood ratio for a positive test is: sensitivity/(1-specificity), or, for a negative test, (1-sensitivity)/specificity. Therefore, the post-test probability is equal to the pre-test probability multiplied by the likelihood ratio.

The choice of test should therefore be based on:

- Prevalence of the infection in the population
- Symptoms, such as the presence of alarm symptoms
- 'Likelihood ratio' for a positive and negative test
- Costs
- Availability of tests in different settings

Invasive tests

Endoscopy

Endoscopy has been commonly used in diagnostic units, increasing costs and waiting lists. Upper gastrointestinal endoscopy is an expensive and unpleasant procedure that carries the risk of haemorrhage and perforation, and has a reported mortality and morbidity of 0.008% and 0.432%, respectively. The European Helicobacter Study Group (EHSG) Maastricht II Report recommended that, in the primary care environment, patients presenting with dyspepsia, who were under 45–50y, in the absence of alarm symptoms (weight loss, anaemia) or symptoms of GORD (heartburn, regurgitation), and who were not taking non-steroidal anti-inflammatory drugs, should be offered a 'test and treat' intervention (TTI) strategy using the non-invasive urea breath test or faecal antigen test.

Biochemical endoscopy

To avoid endoscopy and yet assess whether *Helicobacter pylori* and inflammation are present, a 'biochemical' endoscopy has been suggested to quantify the levels of pepsinogen (PSGN) I and II, the PSGN I/II ratio, gastrin and presence of antibodies to *Helicobacter pylori*. Infection with *Helicobacter pylori* increases plasma gastrin

(e.g. 150 ng/ml) compared with control levels (e.g. 50 ng/ml) as a consequence of the inhibition of somatostatin production.

Variation of PSGN I and II and their ratio occurs with age, weight, smoking and chronic renal failure. Elevation of both PSGN I (e.g. 70 ng/ml compared with 50 ng/ml); PSGN II (e.g. 25 ng/ml compared with 10 ng/ml) with a reduction of the PSGN I/II ratio (e.g. 3.5 compared with 6.2) is found in *Helicobacter pylori*-associated gastritis compared with *Helicobacter pylori*-negative individuals. Some studies have shown that PSGN I levels are even further elevated in peptic ulcer disease compared with gastritis. A low PSGN I level is correlated with gastric atrophy, and a PSGN I <50 ng/ml with the presence of IgA to *Helicobacter pylori* has been reported to be a risk factor for gastric cancer. Current opinion is that these assays do not replace the need for endoscopy.

A 'test and treat' strategy was recommended for peptic ulcer patients who were on long-term acid suppressive treatment. Endoscopy should only be performed in patients less than 45–50y old with symptoms. In patients over this age limit, endoscopy should be performed irrespective of alarm symptoms. This strategy was endorsed by the EHSG Maastricht III guidelines and has been supported by a number of publications, including a Cochrane Systematic Review. Colonization by *Helicobacter pylori* is interpreted in the clinical context of investigation for dyspepsia. The majority of persons colonized by *Helicobacter pylori* are asymptomatic. There is currently no indication to determine the presence of the organism in asymptomatic persons unless they are concerned about the risk of developing gastric malignancy. However, population studies with high gastric cancer prevalence rates may in the future provide indications for screening and eradication. The patient populations for whom eradication of *Helicobacter pylori* is indicated are set out in the Maastricht Consensus Report and it is within these groups of patients that *Helicobacter pylori* infection should be investigated. Dyspepsia is a very common complaint, which may be caused by a number of conditions, only some of which are unambiguously linked to colonization by *Helicobacter pylori*. Peptic ulcer disease can be cured by eradication of *Helicobacter pylori* but in non-ulcer dyspepsia the role of *Helicobacter pylori*, and hence its eradication, is more controversial. Currently, ulceration can only be diagnosed by endoscopy; however, as endoscopy is unpleasant and expensive there are four principal strategies for managing patients with dyspepsia:

1. Empirical treatment with eradication therapy
2. Endoscopy and eradication if colonization is confirmed
3. Testing for colonization by non-invasive screening and treating if colonization is confirmed—the 'test and treat' intervention (TTI) approach
4. Testing for colonization with non-invasive screening and followed by endoscopy and subsequent treatment if indicated

These approaches are conditional upon the age of the patient, where the consultation is taking place, and the clinical group to which the patient belongs. Patients with alarm symptoms (weight loss, bleeding, anaemia) of any age and patients aged >55 y, irrespective of the presence of alarm symptoms, should be offered upper gastrointestinal endoscopy. Most patients with dyspepsia are managed in the community by primary care physicians and the commonest approach is the 'test and treat' approach. The only disadvantage of the TTI approach is that a definitive diagnosis of ulceration as opposed to non-ulcer dyspepsia cannot be made, although a proportion of patients with non-ulcer dyspepsia do improve after eradication of *Helicobacter pylori*. The recommended non-invasive tests with the highest accuracy are the urea breath test and the faecal antigen test (**5.1**). The most significant findings were of a reduction in the number of endoscopies, and of a cost saving: £160 for the 'test and treat' approach compared with £400 for the endoscopy strategy. Endoscopies had a marginal advantage in the older patient, but even here there was a definite cost saving. Further recommendations of the Maastricht III guidelines were that a 'test and treat' strategy was optimal in all adult patients with functional dyspepsia in areas of high *Helicobacter* prevalence, but its efficacy was less in low *Helicobacter* prevalence areas—an option here was empirical acid suppression. Endoscopy has also been used as a follow-up procedure for patients with gastric ulcer.

In recent years, there has been increasing interest in the goal of endoscopic *in vivo* histology using narrow-band imaging, chromoendoscopy and confocal laser endomicroscopy. In chromo- and microendoscopy, the mucosal surface and subsurface can be examined in detail for the presence of characteristic pathological features and the detection of *Helicobacter pylori*. Narrow-band imaging endoscopy is based upon the principle of splitting white light into red, green and blue components by narrow-band filters (thus preventing wavelength overlap), with each wavelength being reflected from the mucosal surfaces at different depths. The integrated final image has the majority contribution from the blue part of the spectrum and reveals the surface microvasculature. Confocal laser endomicroscopy was developed by including a confocal laser microscope in the tip of a video endoscope. The diameter of the insertion tube is 12.8 mm, indicating a high degree of miniaturization. Images can be viewed at a resolution of 1024 pixels with a field of view of $500 \mu m^2$ and at a depth of $250 \mu m$. A contrast agent (either acriflavin or fluorescein) has to be used to see the cellular details. Fluorescein (given intravenously) does not stain nuclei, whereas acriflavin (a topical agent) does; the latter is thus useful for determining nuclear abnormalities and has been used in combination with fluorescein to detect the presence of *Helicobacter pylori* on the mucosal surface. The endoscopic appearance of the normal stomach is of a regular arrangement of epithelial cells, gastric pits and the subepithelial capillaries, giving a honeycomb appearance. In *Helicobacter pylori* gastritis, the collecting venuoles cannot be seen or the gastric pits are enlarged with surrounding erythema and the normal capillary network is lost. In atrophic gastritis, both the gastric pits and capillary network are lost. In gastric cancer, there is loss of the capillary network, irregular branched tubules and loss of polarity and pleomorphism of the nuclei (**5.2**).

Several conditions are characterized by prominent mucosal folds, which can be seen by endoscopy. In lymphocytic gastritis, thought to be an unusual reaction to *Helicobacter* and also found in coeliac disease, the surface mucosa can appear normal although a typical appearance is varioliform, having prominent rugal folds carrying nodular elevations with white erosions at the apex and surrounded by a hyperaemic margin. In Ménétrier's disease, there are also prominent folds, which, on endosonography, reveal hyperplasia of the deep mucosa. The regularity of the epithelial cells, arrangement of the gastric pits and nuclear morphology can thus all be used to make a real-time pathological diagnosis. Additionally, this advance in endoscopic technique opens the way for the development of real-time *in vivo* sensitivity testing. Endoscopists should, of course, should be specially trained in gastric histopathology. A shortcoming of these endomicroscopic techniques is the inability to view very far below the mucosal surface. In addition, endoscopy provides biopsy specimens that can be used in different diagnostic tests such as culture, histology, rapid urease test and polymerase chain reaction (PCR).

Histology

Histology can reveal the presence of bacteria as well as the grading of gastritis and presence of cancer. Many

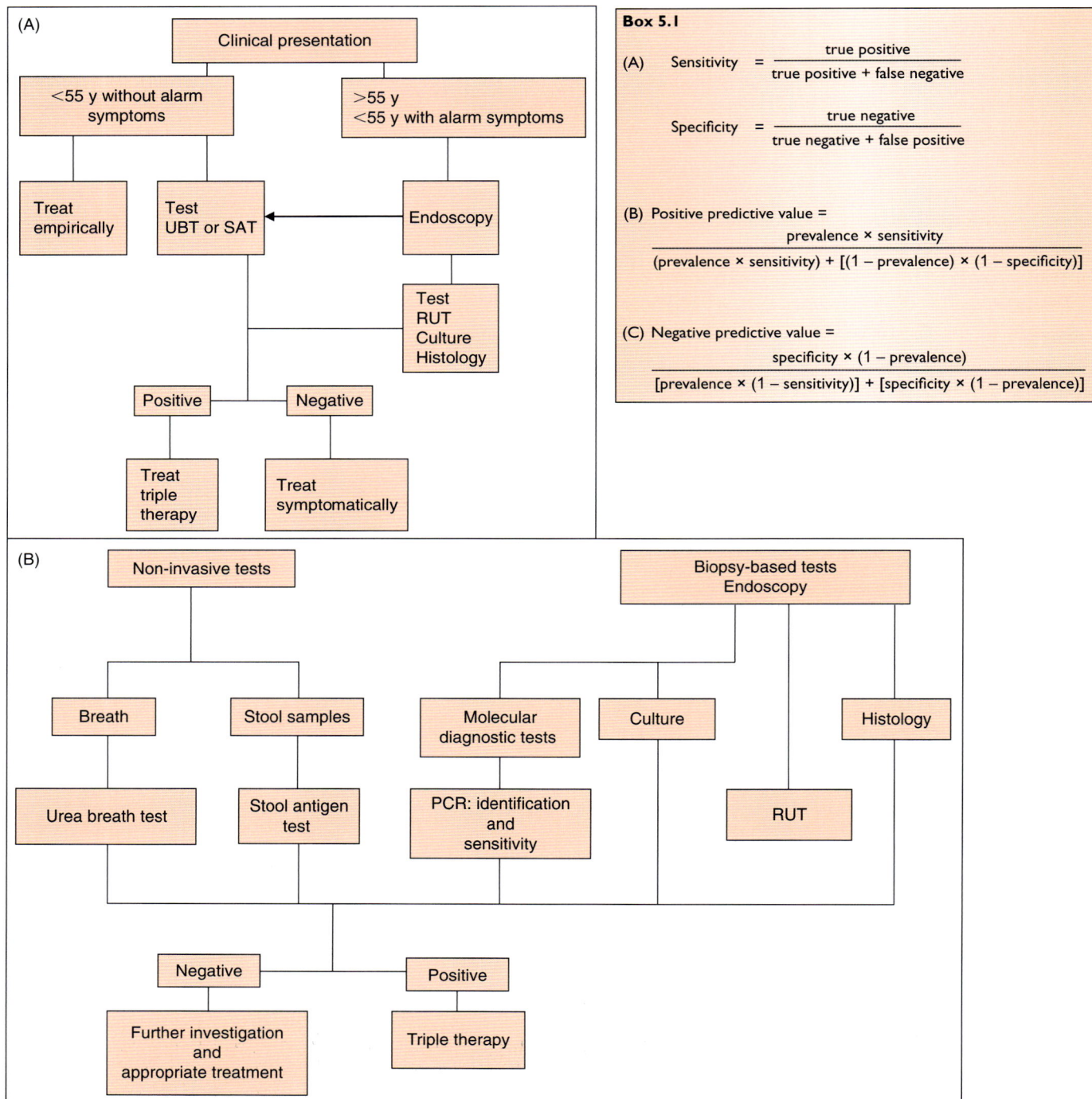

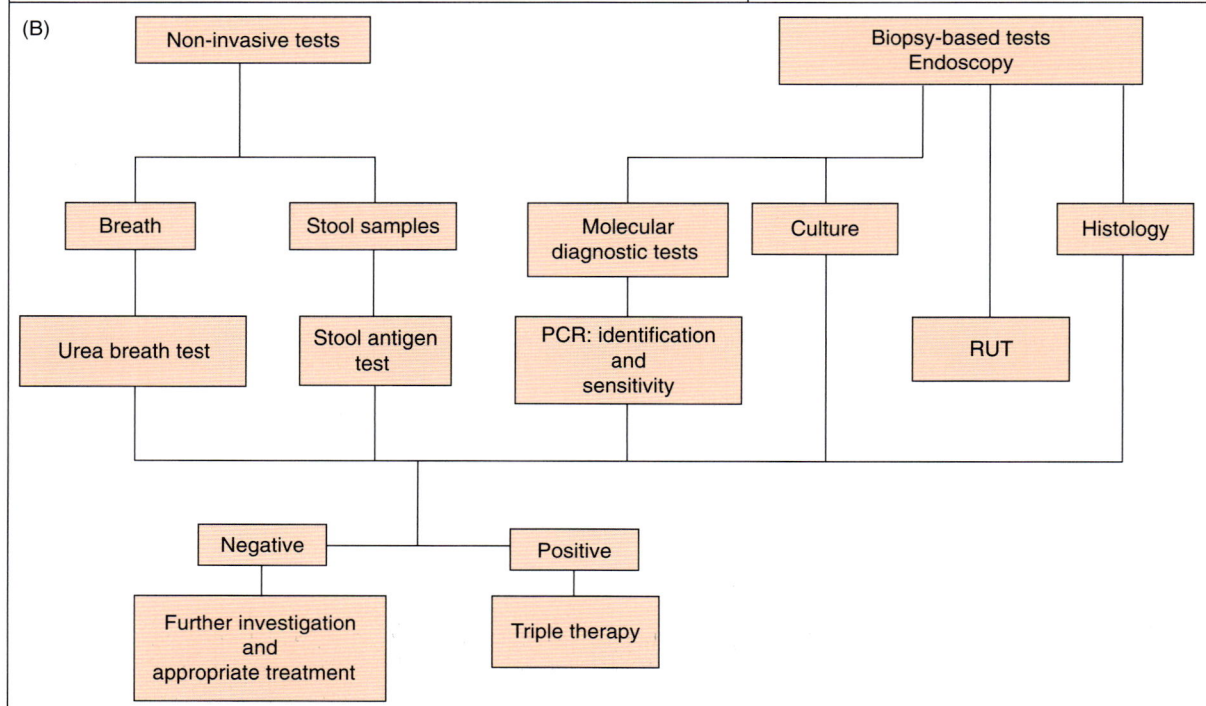

5.1 Management algorithm for dyspepsia (A). Choosing diagnostic test to confirm Helicobacter pylori (B). PCR = polymerase chain reaction; RUT = rapid urease test; SAT = stool antigen test; UBT = urea breath test.

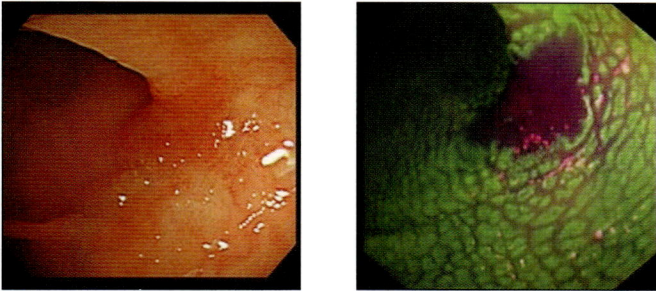

5.2 Abnormal lesions in narrow-band endoscopy.

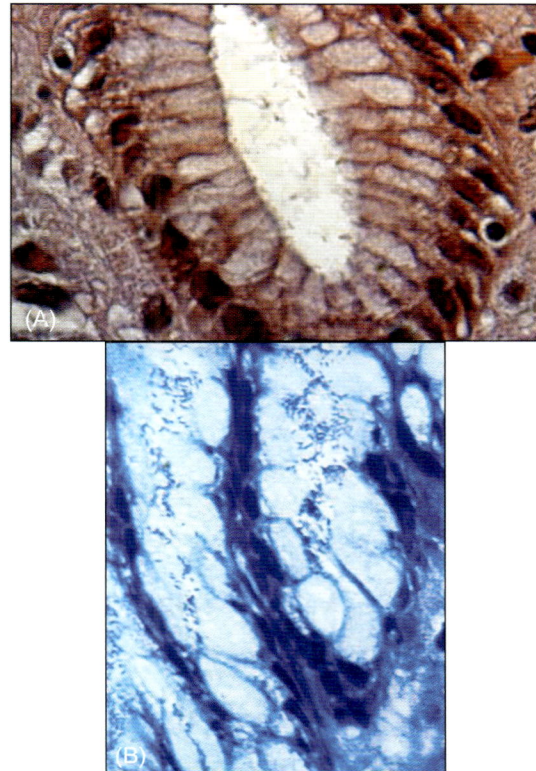

5.3 (A) Haematoxylin and eosin stain showing morphology of stomach section. (B) Giemsa stain showing *Helicobacter*.

staining techniques have been used to detect *Helicobacter pylori*, e.g., Warthin–Starry silver stain, Dieterle, Giemsa, Gimenez, acridine orange, McMullen and immunostaining. Generally, specificity is high due to the organism's peculiar morphology and its close relation to gastric mucosa.

Current guidelines suggest that at least two stains are used: haematoxylin and eosin (**5.3A**), to evaluate the inflammatory cells; and Giemsa (**5.3B**) or Genta stains for detecting *Helicobacter pylori*. The Genta stain has the advantage of visualizing both the inflammatory cells and *Helicobacter pylori* by combining a silver stain, haematoxylin and eosin, and alcian blue, although it is technically complex and in its original formulation uses uranyl nitrate. Overall, the Giemsa stain is the preferred stain for detecting *Helicobacter pylori* because of its technical simplicity, high sensitivity and low cost. Despite the high sensitivity of histology, the site, number and size of the biopsy will affect diagnostic accuracy. Patchy colonization can also result in misdiagnosis. Investigators should be aware that although a single biopsy taken in the lesser curve, close to the angulus, can detect *Helicobacter pylori* presence in more than 90% of patients, it is possible to increase accuracy with multiple biopsies from the greater curve and corpus.

The histological appearance of gastritis uses the updated Sydney system (**5.4**). The Sydney system combines aetiology, morphology, topography and histology into a scoring system that has a visual analogue scale; semiquantitative scoring of mild, moderate and marked can score the density of *Helicobacter pylori*, granulocyte infiltration (acute gastritis), mononuclear cell infiltration (chronic gastritis), atrophy and intestinal metaplasia. Other than provision of the visual analogue scale, the main difference in the updated system from the original Sydney system is a greater emphasis on

atrophic gastritis. In acute gastritis, there is a marked infiltration of the lamina propria with granulocytes, which in chronic gastritis becomes a predominant mononuclear infiltration. In atrophic gastritis, there is loss of gastric glandular tissue, fibrosis and appearance of an intestinal-type epithelium. A further development in the staging of gastritis is the development of an Operative Link for Gastritis Assessment (OLGA), which grades gastritis according to an increased risk of developing gastric cancer.

In a histological section, *Helicobacter pylori* is recognized by its appearance as a short curved or spiral bacillus resting on the epithelial surface or in the mucus layer. The organism is also found deep in the gastric pits. Other *Helicobacter* spp., such as *H. heilmannii* or *H. bizzozeroni* are also detected in the human stomach. *Helicobacter heilmannii* is prevalent in about 0.1% of gastric biopsies. Its appearance differs from that of *Helicobacter pylori*, as it is longer with tight spirals giving it a corkscrew shape. Gastritis associated with *Helicobacter heilmannii* has a characteristic histology of

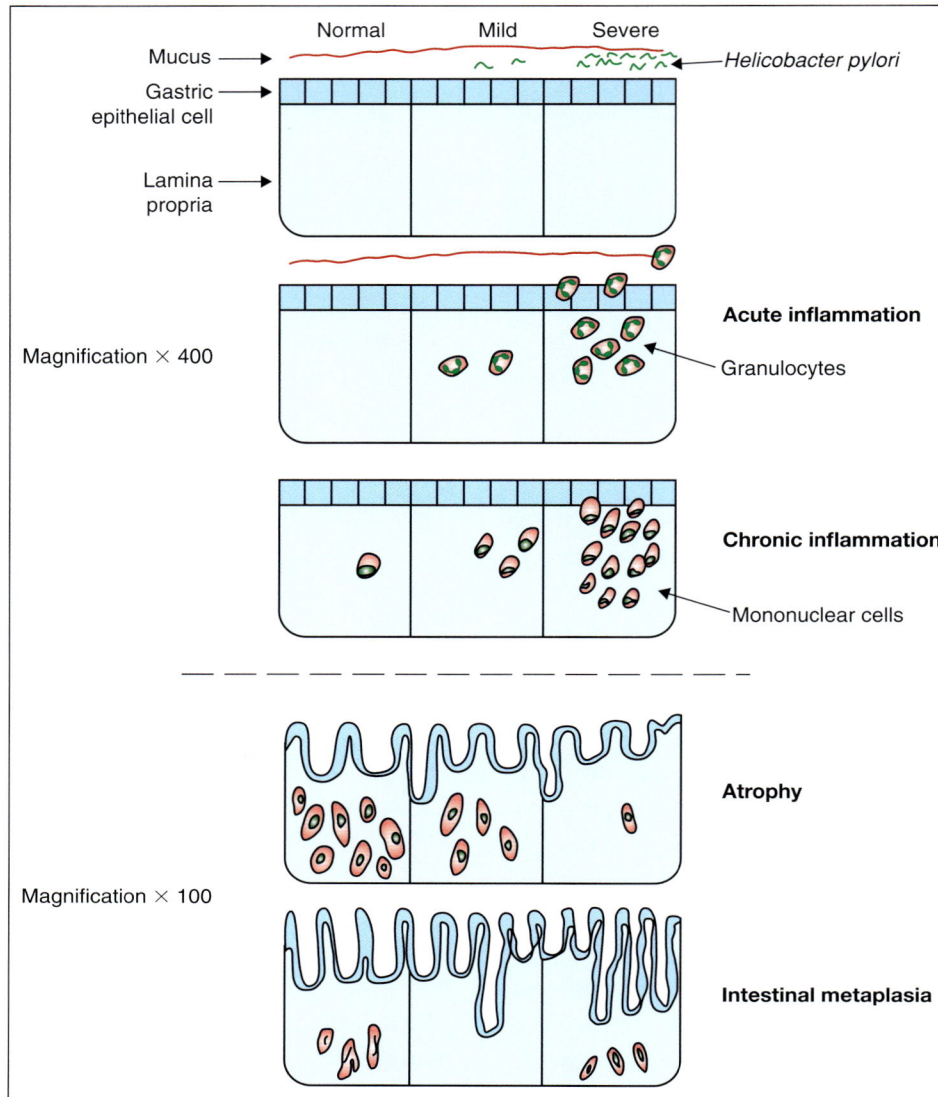

5.4 Sydney system for the classification of gastritis.

lymphocyte infiltration into gastric foveolae with lack of mucus depletion.

Helicobacter heilmannii is similar to *Helicobacter bizzozeroni*, but distinguishable from *Helicobacter pylori*, and can be clearly recognized in histological sections. *Helicobacter heilmannii* is a zoonotic infection in humans, derived from cats or dogs, and can give rise to chronic gastritis and possible mucosal-associated lymphoid tissue lymphoma. The sensitivity and specificity of histology for the diagnosis of *Helicobacter pylori* varies from 53% to 90%, which in part depends upon clinical setting, density of colonization and experience of the histopathologist. In general, a histological diagnosis can be made in about 90% of cases. Although the average time

for a histological diagnosis is just 2–3 days, as multiple biopsies are taken this will increase the processing costs of the biopsies and overall cost of the diagnosis. Further, prior treatment to reduce the numbers of *Helicobacter pylori* will adversely affect the sensitivity of histology.

In addition to the typical appearance of acute or chronic gastritis associated with *Helicobacter pylori* or non-pylori *Helicobacter,* other forms of gastritis are also associated with *Helicobacter* infection, such as lymphocytic gastritis and Ménétrier's gastritis.

Lymphocytic gastritis
Lymphocytic gastritis is characterized by the accumulation of small lymphocytes in the surface and

foveolae epithelium. A value of >25 intraepithelial lymphocytes per 100 epithelial cells is the diagnostic criterion. It is present in about 1% of unselected endoscopies and about 4% of patients with chronic gastritis. The histological appearance correlates well with the endomicroscopic appearance of varioliform gastritis.

Ménétrier's gastritis

In Ménétrier's gastritis—thought to be associated with *Helicobacter pylori*—there is a hyperplastic epithelium with elongated, dilated and tortuous gastric glands penetrating the muscularis mucosae, cyst formation, and oedematous lamina propria with an inflammatory cell infiltrate when in the presence of *Helicobacter pylori*.

Mucosal-associated lymphoid tissue lymphomas

Mucosal-associated lymphoid tissue lymphomas, the majority of which are B cell in origin, have been defined as infiltrates of centrocytoid cells with the appearance of plasma cells, destroying the foveolae or gastric glands. The lymphomatous cells infiltrate all layers of the stomach. In low-grade lymphomas architecture is maintained, and cell lineage spans the histological range from small lymphocytes to centrocyte-like cells and monocytic-like B cells.

Culture

Helicobacter can be cultured from gastric biopsies. Although reported to be difficult, *Helicobacter* grows very well on 5% horse blood Columbia agar and its isolation is quite easy (**5.5**). *Helicobacter pylori* soon loses viability when exposed to the environment and biopsies should be cultured quickly to maximize the recovery of bacteria. A study of three transport media using laboratory adapted strains showed that Stuart's medium (a standard bacteriological transport medium) did not support viability, but the organism could be recovered after 10 days from brain–heart infusion medium (containing brain–heart infusion broth, 0.5% agar and 7% horse blood) whether kept at 4°C or room temperature. However, *Helicobacter pylori* was recoverable from biopsy material stored in Stuart's transport medium for 24 h at 4°C with the same frequency as when the biopsy was processed within 2 h. A comparison of Stuart's transport medium with isotonic saline and urea-containing isotonic saline showed increased recovery from Stuart's transport medium compared with isotonic saline, with

a greater loss of viability if urea was present. Longer periods of viability were possible with a temperature of 4°C. Above 15°C, viability was poor after 6 h. The use of Stuart's transport medium gives good recovery of *Helicobacter pylori* for up to 48 h if the storage is between 4°C and 15°C.

Provided certain precautions are taken to ensure rapid processing of the biopsy, the yield of positive cultures can be high. The agar plates are incubated in a micro-aerobic environment obtained by using a jar with a gas-generating kit for a microaerobic atmosphere (5% oxygen and 5–10% carbon dioxide). The plates are incubated for at least 5 days at 37°C, even if *Helicobacter* colonies appear after just 3 days, as sometimes happens.

Helicobacter pylori was first isolated from biopsies using chocolate agar and, subsequently, several selective and differential media have been proposed (*see also* p. 12). The media are usually, but not exclusively, based upon either Columbia or brain–heart infusion agar (BHIA) base containing either, blood or blood products, or an additive such as starch, charcoal, cyclodextrin or bovine serum albumin, thought to act like a serum and to inactivate toxic metabolites in the medium. Selectivity is provided by the addition of different combinations of antibiotics. Addition of triphenylterazolium chloride to the media imparts a characteristic golden sheen to the *Helicobacter pylori* colonies. L-lactic acid seems to be a specific growth factor for the organism.

The ideal method of comparison of solid media is probably the relative bacterial covered area, where not

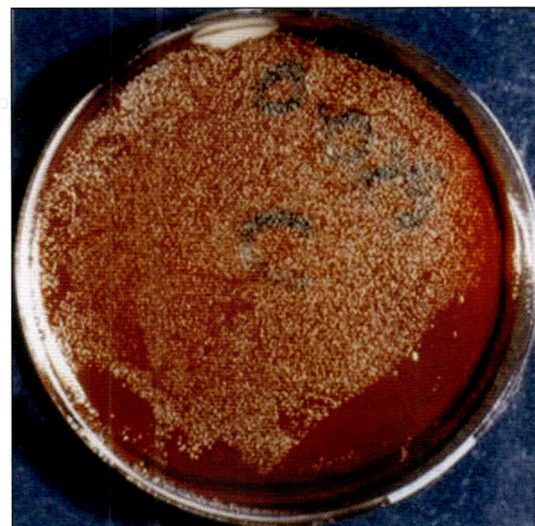

5.5 Culture of *Helicobacter pylori* from a biopsy specimen.

only the number of colonies produced by comparable bacterial dilutions, but also the size of the colonies is taken into account, and the area of the plate covered by bacterial growth calculated using a simple mathematical formula. All values are expressed as a percentage of the maximal value produced by any one medium under test. One such study compared Skirrow's medium with a charcoal agar-based medium containing 10% horse blood—the latter was modified by, for example, the addition of antibiotics or Isovitalex, or substitution of the blood by 10% serum or egg yolk emulsion. In this study, the medium supporting the most luxuriant growth at both 3 and 5 days was the charcoal agar base supplemented with 10% horse blood, 1% Isovitalex and an antibiotic cocktail. In a similar comparison of some of the more commonly used media, egg yolk emulsion agar (EYA) was demonstrated as the best after 7 days incubation. The discrepancy between these two studies regarding the efficacy of EYA probably relates to the addition of Isovitalex in the original description of the medium. Comparison of the isolation of *Helicobacter pylori* from biopsies rather than laboratory-adapted isolates, demonstrated BHIA with 7% lysed horse blood to be more effective than either tryptone soy agar, EYA or Columbia agar base with cyclodextrin.

The clinical relevance of isolating *Helicobacter pylori* from any specimen other than the stomach is unknown, except that detecting it in oral or faecal specimens does suggest that it may also be present in the stomach. This is a topic that requires further study because of the ease of collecting these specimens and their potential utility in diagnosis. Modification of a standard non-selective media for isolation of *Helicobacter pylori* from the stomach (Columbia agar base + 5% horse blood + 1% Isovitalex) by the addition of vancomycin (100 mg/l), colistin (2500 iu/l), amphotericin (12 mg/l) and cefsulodin (5 mg/l) does support the growth of *Helicobacter pylori*; they also inhibit most of the oropharyngeal flora and may prove useful for culturing *Helicobacter pylori* from oral specimens. Techniques for the isolation of *Helicobacter pylori* from faeces have been developed. One such technique is the preparation of a faecal slurry in phosphate buffer, separation of faecal material by sieving, concentration of a bacterial pellet by centrifugation and plating on Dent and McNulty's selective medium. Using this technique, *Helicobacter pylori* have been isolated from 18 of 36 (50%) volunteers.

Cholestyramine treatment of faeces appears to increase the isolation of *Helicobacter pylori*.

Helicobacter pylori has been isolated from a blood culture of a patient on one occasion as an incidental finding rather than being deliberately sought. This lack of isolation may be partly due to the inability of *Helicobacter pylori* to grow in several conventional blood culture media (e.g. SeptiCheck). However, comparisons using three other commercial blood culture media— Brucella broth, biphasic brain–heart infusion broth and supplemented peptone broth—all supported the growth of *Helicobacter pylori*. Culture of *Helicobacter pylori* might be clinically relevant, for example, in cases of pyrexia of unknown origin in immunocompromised patients or patients in intensive care, pyrexia following gastroduodenoscopy, or in patients with gastric cancer. Finally, *Helicobacter pylori* has been isolated from the peritoneum in a case of peritonitis, and from a tracheal aspirate in a respiratory infection case.

Colonies are identified by Gram staining and biochemical tests: *Helicobacter pylori* are Gram-negative and positive for urease, oxidase and catalase. Although culture has a high specificity (100%), the sensitivity can be lowered by: an insufficient number of biopsies being taken; delays in transport to the laboratory; exposure to an aerobic environment; and microbiologists' inexperience in recognizing the colonies. Moreover, antibiotics, proton pump inhibitors and H_2 receptor antagonists must not taken in the preceding two weeks as these also reduce the sensitivity of culture.

Culture is typically done to determine antibiotic sensitivities, and often only in research centres particularly dedicated to *Helicobacter pylori* infection. As the prevalence of antibiotic resistance increases globally there is a strong argument for performing culture and sensitivity testing after the first treatment failure (to prevent emergence of double resistance to clarithromycin and metronidazole) and certainly after the second; indeed, some would argue that it should be performed at the initial diagnosis in areas of high resistance prevalence. Moreover, it has to be emphasized that susceptibility to a full range of antibiotics can only be tested on cultures. When testing for antibiotic sensitivity on a routine basis, the two most used tests are disc diffusion and the epsilometer test (E-test), with the agar dilution test as the reference (**5.6**). For clarithromycin and amoxicillin there is a good correlation between the E-test and agar dilution, but for metronidazole the E-test tended to give higher minimum inhibitory concentrations compared with the reference method or the disc test. An additional important reason that *Helicobacter pylori* should be cultured is for research purposes, such as correlating specific virulence characteristics with different clinical outcomes, and investigation of the molecular events after binding of the organism to gastric epithelial cells.

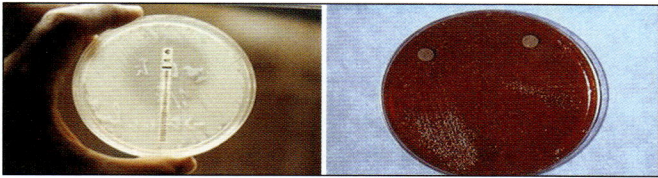

5.6 E-test and disc diffusion tests.

Rapid urease test

This gastric biopsy test (**5.7**) is based on the activity of the *Helicobacter pylori* urease enzyme (*see* Chapter 4), which splits the urea test reagent to form ammonia. Ammonia increases pH, which is detected by the indicator phenol red. Although some of the commensal flora of the oropharynx produce urease that is swallowed in the saliva, this weaker enzyme is denatured rapidly in the acid lumen of the stomach, where pH <2.0.

Many different commercial rapid urease tests are available, including ones that are gel-based (CLOtest, HpFast), paper-based (PyloriTek, ProntoDry HpOne) and liquid-based (CPtest, Endosc Hp). The tests produce results after 1 h or up to 24 h depending in part on the format of the test and the number of *Helicobacter* in the biopsy specimen. In some tests, such as PyloriTek, the suggested advantage is the built-in positive and negative control with each test strip and the fact that results are obtained within an hour, whereas some can take 24 h. A more rapid (1 min) urease test (HUT A1) is also now available. Unbuffered tests can give results in <1 h (e.g. CPtest) and these liquid tests can be performed cheaply in-house by preparing a solution of urea, adding phenol red and adjusting the pH to 6.6. At pH 6.6 the indicator is yellow and, on addition of a positive biopsy sample, will convert the solution to a red colour. One disadvantage of in-house tests, apart from quality control, is a short shelf-life. All the commercial rapid urease tests have specificities of 95–100% but the

sensitivity is slightly less at 85–95% (*see also* discussion on pp. 95–6). In comparison with histology, culture or PCR, the urease tests are more rapid and much cheaper with comparable sensitivity and specificity, except for culture, which has 100% specificity.

The sensitivity is affected mainly by the number of bacteria present in the biopsy. It has been calculated

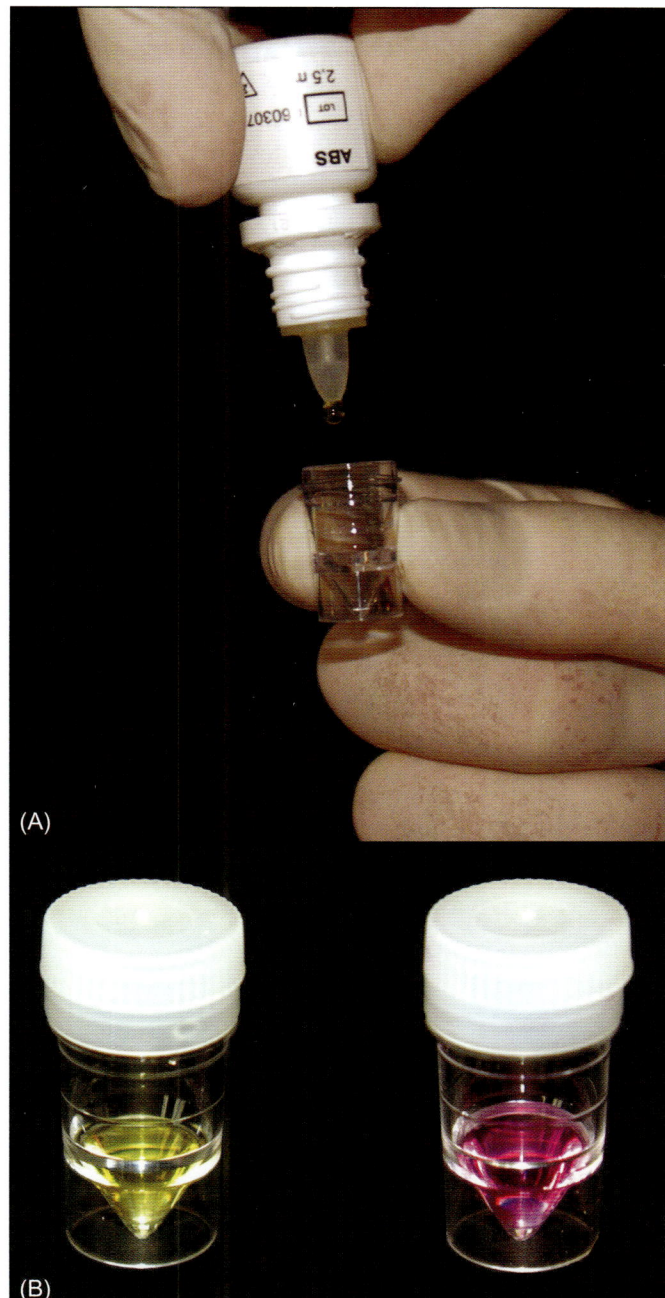

5.7 Rapid urease biopsy test. (A) Addition of reagent to biopsy. (B) Negative (left) and positive (right) test.

that approx. 1×10^4 organisms are required for a positive result, and a proportion of patients can harbour densities lower than this. Low sensitivity and specificity are also reported in post-treatment and in bleeding patients—for these reasons their use is not advised in these clinical settings.

False-negative urease tests can also occur in patients with achlorhydria and in patients on proton pump inhibitors, because the increased luminal pH can lead to extremely high pH adjacent to the organism, enough that *Helicobacter pylori* is destroyed by the action of its own urease. In addition, proton pump inhibitors have an anti-urease and antimicrobial activity, which may reduce the bacterial density to under the threshold level of detection.

Molecular tests

Two molecular tests that are available are *in situ* hybridization and PCR.

Mechanics of the polymerase chain reaction (5.8)

Within any organism there are DNA nucleotide sequences that are unique for any particular species. In a specimen, low numbers of bacteria can be detected by amplifying the specific nucleotide sequence to a sufficient number to allow presence of the organism to be detected. This amplification process requires the presence of DNA from the target organism in the specimen. To this are added the four DNA nucleotides (G-C-A-T) along with DNA polymerase and two DNA primers, i.e., two sequences that are complementary to a specific region of the target organism. By manipulation of the physical conditions in the reaction mixture in repeated cycles, a series of chemical reactions occur that massively amplify the amount of the target sequence. The amplified DNA sequence strand can then be detected by electrophoresis and staining of the gel with ethidium bromide, or by colorimetric detection using biotinylated PCR probes and horseradish peroxidase-labelled streptavidin followed by

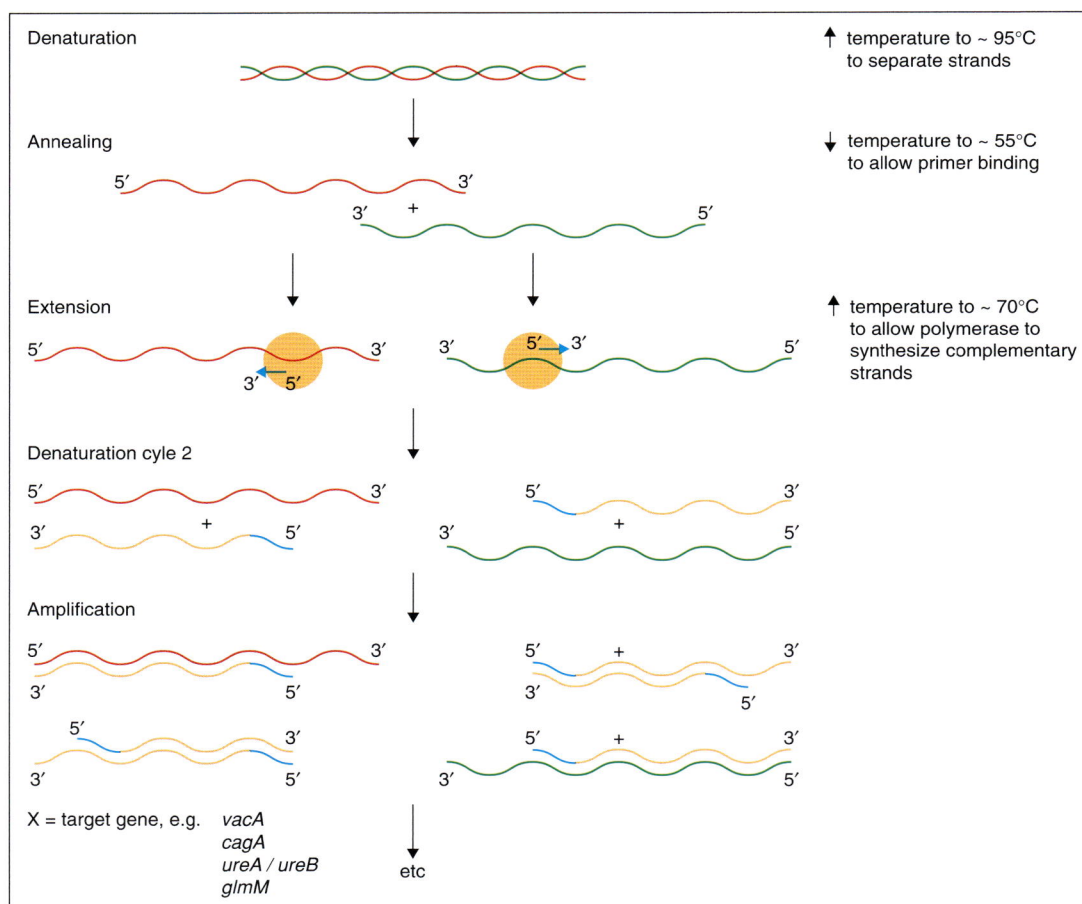

5.8 The basic mechanics of the polymerase chain reaction.

a chromogenic or chemiluminescent substrate. More rapid detection and quantification of the DNA can be obtained by using a reporter probe carrying a reporter molecule and quencher fluorophore. Once the probe is bound to the DNA, the DNA polymerase synthesizes a complementary strand on the target and in so doing displaces the fluorescent reporter molecule, which can be quantified. An isothermal helicase-dependent DNA amplification method has also been used to detect *Helicobacter pylori*.

In situ hybridization and PCR have both been used to detect the presence of *Helicobacter pylori* or the presence of specific virulence markers in archival specimens, but have more often been used to detect clarithromycin resistance. The sensitivity and specificity for the diagnosis of *Helicobacter pylori* infection, using *in situ* hybridization with biotinylated probes, or PCR, has been reported at 95% and 100%.

PCR yields information on the presence of the organism as well as potential virulence markers present in the strain, which may have implications for the development of severe disease or efficacy of eradication. A number of different primers have been used and some have been developed into commercial kits (*Table 5.1*). Different loci have been used as targets for amplification: 16S rRNA, *ureA*, *-B*, *-C*, *flaA*, *cagA*, *vacA* and heat shock protein. Real-time results can be obtained using LightCycler technology, where the PCR reaction takes place within a sealed glass ampoule in which the accumulation of amplified duplex DNA is continuously measured by fluorophor emission (SYBR Green, Applied Biosystems, UK). The use of a LightCycler can significantly shorten the time for a result to be obtained.

PCR detection in faeces is less generally used, partly because there are cheaper, technically easier and more reliable tests available, particularly as some faeces are replete with inhibitors of the PCR reaction. PCR has also been used to test the chemosusceptibility of *Helicobacter* to clarithromycin (used in the standard eradication regimen), because resistance to clarithromycin is caused by point mutations (A-G transition) in 23S rRNA. It is more difficult to detect multiple mutations, but they can be detected with a line probe assay using biotinylated probes for the different mutations, or after amplification with a preferential homoduplex formation assay.

The disadvantages of PCR as a routine test are that it is both technically demanding and an expensive test when compared with culture, histology and rapid urease tests. It requires special laboratory conditions with separate areas for each stage of the technique and, as it is highly sensitive, it is subject to false-positive results by contamination. Any of the molecular techniques will not only give an indication of current active infection but will also detect the DNA of dead organisms.

Although currently a research tool, microarrays may in the future be used diagnostically for *Helicobacter pylori*. These tests are not generally used in routine diagnosis but are more likely to be used in research studies.

Non-invasive tests

Non-invasive tests comprise serology (antibody or antigen detection) and breath analysis (urea breath test). These tests can be either direct or indirect. Direct tests detect the presence of *Helicobacter pylori* (i.e., provide evidence of a current infection). Antigen detection tests in the faeces are direct tests and they detect the presence of bacterial antigens of *Helicobacter pylori* in stools; these antigens disappear when *Helicobacter pylori* infection is cured. The urea breath test is another direct test based on the detection of urease activity, which is demonstrated in individuals with active *Helicobacter pylori* infection. Indirect tests only provide evidence of exposure to *Helicobacter pylori* at some time and do not indicate whether the infection is currently active. These tests are based on the detection of antibodies to *Helicobacter pylori*.

Serological tests

There are three main formats for these tests: the commonest is the enzyme-linked immunosorbent assay (ELISA) test, which detects the totality of the immunoglobulin in a patient's serum and can detect any of the immunoglobulin isotypes. If the antibody response to specific antigens is important, a separate ELISA test has to be done for each antigen. This test is usually laboratory based as it requires an ELISA reader. Latex agglutination tests, which require only minimal equipment, can also detect any of the immunoglobulin isotypes, can be performed more rapidly than an ELISA test, and are commonly used for near-patient tests. The third type of test is based upon Western blotting, where the specific antigens are separated by gel electrophoresis,

Table 5.1 Some primer sequences for various markers of *Helicobacter pylori* and virulence markers: where available, names listed in literature are given. For discussion of *vacA* regions see Chapter 1 (p.13).

Locus	Gene region	Forward sequence (name)	Reverse sequence (name)	Size (bp)
16S rRNA		GCGACCTGCTGGACCATTAC	CGTTAGCTGCATTACTGGAGA	139
1.9kDa cloned fragment		CATCTTGTTAGAGGGATTGG	TAACAAACCGATAATGGCGC	203
Species-specific antigen		TGGCGTGTCTATTGACAGCGAGC	CCTGCTGGGCATACTTCACCATG	298
ureA		GCCAATGGTAAATTAGTT	CTCCTTAATTGTTTTAC	411
ureB		TGGGATTAGCGAGTATGT	CCCATTTGACTCAATG	132
		AATTGCAGAAATATCAC	ACTTTATTGGCTGGTTT	115
glmM		AAGTTTTAGGGGTGTTAGGGGTTT	AAGCTTACTTTCTAACACTAACGC	293
		CTTTCTTCTCCAAGCAATTGTC	CAAGCCATCGCCGGTTTTAGC	252
cagA		TTGGACCAACAACCACAAACCGAAG	CTTCCCTTAATTGCGAGATTCC	183
		AATACACCAACGCCTCCAAG	TTGTTGCCGCTTTTGCTCTC	396
		GGAATTGTCTGATAAACTTG	CCATTATTGTTATTGTTATTG	612–615
		GGAACCCTAGTCGGTAATG	ATCTTTGAGCTTGTCTATCG	450–558
vacA	s1/s2	ATGGAAATACAACAAACACAC (VA1F)	CTGCTTGAATGCGCCAAAC (VA1R)	259/286
	s1a	GTCAGCATCACACCGCAAC	(VA1R)	190
	s1b	AGCGCCATACCGCAAAATGATCC	(VAIR)	187
	s2	GCTAACACGCCAAATGATCC	(VA1R)	192
	m1	GGTCAAAATGCGGTCATGG (VA3F)	CCATTGGTACCTGTAGAAAC (VA3R)	290
	m2	GGAGCCCCAGGAAACATTG (VA4F)	CATAACTAGCGCCTTGCAC (VA4R)	352
	s1/s2	GAAATACAACAAACACACCGC (VAC1F)	GGCTTGTTTGAGCCCCCAG (VAC1R)	201/228
	m1	(VA3F)	CATCAGTATTTCGCACCACA (VAC3R)	388
	m2	CCAGGACCAATTGCCGGCAAA (VAC4F)	(VA4R)	346

transferred to nitrocellulose paper and then exposed to the patient serum sample. These immunoblots again detect all the immunoglobulin isotypes but have the advantage of detecting specific antigens in one assay (*Table 5.2*).

Since the appearance of the first serological tests for the diagnosis of *Helicobacter pylori* infection, these tests have become the most frequently used in routine practice because of their accuracy, low cost and for their availability. Serological tests are based on the detection of specific anti-*Helicobacter pylori* IgG antibodies in a patient's serum. Some tests also detect the presence of IgA in the saliva or IgG in the urine.

However, the sensitivity and specificity of the tests depends upon the antigen used, clinical context, gold standard comparator, as well as the prevalence of *Helicobacter pylori* in the community. Overall, the sensitivity has been reported (mostly for the ELISA-based format) as ranging between 90% and 97% and the specificity between 50% and 96%.

The most important disadvantage is that serological tests are not able to distinguish between active infection and previous exposure to *Helicobacter pylori*. Antibody levels can persist in the blood of individuals cured of *Helicobacter pylori* infection for long period of time. Therefore, as the numbers of patients successfully treated for *Helicobacter pylori* increase in a population, the prevalence of false-positive tests with serology increases. Thus, a positive serological test can mean:

1. The patient is infected at the time of the test.
2. The patient was once infected, but by the time of the test infection has resolved.
3. The patient is detecting non-specific cross-reacting antibodies.

CagA and VacA antibodies

CagA is a 120-kDa protein of *Helicobacter pylori* with high immunogenicity, and the *cagA* gene is found within the pathogenicity island (PAI) of the chromosome of *Helicobacter pylori*. The vacuolating toxin (VacA) is an 87 kDa protein not located in the *cag*PAI but secreted by *Helicobacter* strains that contain the *cag*PAI. Individuals infected with CagA/VacA-positive strains tend to have more severe gastritis, a higher likelihood of developing gastric atrophy and intestinal metaplasia, and a higher incidence of duodenal ulcer and intestinal-type gastric

cancer (*see* Chapters 3 and 4). Thus, specific serological assays have been developed to help assess the likelihood of more severe disease.

Although these tests are of limited value in the clinical setting, they have increased our understanding of the pathogenesis of disease caused by *Helicobacter pylori*. Antibodies against the *Helicobacter pylori*, CagA and VacA proteins can be detected using different immunological techniques. After eradication of *Helicobacter pylori*, the antibodies disappear at different times and some, such as anti-CagA antibodies, may persist for years. Although the antibody response to CagA can be detected using ELISA, immunoblots have a particular advantage in that they are more sensitive and, as discussed above, can provide evidence of immunological reactions to several antigens all at once, which may have clinical relevance.

Tests on saliva and urine

Tests on saliva and urine are attractive because samples can be easily obtained. They share the same sensitivity and specificity as other antibody tests in the serum. One disadvantage is that the concentration of the antibody being detected is lower than in serum, making detection more difficult. Individual centres have reported promising results (sensitivity 81%; specificity 95%). However, these data were not confirmed in a multicentre trial using the same urine assay kit, in which a sensitivity of 89% and specificity of 69% were reported.

Near-patient tests

Near-patient tests are technically simple to perform and the most convenient of them uses a drop of whole blood obtained by finger-prick. Other near-patient tests require serum, which involves venepuncture followed by centrifugation to separate the serum. The results of finger-prick tests can vary significantly when the flow of blood is poor and there is difficulty in obtaining a drop of blood. Squeezing the finger can express tissue fluid into the blood sample, thereby changing the concentration of the antibody sample being studied. Whole-blood tests are affected by circulating chylomicrons, which change the permeability of the blood sample to the various antigens through the various membranes used in diagnostic tests. Studies have reported a lower sensitivity and specificity than was originally suggested. The mean sensitivity was 71% and specificity 87%. A Canadian study of serology found that 33% of positive near-patient tests in

Table 5.2 Commonly available immunological tests for *Helicobacter pylori*

Test	Manufacturer
ELISA	
GAP™ IgA *H. pylori*	BioRad, USA
GAP™ IgG *H. pylori*	
GAP™ IgM *H. pylori*	
H. pylori-IgG	Biousa, USA
H. pylori-IgM	
Helori-Test	Eurospital, Italy
CagA IgG	Genesis Diagnostics, UK
H pylori IgA	
H pylori IgG	
H pylori IgM	
H. pylori IgA	Gold Standard Diagnostics, USA
H. pylori IgG	
H. pylori IgA	Hycor Biomedical, USA
H. pylori IgG	
H. pylori IgM	
Premier™ *H. pylori*	Meridian Biosciences, USA
Pyloriset® EIA A III	Orion Diagnostica, Finland
Pyloriset® EIA G III	
Helicobacter pylori Antigen EIA	Quest Diagnostics, USA
Immunochromatographic assay	
H. pylori Dipstick	Biousa, USA
H. pylori IgA Line immunoblot	Gold Standard Diagnostics, USA
H. pylori IgG Line immunoblot	
Immunocard STAT!® HpSA	Meridian Biosciences, USA
Immunocard® *H. pylori*	
QuickVue H. pylori gII®	Quidel Corporation, USA
Latex agglutination	
Pyloriset® Dry	Orion Diagnostica, Finland
Western blot	
HELICO BLOT 2.1	GeneLabs Diagnostics, USA

patients with dyspepsia in the primary care setting were false positives. The current near-patient tests are not recommended for diagnosis, as they are likely to have false-positive results if prevalence of the disease is low, even though the sensitivity may be high.

Active tests

These tests are useful for the initial detection of *Helicobacter pylori* and for confirming eradication.

Urea breath test

The urea breath test is one of the main methods for diagnosis (**5.9**). The breath test can be performed with either ^{13}C- or ^{14}C-labelled urea. *Helicobacter pylori* produces urease, an enzyme that splits urea into ammonia and carbon dioxide. The organism may use urease activity to regulate pH in its micro-environment (*see* Chapter 4). The urea breath test is based on the principle that urease activity is present in the stomach of individuals infected with *Helicobacter pylori*. Hydrolysis of urea occurs within the mucus layer and results in the production of labelled carbon dioxide. The carbon

dioxide diffuses into the epithelial blood vessels and, within a few minutes, it appears in the subject's breath.

The isotopic labelled urea is usually given to the patient with a test meal to delay gastric emptying and increase contact time with the mucosa. Some protocols, however, omit the test meal. After ingestion of the urea, breath samples are collected for up to 20 min by exhaling into a CO_2-trapping carbon dioxide trapping agent (hyamine). The urea breath test has a very high sensitivity and specificity, ranging from 95% to 97%; however, it may not be reliable in assessing patients who have had gastric surgery, or in patients who have been on proton pump inhibitors. The ^{13}C-urea breath test is similar to the ^{14}C-urea breath test, except that ^{13}C is a non-radioactive isotope of ^{12}C and its detection requires a mass spectrometer rather than a scintillation counter. An alternative detection method is infrared spectroscopy, which is technically simpler and also cheaper than a mass spectrometer. Because ^{13}C is a naturally occurring stable isotope, there are no nuclear regulatory concerns and the test can be used in children and pregnant woman. Since the initial report of this test, it has been extensively modified, including variations in dose-labelled urea, sampling time and test meal,

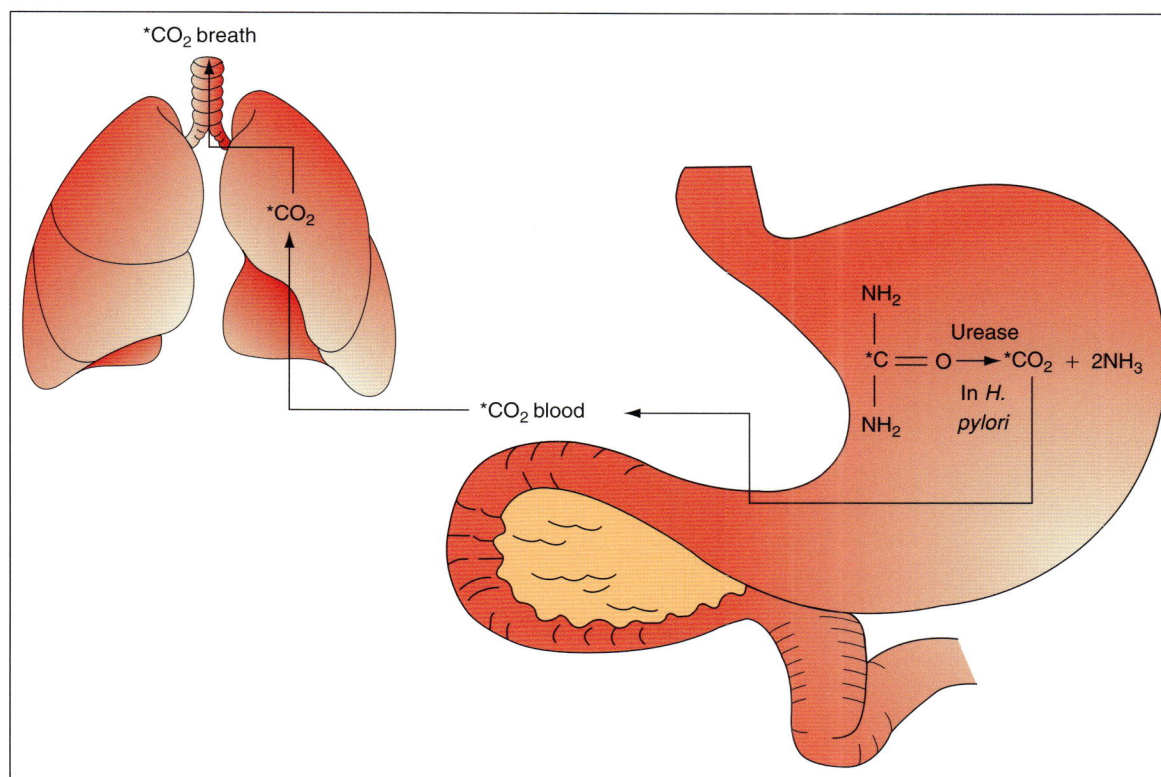

5.9 Urea breath test. The asterisk denotes the carbon isotope label.

and cut-off values. A rapid low-dose test, formulated as a tablet containing citric acid and 50 mg ^{13}C, was compared with the standard test (75 mg ^{13}C). The rapid test used to diagnose *Helicobacter pylori* and evaluate its clearance after eradication gave the same sensitivity and specificity as the standard test, i.e., 100%. Doses of ^{13}C as low as 10 or 15 mg also gave sensitivity and specificity of 89–96% and 100%, respectively, and the 15 mg dose was sufficiently accurate for assessing eradication.

Future urea-less test

A urea-less breath test based upon a quartz crystal microbalance has also been developed (5.10). A quartz crystal microbalance is a sensor that weighs volatile products partitioned on a coated vibrating quartz crystal. Specifically, seven quartz crystals, each coated with a different gas chromatographic stationary phase, and each selectively adsorbing different chemical groups, were used. The design of specific sensors that maximize all of the common types of chemical interactions would produce a general purpose, profiling array. The array instrument incorporated on-line data processing based upon principal components analysis, discriminant function analysis and Kohonen and Back-propagation networks. Preliminary work using this instrument could distinguish between *Helicobacter pylori*-colonized and non-colonized individuals with 70% sensitivity and specificity. Further work is needed to increase the sensitivity/specificity to that of the urea breath test but would be perfectly possible by temperature regulating the vibrating crystals and optimizing the stationary phases. There are several advantages in developing such an instrument: (a) the instrument itself is relatively affordable (approx. £2000, or $3100) (b) it does not need a urea test meal; (c) it gives a rapid yes/no answer, which could be used in near-patient testing; and (d) it could be applied to other conditions.

Stool antigen test

An enzymatic immunoassay that detects the presence of *Helicobacter pylori* antigen in stool specimens has recently become available. This assay has undergone extensive testing for use in initial diagnosis of *Helicobacter pylori* infection and for confirming eradication after treatment. Polyclonal antibody tests are the most widely used and have been extensively evaluated in the diagnosis of *Helicobacter pylori* infection before therapy. Most of the studies have suggested that the accuracy of this test is

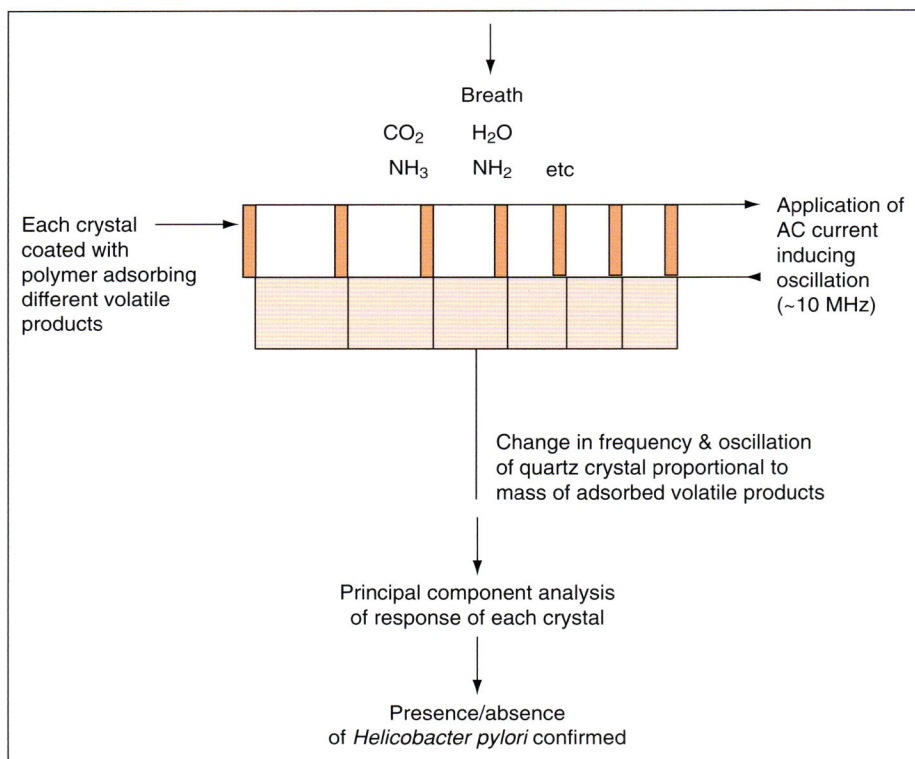

5.10 Detecting volatile products in breath using quartz crystal microbalance.

similar to that of the urea breath test for initial diagnosis of infection. The urea breath test and stool antigen test are equally accurate in confirming active infection and are recommended for diagnosis by both the National Institute for Health and Clinical Excellence (NICE) in the UK and in the EHSG Maastricht III Consensus Statement.

An immunochromatographic assay is also available for near-patient testing of the presence of *Helicobacter pylori* in faeces (**5.11**). Detection of antigens can be either in a well-based system (**5.11A–B**) or using an immunochromatographic membrane (**5.11C**). In the well-based system, if a binary enzyme is used, the reaction can be a one-step process, the functioning enzyme formed by antigen binding to both antibodies (**5.11A**). Alternatively, it can be performed as a three-step process with sequential addition of specimen, conjugated antibody and substrate (**5.11B**). The current test uses a monoclonal antibody compared with polyclonal antibody and is superior both for the initial diagnosis of *Helicobacter pylori* and for confirmation of its eradication after treatment. A positive stool test 7 days after completion of treatment is predictive for failed eradication.

A new rapid monoclonal one-step lateral flow immunoassay stool test has recently been released, requiring only 5 min to be performed. Faeces is placed in a diluent vial and then a drop of the liquid is placed in the well of the test. Early results are promising, with a sensitivity and specificity of 92%. This test may be useful as a near-patient test in primary care settings. It has a particular advantage in needle-phobic patients and children (who are generally averse to venepuncture). In principle, the test can be amended to pick out specific proteins such as CagA and VacA, which may be used to determine the virulence type of the infecting strain.

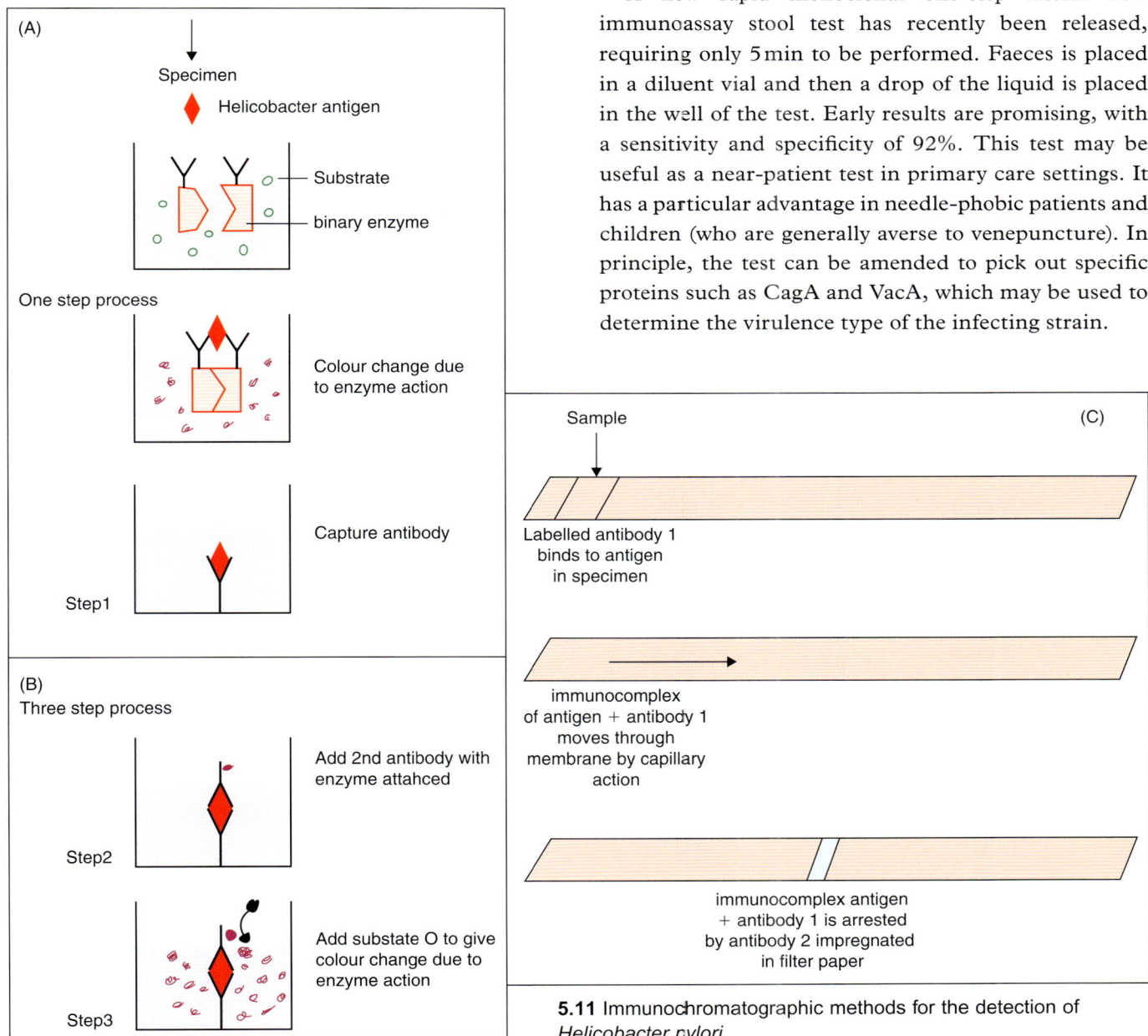

5.11 Immunochromatographic methods for the detection of *Helicobacter pylori*.

Cost-effectiveness and strategies based on pre-test probability of infection

The choice of an initial test for *Helicobacter pylori* detection depends on the prevalence of *H. pylori* infection and the value placed on increased diagnostic accuracy. A recent cost analysis evaluated the single test and sequential testing strategy costs in the US healthcare system. The serology test had the lowest cost at $90–$95 per correct diagnosis at low (30%), intermediate (60%) and high (90%) prevalence; but, its diagnostic accuracy was low at just 80–84%. At low and intermediate prevalence, the stool test was more accurate (93%), with an average cost of $126 per correct diagnosis and an incremental cost of $336–$381 per additional correct diagnosis. ELISA testing was preferable when prevalence rates were very high (90%), and using a confirmatory urea breath test for a negative ELISA test increased the diagnostic accuracy to 96% with modest incremental costs. If the cost of the breath test was less than $50, or if the cost of the stool test was greater than $82, breath testing became preferable to stool testing. In patients who have a less than 60% pre-test probability of infection, as is the case in dyspeptic patients in much of the Western world, the stool test provides increased accuracy with modest incremental costs.

Further reading

Anon. DNA microarray methodology Flash animation. http://www.bio.davidson.edu/Courses/genomics/chip/chipQ.html [Accessed Nov 2011] (An introductory animation to microarrays.)

Kawai T, Kawakami K, Kataoka M, *et al*. A study of the relationship between *Helicobacter pylori* microbial susceptibility, ^{13}C urea breath test values. *Hepatogastroenterology* 2008; 55: 786–90.

Krausse R, Müller G, Doniec M. Evaluation of a rapid new stool antigen test for diagnosis of *Helicobacter pylori* infection in adult patients. *J Clin Microbiol* 2008; 46: 2062–5.

Leodolter A, Vaira D, Bazzoli F, *et al*. European multicentre validation trial of two new non-invasive tests for the detection of *Helicobacter pylori* antibodies: urine-based ELISA and rapid urine test. *Aliment Pharmacol Ther* 2003; 18: 927–31.

Makristathis A, Hirschl AM, Lehours P, Mégraud F. Diagnosis of *Helicobacter pylori* infection. *Helicobacter* 2004; 9(Suppl 1): 7–14.

Malfertheiner P, Megraud F, O'Morain C, *et al*. The European Helicobacter Study Group (EHSG). Current concepts in the management of *Helicobacter pylori* infection: the Maastricht III Consensus Report. *Gut* 2007; 56: 772–81.

Nguyen TV, Bengtsson C, Nguyen GK, Granström M. Evaluation of a novel monoclonal-based antigen in stool enzyme immunoassay (Premier Platinum HpSA PLUS) for diagnosis of *Helicobacter pylori* infection in Vietnamese children. *Helicobacter* 2008; 13: 269–73.

Peng NJ, Lai KH, Lo GH, Hsu PI. Comparison of non-invasive diagnostic tests for *Helicobacter pylori* infection. *Med Princ Pract* 2009; 18: 57–61.

Raţiu N, Rath HC, Büttner R, *et al*. The effects of chromoendoscopy on the diagnostic improvement of gastric ulcers by endoscopists with different levels of experience. *Rom J Gastroenterol* 2005; 14: 239–44.

Ricci C, Holton J, Vaira D. Diagnosis of *Helicobacter pylori*: invasive and non-invasive tests. *Best Pract Res Clin Gastroenterol* 2007; 21: 299–313.

Rugge M, Correa P, Di Mario F, *et al*. OLGA staging for gastritis: a tutorial. *Dig Liver Dis* 2008; 40: 650–8.

Saini SD, Eisen G, Mattek N, Schoenfeld P. Utilization of upper endoscopy for surveillance of gastric ulcers in the United States. *Am J Gastroenterol* 2008; 103: 1920–5.

Stenstrom B, Mendis A, Marshall B. *Helicobacter pylori* – the latest in diagnosis and treatment. *Aust Fam Physician* 2008; 37: 608–12.

Yao K, Takaki Y, Matsui T, *et al*. Clinical application of magnifying endoscopy and narrow-band imaging in the upper gastrointestinal tract: new imaging techniques for detecting and characterizing gastrointestinal neoplasia. *Gastrointest Endosc Clin N Am* 2008; 18: 415–33.

Zuniga-Noriega JR, Bosques-Padilla FJ, Perez-Perez GI, *et al*. Diagnostic utility of invasive tests and serology for the diagnosis of *Helicobacter pylori* infection in different clinical presentations. *Arch Med Res* 2006; 37: 123–8.

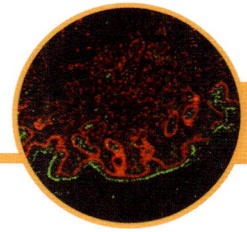

Management

Populations requiring treatment

To determine optimal treatment, it is necessary to conduct clinical trials. Although *Helicobacter pylori* is very sensitive *in vitro* to many antibiotics, anti-ulcer agents and homeopathic remedies, not all may lead to a clinically effective treatment because of pharmacokinetics, pharmacodynamics or the effects of acidity on the agent. Ideally, clinical trials should:

1. Define a population.
2. Define inclusion and exclusion criteria.
3. Define an endpoint.
4. Record the reasons and number of patients who withdraw from the trial or who cannot be evaluated because of protocol violations.
5. Be conducted using a randomized, double-blind placebo controlled methodology.

In the UK, advice on clinical trials can be obtained from the UKCRC Clinical Trials Unit. Inclusion and exclusion criteria and endpoints will vary for *Helicobacter pylori*-related disease, because of the different conditions that can result (peptic ulcer disease, non-ulcer disease, MALT lymphoma, gastric cancer and extra-gastric conditions). Two main endpoints are clinical (resolution of the condition, e.g. ulcer healing) and microbiological (eradication of *Helicobacter pylori*). One significant problem in relation to non-ulcer disease or functional dyspepsia is the nebulous and varied nature of the symptoms, making scoring and diagnosis difficult. Most clinical trials on *Helicobacter pylori* include an initial diagnostic test of active infection (urea breath test or faecal antigen test) followed by the same test at 4 and 8 weeks after the cessation of treatment.

The recommendations for which people require treatment are shown in *Table 6.1* and given in the EHSG Maastricht III Consensus statement. For high-risk patients, it is strongly recommended that the organism be eradicated. Similarly, in patients excessively worried about developing gastric cancer, the organism should be eradicated after an explanation of the treatment side effects.

Eradication of *Helicobacter pylori* in functional dyspepsia is controversial and the evidence is contradictory; however, a small subgroup of patients do benefit (approximately 10% may have improvement or resolution of symptoms). Moreover, in the absence of any other explanatory factor, it is advisable to give a course of eradication therapy—the level of improvement is comparable with other management modalities and the chances of developing peptic ulcer disease (PUD) or gastric cancer are diminished. In areas of low *Helicobacter pylori* prevalence (<20%), proton pump inhibitor (PPI) empirical therapy or a 'test and treat' strategy (*see also* Chapter 5) are considered to be equivalent options and the use of this approach has been justified on economic grounds.

The relationship between gastro-oesophageal reflux disease (GORD) and colonization by *Helicobacter pylori* is controversial but, on balance, there is no good evidence that eradicating the organism causes or exacerbates GORD. However, in patients on long-term acid suppressive therapy, it is advisable to eradicate *Helicobacter pylori* in case there is development of atrophic gastritis caused by bacterial overgrowth.

Table 6.1 Population groups in which *Helicobacter pylori* eradication should or should not be undertaken

Condition	Strength of evidence
Peptic ulcer disease	Level 1*
Mucosal-associated lymphoid tissue lymphoma	Level 2*
Atrophic gastritis	Level 2*
Post-gastric cancer resection	Level 3*
First-degree relatives of gastric cancer patient	Level 3*
Cancerophobes after consultation	Level 4*
Functional dyspepsia	Level 2
GORD on long-term acid suppressive therapy	Level 3
Planned long-term NSAID therapy	Level 2
Patients with history of PUD on low-dose aspirin	Level 3
Extra-gastric disease	Not recommended
Asymptomatic cancer prevention	Not recommended

*Strongly recommended, the remainder are advisable.
The strength of the evidence supporting the recommendation is ranked according to one of the following levels: (1) well-designed and appropriately controlled studies; (2) well-designed cohort or case-controlled studies, or persuasive indirect evidence; (3) case reports or suggestive indirect evidence; (4) clinical experience.

The relationship between *Helicobacter pylori* infection and non-steroidal anti-inflammatory drugs (NSAIDs) in gastroduodenal pathology is complex: *Helicobacter pylori* and NSAIDs independently and significantly increase the risk of peptic ulcer bleeding by 1.79- and 4.86-fold, respectively. The risk of ulcer bleeding is increased by 6.13-fold when both factors are present. Results of *Helicobacter pylori* eradication in NSAID users are conflicting: part of the problem is that both NSAIDs and *Helicobacter pylori* can cause peptic ulcers. *Helicobacter pylori* eradication can only be expected to prevent recurrence of *Helicobacter pylori* ulcers and, while it may also reduce the incidence of ulcers among those with both *Helicobacter pylori* and NSAID use, the effect will vary depending on the proportion with true *Helicobacter pylori* ulcers in the population studied. In chronic NSAID users with peptic ulcer, *Helicobacter pylori* eradication was no better than placebo for maintaining a remission of peptic ulcer with PPI therapy; however, 6 months of PPI maintenance therapy is superior to *Helicobacter pylori* eradication alone in preventing upper gastrointestinal bleeding. In contrast, in patients with *Helicobacter pylori* infection who are naïve NSAID users, *Helicobacter pylori* eradication is superior to placebo in preventing peptic ulcer and upper gastrointestinal bleeding at 6 months.

Philosophy of current treatment

For many years, the primary objective of ulcer therapy was to control acid output either initially by surgical intervention or latterly by pharmaceuticals. This approach was based on the concept of 'no acid–no ulcer' and pre-dated the recognition of *Helicobacter pylori's* role in ulcer development. With this approach, because the organism had not been eradicated and only the level of gastric acid suppressed, once the drug was withdrawn, the ulcer recurred. Since the discovery of the role of *Helicobacter pylori*, the emphasis has changed to 'no *Helicobacter*–no ulcer'. The current approach to ulcer management is to eradicate *Helicobacter pylori* in addition to suppressing acid production, which facilitates ulcer healing. This can be achieved by a number of different therapeutic regimens, with varying degrees of success as assessed by the endpoints of *Helicobacter* eradication rates, ulcer healing rates and ulcer relapse rates.

Because PUD is caused by *Helicobacter pylori* inducing excess acid plus other aggressins, and by decreasing mucosal protection, the therapeutic aim is to eradicate the organism, thereby decreasing the former and enhancing the latter. Consequently, there are several potential targets for PUD therapy. While antibiotics can eradicate the organism, PPIs, H_2-receptor antagonists, cholecystokinin antagonists and inhibitors of gastrin receptors can diminish acid secretion. Enhanced mucosal protection is brought about by increasing the synthesis of, or replacing, mucosal prostanoids (agents that promote epithelial cell growth or mucus secretion) and agents that act as a physiochemical mucosal barrier.

The ideal therapeutic agent for PUD is one that combines antimicrobial, acid reducing and cytoprotective activities. It should have a long half-life, high penetration to the site of infection, high stability and bioavailability, and minimal side effects. It should be cheap to produce and have no cross-resistance to other antibiotics.

Therapeutic targets

The potential therapeutic targets for the management of *Helicobacter*-related gastric disease are shown in **6.1**. The main therapeutics currently in use, or potentially useful for these particular targets, are:

- Antimicrobials: antibiotics, bismuth, probiotics, natural and homeopathic products, and vaccines

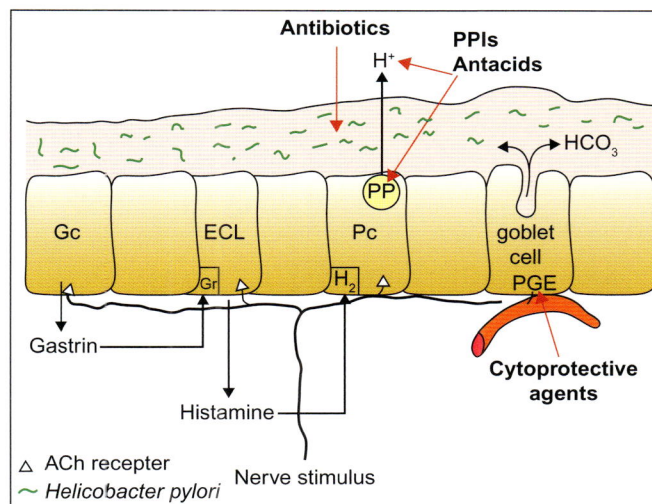

6.1 Diagram of therapeutic targets to treat *Helicobacter*-related gastric disease. Gastrin is released from gastrin-producing G cells (Gc) and acts upon the gastrin receptor (Gr) of enterochromaffin-like cells (ECL) to release histamine. The histamine in turn binds to histamine receptors (H_2) on parietal cells (Pc). Intracellular signal transduction within parietal cells stimulates the H^+/K^+ ATPase proton pump (PP) which releases hydrogen ions (H^+) into the extracellular space. The release of gastrin, histamine and hydrogen ions is modulated by nerve stimuli and the inhibitory effects of somatostatin. Colonization by *Helicobacter pylori* leads to excessive gastrin and hence H^+ release. Locally-produced prostaglandins (PGE) are involved in cytoprotection by stimulating mucus and bicarbonate production. The three main therapeutic targets are: (i) eradication of *Helicobacter pylori*, (ii) reduction of acid secretion and (iii) enhancement of cytoprotection.

- Acid reduction: H_2-receptor antagonists, PPIs, gastrin antagonists, cholecystokinin antagonists
- Cytoprotection: barrier products and prostaglandins

Antibiotics

Helicobacter pylori is very sensitive to many antibiotics, although over the past two decades there has been an increasing problem with the development of resistance. The antibiotics commonly used to treat *Helicobacter pylori* are amoxicillin, clarithromycin and metronidazole as first-line agents; and tetracycline, levofloxacin, moxifloxacin, rifabutin, rifaxamin, furazolidone and tinidazole as second-line agents (*Table 6.2*).

Amoxicillin

Amoxicillin binds to cell wall transpeptidases (penicillin-binding proteins) inhibiting synthesis of

Table 6.2 Some antibiotics currently used to eradicate *Helicobacter pylori*

Antibiotic	MIC Range (µg/ml)	MIC$_{90}$ (µg/ml)
Amoxicillin	0.015–0.25	0.125
Clarithromycin	0.015–32.0	0.03
Metronidazole	0.5–32.0	4.0
Levofloxacin	–	1.0–32.0
Tetracycline	0.063–0.25	0.125
Rifabutin	0.004–0.016	0.008
Furazolidione	0.03–0.5	0.25

MIC = minimal inhibitory concentrations.

the peptide bond between adjacent GlcNAc:MurNAc heteropolymers (*see* Chapter 1). Resistance to β-lactam antibiotics is due to β-lactamase production or an altered penicillin-binding protein target. In *Helicobacter pylori* there are at least seven penicillin-binding proteins (Pbp) and mutations in the *pbp1A* gene lead to amoxicillin resistance. Amoxicillin resistance is very uncommon.

Clarithromycin

Clarithromycin is a macrolide and inhibits protein synthesis by binding to the 23S rRNA component of the 50S subunit of the prokaryotic ribosome, thereby preventing the peptidyltransferase reaction. Clarithromycin resistance is due to point mutations in the 23S rRNA gene which include A2124G, A2142C, A2143G, C2147G, G1929A and A2144T. Resistance varies between 1–30% and leads to failure of treatment.

Metronidazole

Metronidazole is a 5-nitroimidazole and is activated by *Helicobacter pylori* nitroreductase enzymes, inducing single-stranded breaks in the DNA. Metronidazole resistance is due to inactivation of nitroreductase and/or falvadoxin oxidoreductase by frameshift mutations in *rdxA* or *frzA* genes, respectively. Resistance varies between 15% and 78% and leads to failure of treatment.

Levofloxacin

Levofloxacin is a fluoroquinolone that interacts with type II topoisomerases (e.g. DNA gyrase), preventing the unwinding of DNA and DNA replication. Resistance mechanisms consist of point mutations in *gyrA* or -*B* genes. Resistance may also occur in the presence of fluoroquinolone-resistance (*qnr*) genes carried on plasmids; an inactivation enzyme, *aac(6′)*, has also been described. Levofloxacin is normally used as a second-line agent.

Tetracyclines

Tetracyclines inhibit protein synthesis by binding to the 30S subunit of ribosomes, thus preventing binding of the charged acyl-tRNA to the acceptor site on the ribosome. Resistance is principally due to an efflux pump.

Other antibiotics

Helicobacter pylori is also resistant to trimethoprim, polymyxins and glycopeptides. Because the organism is relatively slow-growing, there are some problems in determining the sensitivity of an isolate using disc diffusion, particularly with the nitroimidazoles (e.g. metronidazole). The broth or agar dilutions are more accurate but more labour-intensive than diffusion assays. An acceptable alternative for most of the antibiotics is the E-test (*see* Chapter 5). Antibiotic sensitivity testing is important for two reasons:

1. To check sensitivity before treatment
2. To assess local, national or international resistance rates

In the former case, it is probably better to test the sensitivity of an isolate in areas of high resistance before initial therapy and certainly after a patient has failed a rescue regimen.

Apart from resistance of the organism, failure of eradication can be due to: lack of compliance on the part of the individual; inactivation of the antibiotic by the acidic conditions of the stomach; or failure to achieve sufficient antibiotic at the site of infection (pharmacological resistance). In acid conditions, the minimal inhibitory concentrations of amoxicillin (and erythromycin) are increased, and clarithromycin is degraded. The addition of a PPI during treatment ameliorates these pharmacological problems.

Proton pump inhibitors

These agents are substituted benzimidazoles, including omeprazole, esomeprazole (an enantiomer of omeprazole), lansoprazole, pantoprazole and rabeprazole. They have antisecretory activity as well as some antimicrobial activity against *Helicobacter pylori*.

PPIs inhibit acid secretion by blocking the H^+/K^+ ATPase proton pump in the parietal cell (**6.1**, **6.2**; *see also* Chapter 4). They require conversion to the sulphonamide form intracellularly. Inhibition of acid secretion correlates with binding of the PPI to a cysteine residue on one or more transmembrane loops of the ATPase. Not only do PPIs inhibit acid secretion but they also have some degree of antimicrobial activity against *Helicobacter pylori*. Due to their inhibitory effect on acid secretion PPIs also enhance the pharmacodynamics of some antibiotics in the stomach.

The side effects of PPIs include diarrhoea and rashes. An important side effect of current concern is the role of PPIs in predisposing to *Clostridium difficile*-associated diarrhoea. Also of concern is the possibility, associated with long-term use for the treatment of GORD, of stimulation of enterochromaffin-like (ECL) cells and gastrin cells, leading to tumour development. Studies have demonstrated elevation of gastrin levels after 6 months of treatment, although ECL cell hyperplasia was not noted. However, carcinoid tumours have been noted in association with long-term PPI treatment. A further possible side effect of long-term use is the development of gastric atrophy. Altered bile metabolism has been noted due to an altered small bowel microflora, although the significance of this is not clear. Finally, there is some evidence that Ca^{2+} metabolism may be disturbed, leading to an increased incidence of hip fractures.

Metabolism of PPIs is dependent upon polymorphisms in the cytochrome P450 2C19 (CYP2C19), leading to high and low metabolizers. The particular genotype carried by an individual is related to the eradication rate when given standard triple therapy, with high metabolizers having a lower eradication rate. PPIs are used to treat PUD, GORD, Zollinger–Ellison syndrome and ulceration due to NSAIDs.

H₂-receptor antagonists

The general structure of these agents is an aromatic ring linked to a flexible chain with a terminal polar group.

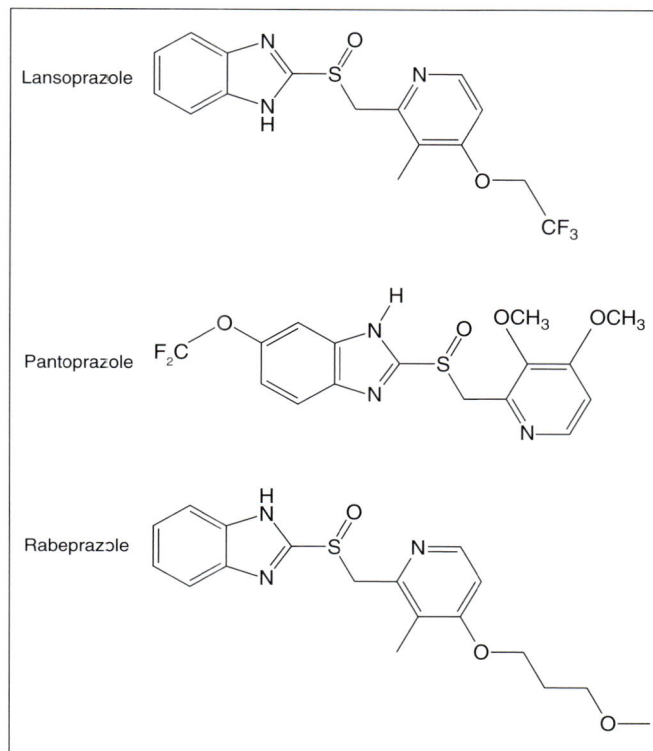

6.2 The structure of some PPIs.

The aromatic ring can be an imidazole (cimetidine), dimethyl amino furan (ranitidine), guanidinothiazole (nitazidine, famotidine) or piperidimethylphenoxy (roxatidine). Ebrotadine has been withdrawn because of hepatic toxicity. They inhibit acid secretion by blocking histamine (H_2) receptors on the parietal cell (**6.1**, **6.3**). H_2-receptor antagonists are used to treat PUD and GORD. Unlike PPIs, they do not have any activity against *Helicobacter pylori*. They have few side effects, the most notable being gynaecomastia. They are less effective than the PPIs as they only inhibit one of the three pathways of acid secretion.

Other agents
Antacids

The pH of the stomach can be buffered with the use of antacids such $Mg(OH)_2$ or $Al(OH)_3$. These agents are used to take away the feeling of 'heartburn' and are probably one of the most common over-the-counter medications bought by the general public. They do have a healing effect on duodenal ulcer, but less so on gastric ulcer because less acid is present. The major disadvantage

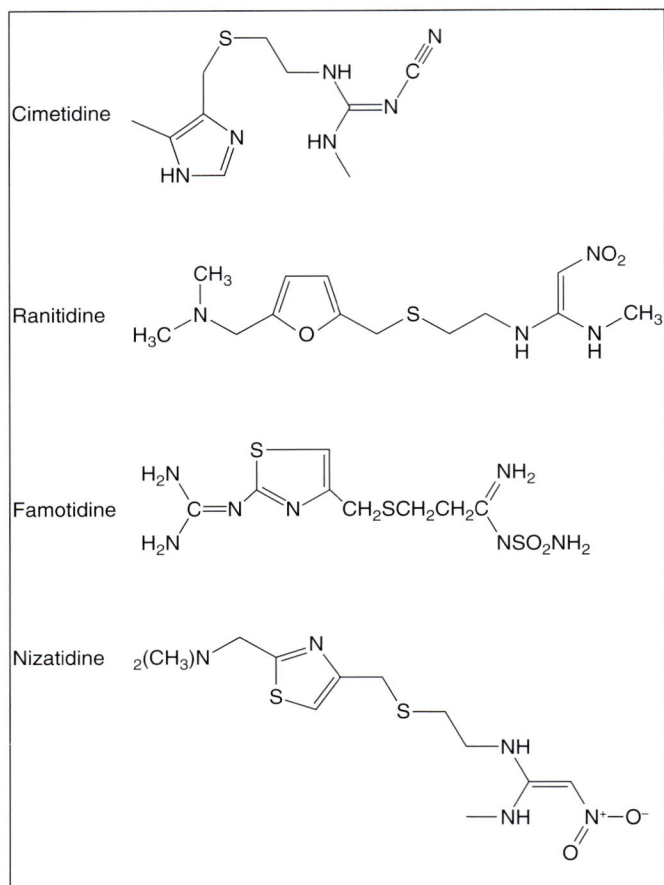

6.3 The structure of H$_2$ receptor antagonists.

is the side effects of diarrhoea or constipation. Antacids also affect absorption of some other drugs. They are frequently used for dyspepsia as a primary medication.

Cytoprotective agents

Cytoprotective agents include prostaglandins, agents that stimulate the production of prostaglandins, or barrier agents acting as a surrogate mucus layer (**6.4**).

Bismuth is a pinkish-grey metal (the pink hue due to surface oxidation) that has been used for diarrhoea since antiquity. Sucralfate is an aluminium sulphate salt of sucrose that increases growth factor release. Sulglycotide, ecabet and plaunotol exert gastroprotective effects by stimulating prostaglandin synthesis or release.

Several other cytoprotective agents exist, such as benexate, sofalcone, trepenone and cetraxate that affect

prostaglandin synthesis and mucus secretion. They are more commonly used in Japan than in the UK.

Prostaglandins

Prostaglandin E$_2$ (PGE$_2$) synthesis is catalysed by two cyclo-oxygenase enzymes: COX-1 (constitutive in most tissues) and COX-2 (inducible in inflammatory sites). The prostaglandins inhibit gastric acid secretion and stimulate mucosal resistance by increasing bicarbonate and mucus secretion and increasing blood flow, thus maintaining the integrity of the barrier function of the gastric epithelium. Lack of production of prostaglandins is caused by NSAIDs due to inhibition of COX-1 and COX-2 activity. This can lead to ulceration. On the other hand, *Helicobacter pylori* increases PGE$_2$ synthesis by upregulating COX-2. The role of PGE$_2$ analogues in relation to ulceration by *Helicobacter pylori* is doubtful, although they are useful in healing peptic ulcers induced by NSAIDs. Some prostaglandins that have been investigated for use in PUD are misoprostol, enprostil, nocloprost and rioprostil. Only misoprostol is available in the UK, as rioprostil and enprostil have been withdrawn due to side effects, although they may be available in other countries.

Bismuth compounds

There are several bismuth compounds (bismuth subcitrate, bismuth subsalicylate, bismuth nitrate, bismuth tartrate, bismuth oxychloride, bismuth sulphate and ranitidine bismuth citrate) that have a cytoprotective action by stimulating endogenous prostaglandins and mucus production, forming a viscid barrier to H$^+$ diffusion. Additionally, bismuth acts as a scavenger of reactive oxygen species and is directly bactericidal to *Helicobacter pylori*. Bismuth compounds are active at healing gastric or duodenal ulcers. There are several side effects, including renal and liver failure, encephalopathy, osteoporosis and erythroderma. Consequently, bismuth compounds are now used in rescue regimens rather than first-line regimens for *Helicobacter* eradication.

Sucralfate

Sucralfate forms a physicochemical barrier over the gastric epithelium and has multiple effects: it induces upregulation of epidermal and fibroblast growth factors and their receptors; it reduces epithelial cell apoptosis,

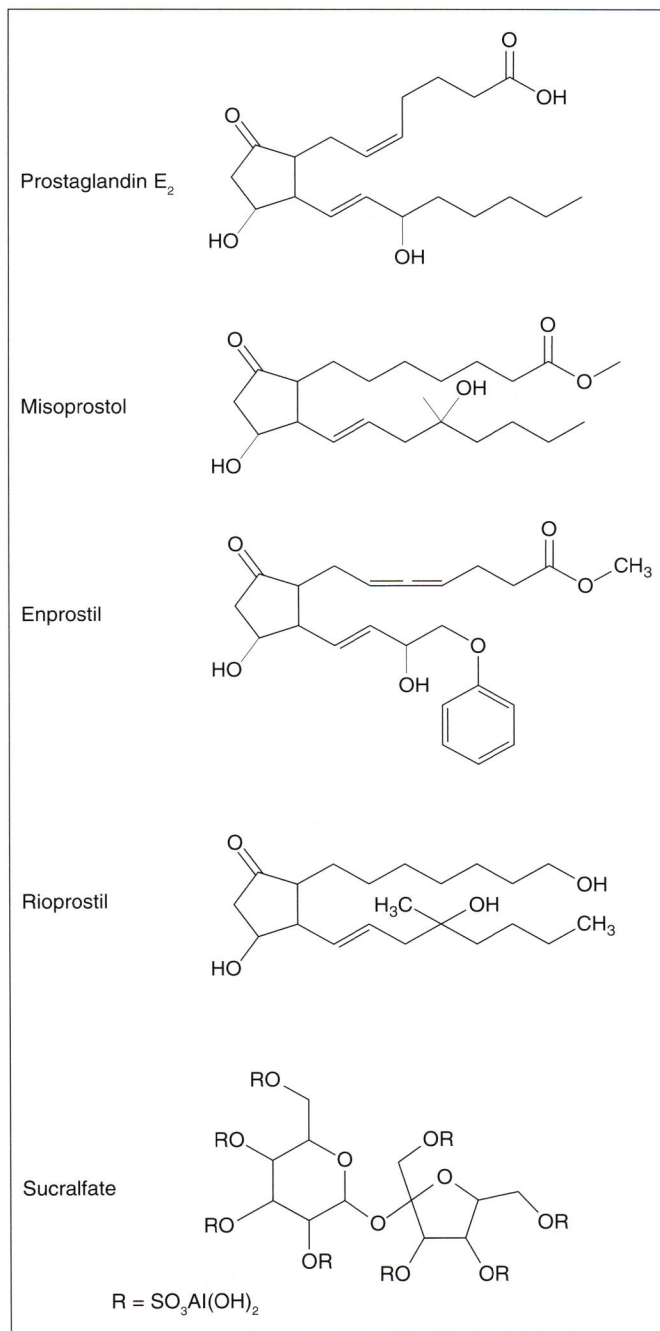

6.4 Chemical structure of PGE$_2$ analogues and surface acting agents.

inducible nitric oxide synthase and the activity of caspase-3; it inhibits the adherence of *Helicobacter pylori*; it also inhibits the degradation of transforming growth factor-β and platelet-derived growth factor by *Helicobacter* protease; it causes inhibition of *Helicobacter* urease and

vacuole formation; and sucralfate blocks the inhibitory action of *Helicobacter* lipopolysaccharide on somatostatin production. Finally, in addition, sucralfate has been complexed with tetracycline as a slow-release carrier for the antibiotic in the treatment of *Helicobacter pylori*.

Sulglycotide

Sulglycotide is a sulphated glycopeptide similar to mucus. It stimulates prostaglandin synthesis and mucosal blood flow. It also increases expression of cyclin-dependent kinase-2 and growth factor receptors during ulcer healing. Sulglycotide diminishes epithelial cell apoptosis, and reduces the expression of TNF-α, caspase 3 and inducible nitric oxide synthase in the mucosa. It also prevents the inhibitory action of *Helicobacter* lipopolysaccharide on somatostatin release and binding of gastric mucus to its receptor, as well as inhibiting the mucolytic activity of *Helicobacter pylori*. Like sucralfate, sulglycotide also inhibits *H. pylori* urease activity. Additionally, it reduces the minimal inhibitory concentrations of amoxicillin and tetracycline for *H. pylori* four- and fivefold, respectively.

Ecabet disodium

Ecabet disodium is a salt of 12-sulphodehydroabietic acid, and is a long-acting gastric cytoprotective agent that increases PGE$_2$ release. It has a bactericidal action against *Helicobacter pylori* as well as inhibiting its urease activity. Addition of ecabet to standard triple therapy increases eradication from 78% to 88%.

Plaunotol

Plaunotol is an oily, locally-acting gastroprotective agent. It increases bicarbonate and mucus secretion, and improves mucosal blood flow as a result of increased prostaglandin synthesis. It has some inhibitory activity against *Helicobacter pylori* and induces autolysis. In combination with clarithromycin, plaunotol has a synergistic activity against clarithromycin-resistant strains of *Helicobacter pylori*.

Vaccines

Because colonization by *Helicobacter pylori* is so extensive in many developing countries and because it is a class I carcinogen, much effort has gone into developing a vaccine against it. Various animal models have been used, from mice to gnotobiotic pigs to primates infected with *Helicobacter pylori* or *Helicobacter felis*, to ferrets naturally infected with *Helicobacter mustelae*. In animal studies, the use of *Helicobacter pylori* vaccine candidates has been encouraging, but little effect has been shown in the few human trials, which have also suffered from the side effects of adjuvants (a suitable adjuvant is still needed). Early vaccine candidates using whole protein or protein subunits are, for example, urease, VacA, CagA and HP-Nap1 (*see* Chapter 4 for further elaboration of these *H. pylori* proteins). Immunoproteomic analysis, however, has identified further potential vaccine antigen candidates, and DNA is also a potential candidate. Alternative approaches include the use of live vectors, nanoparticles and bacterial ghosts. Alternative routes of administration (e.g. nasal application) have also been considered.

The immunological mechanism necessary for an effective vaccine is not clear, and antibodies are evidently not important, as the organism resists eradication despite the presence of antibodies. A CD4$^+$ cellular response seems to be vital for success.

Disease in different population groups

Helicobacter pylori, *dyspepsia and peptic ulcer disease*

Most cases of dyspepsia/PUD are seen in the primary healthcare environment and a 'test and treat' strategy is recommended in adult patients under the age of 45 y presenting with persistent dyspepsia (the age cut-off may vary between countries, depending on the prevalence of gastric cancer). If the patient is over the specified age limit, or if alarm symptoms are present, they should be referred for endoscopy. 'Test and treat' and 'search and treat' strategies (the latter where patients are known to have a diagnosis of PUD but are on long-term acid suppressives) have been validated as cost-effective management algorithms in several healthcare settings.

Helicobacter pylori *and gastro-oesophageal reflux disease*

Screening for *Helicobacter pylori* in patients with GORD is highly recommended before starting PPI treatment, according to the EHSG Maastricht III Guidelines.

Helicobacter pylori *and non-steroidal anti-inflammatory drugs*

Patients on long-term aspirin with ulcer disease and a history of significant bleeding should be tested for *Helicobacter pylori* infection and, if positive, given eradication therapy. Patients who are to receive long-term PPI therapy for prevention of NSAID-induced ulcers should be tested for *Helicobacter pylori* and given eradication therapy.

Prevention of gastric cancer

Gastric cancer is a major public health issue and the global burden of gastric cancer is increasing, particularly in developing countries. *Helicobacter pylori* infection is the major cause of chronic gastritis, a condition that initiates the pathogenic sequence of events leading to atrophic gastritis, metaplasia, dysplasia and subsequently cancer (**6.5**). Pooled analyses of prospective sero-epidemiological studies have shown that individuals with *Helicobacter pylori* infection are at a statistically significant increased risk of developing non-cardiac gastric cancer. It is also well established that both the intestinal and diffuse histological types of gastric cancer are significantly associated with *Helicobacter pylori* infection. Non-randomized clinical follow-up studies in Japan have shown that gastric cancer rates were significantly higher in patients with *Helicobacter pylori* infection than in those in whom the infection had been eradicated. Metachronous tumour rates were also higher in those with persisting infection than those without following endoscopic resection for early gastric cancer.

Furthermore, follow-up studies in Sweden and Denmark of patient cohorts undergoing hip replacement procedures show statistically significantly lower rates of gastric cancer. This can be explained by high doses of prophylactic antibiotics incidentally eradicating *Helicobacter pylori* infection. Thus, it was agreed that *Helicobacter pylori* infection is the most common proven risk factor for human non-cardia gastric cancer.

Infection with *cagA*-positive strains of *Helicobacter pylori* increases the risk for gastric cancer over the risk associated with *Helicobacter pylori* infection alone. Determining *cagA* status in *Helicobacter pylori* infection may confer additional benefit by identifying populations at greater risk for gastric cancer. Interleukin (IL)-1 gene

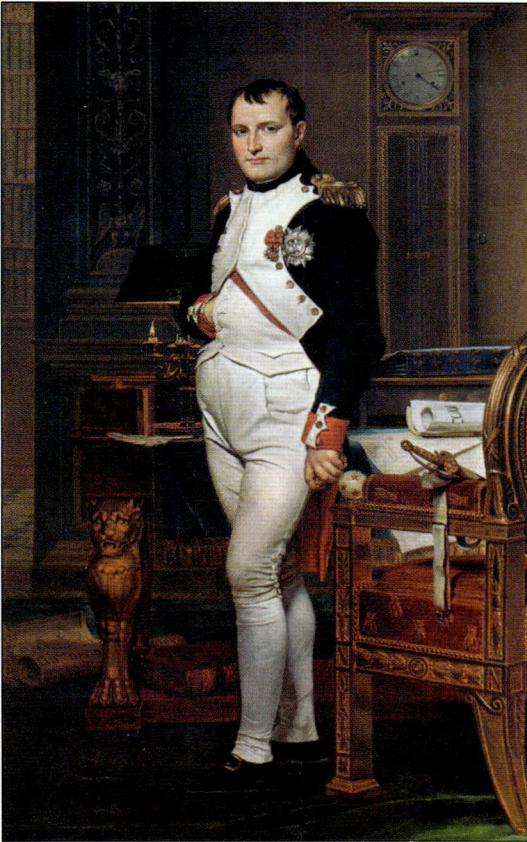

6.5 Napoleon Boneparte (1769–1821). *Phase 1–3:* October 1817–January 1819. Epigastric pain, nausea, headache, constipation/diarrhoea, fever, jaundice and dark urine. *Phase 4:* October 1820–February 1821. Aversion to meat, dysphagia, weight loss and malaise ('to me every activity is a Herculean task'). *Phase 5:* March–May 1821. Abdominal pain, fever, night sweats, haematemesis and melena. It is probable that Napoleon Bonaparte had a long-standing *Helicobacter pylori* infection, a peptic ulcer and eventual gastric adenocarcinoma.

cluster polymorphisms are associated with a higher risk of hypochlorhydria (odds ratio = [OR] 9.1), and of gastric cancer (OR 1.9). Potential extrinsic and intrinsic factors in gastric carcinogenesis include:

- hereditary/family history, both direct and indirect (social inheritance)
- autoimmune (*Helicobacter pylori* may trigger the onset of autoimmune atrophic gastritis in some patients with pernicious anaemia; in diabetes type I, autoimmune atrophic gastritis is frequent and rarely associated with *Helicobacter pylori* infection)

- environmental (occupational exposure/nitrate/nitrite/nitroso compounds)
- nutritional (salt, pickled food red meat, smoking)
- general (low socio-economic status, geography)
- pharmacological (gastric acid inhibition)

All these lines of evidence suggest that bacterial virulence factors, host genetic factors and environmental factors contribute to the risk of developing gastric cancer.

Helicobacter pylori eradication prevents development of pre-neoplastic changes (atrophic gastritis and intestinal metaplasia) of the gastric mucosa. Evidence that *Helicobacter pylori* eradication may reduce the risk of gastric cancer is based on non-randomized controlled studies in animal and humans. Several randomized control studies show regression of pre-cancerous lesions or, at least, slower progression as compared with control groups after *Helicobacter pylori* eradication. One randomized control did not demonstrate reduction of cancer incidence at 5y but showed a significant reduction in the group without pre-neoplastic lesions. The consensus report concluded that eradication of *Helicobacter pylori* has the potential to reduce the risk of gastric cancer development; moreover, the optimal time to eradicate *Helicobacter pylori* is before pre-neoplastic lesions (atrophy, intestinal metaplasia) are present. It was also agreed that the potential for gastric cancer prevention on a global scale is restricted by currently available therapies. Thus, new therapies are desirable for a global strategy of gastric cancer prevention.

Current therapies

Some 25 years after its discovery, *Helicobacter pylori* treatment remains a challenge for the clinician, as no proposed therapy regimen is able to eradicate the infection in *all* treated patients. One-week triple therapies (PPI, clarithromycin plus amoxicillin or metronidazole), as suggested in European guidelines, are the most-used treatments in clinical practice (*Table 6.3*), being currently prescribed by 85%, 84% and 67% of primary care physicians in Italy, Israel and the USA respectively. European guidelines confirmed the use of a standard 7-day triple therapy in those areas where clarithromycin resistance is lower than 15–20%, while

Table 6.3 Eradication regimens for *Helicobacter pylori*

First-line

PPI or RBC (400 mg bid) + C (500 mg bid) + A (1000 mg bid)

or

PPI or RBC (400 mg bid) + M (500 mg bid) + A (1000 mg bid)

or

Sequential first-line

PPI + A (1000 mg bid) 5 days followed by

PPI + C (500 mg bid) + T (500 mg bid) 5 days

Second-line

PPI + BC (120 mg qid) + M (500 mg tds)

or

C (500 mg bid) + T (500 mg qid)

or

(Alternative first line not used initially.)

Rescue

PPI + BC + (240 mg bid) + T (500 mg bid) + F 200 mg bid) 7 days or

PPI + A (1000 mg bid) + BC (120 mg qid) + F (200 mg bid) 14 days

or

PPI + T (500 mg qid) + F (200 mg tds) 7 days

or

PPI + BC + (240 mg bid) + T (500 mg bid) + F 200 mg bid) 7 days

or

PPI + A (1000 mg bid) + BC (120 mg qid) + F (200 mg bid) 14 days

or

PPI or RBC + R (150 mg bid) + A (1000 mg bid) 10 days

or

Rabeprazole (20 mg bid) + T (500 mg bid) + L (500 mg bid) 10 days

A = amoxicillin; BC = bismuth citrate; C = clarithromycin; F = furazolidone; L = levofloxacin; M = metronidazole; RBC = ranitidine bismuth citrate; T = tinidazole

---

a prolonged 14-day regimen or 10–14-day quadruple therapy should be administered when bacterial resistance is higher. However, several studies found that the eradication rates achieved with these therapies are far from promising. A meta-analysis has clearly shown that the 14-day triple therapy disappointingly offers only a modest improvement over the 7-day regimen in terms of *Helicobacter pylori* eradication rates (+5–8%), in spite of a twofold increase in treatment cost. In Italy, a recent multicentre study involving 906 duodenal ulcer patients failed to show even a modest therapeutic gain, *Helicobacter pylori* infection being cured in 79.7% and 81.7% of patients receiving a 7-day or 14-day triple therapy, respectively. Another Italian study, enrolling 486 patients, found an eradication rate as low as 52–57% following 7-day standard triple therapies, only increasing to 56–70% when the same regimens were prolonged to 14 days. As far as quadruple therapy is concerned, a meta-analysis failed to find a significant difference in the success rate between 7-day quadruple and standard triple therapies as a first-line treatment. In addition, bismuth salts are no longer available in several countries, (Italy being one example) so the quadruple therapy is not feasible world-wide.

However, the situation has altered recently with the development of a novel sequential treatment regimen (discussed further below). Eradication rates using this new regimen have achieved an average of 92%, making this an effective first-line treatment option.

Antibiotic resistance is increasing (*Table 6.4*), and the efficacy of these therapies is decreasing world-wide (*Table 6.5*). The success rate in most European and Asian countries, as well as in the USA and Canada, has declined to unacceptable values, with more than one in every five patients failing eradication therapy. Cure rates as low as 20–45% have been recently reported. This phenomenon has been largely related to a world-wide increase in bacterial resistance, particularly against clarithromycin—the key antibiotic in *Helicobacter pylori* treatment. Therefore, an increasing number of patients actually require a second or further therapeutic attempt to eradicate such an infection, with substantial economic implications. All of these observations suggest that other therapeutic approaches to cure *Helicobacter pylori* are needed, the best first-line treatment still being regarded as the best 'rescue therapy'. The most obvious question to be addressed is whether a first-line therapy

Table 6.4 Global resistance rates for clarithromycin and metronidazole

Country	Year	Clarithromycin (%)	Metronidazole (%)
Australia	2003	9	44
Brazil	2003	16	55
China	2004	23	40
Finland	2004	2	38
India	2003	45	78
Italy	2003	23	52
Japan	2004	20	15
Korea	2005	20	42
The Netherlands	2003	5	26
Sweden	2004	1	76
Thailand	2003	19	30
Turkey	2004	18	36
UK	2004	5	32
USA	2003	11	40
(Alaska)	(2003)	(30)	(66)

regimen more effective than the suggested 14-day triple or quadruple therapies is already available.

Sequential therapy

In 2000, the first pilot study using a novel, 10-day sequential regimen, achieving a very high eradication rate, was performed (**6.6**). The sequential regimen is a simple dual therapy (a PPI plus amoxicillin 1 g, both given twice daily) for the first 5 days, followed by a triple therapy (a PPI, clarithromycin 500 mg and tinidazole, all given twice daily) for the remaining 5 days. This novel therapeutic combination was based on a previous observation that, in patients who had failed initial eradication treatment, the eradication rate achieved by a 14-day dual therapy followed by a 7-day triple therapy

course was significantly higher than that obtained when inverting such a treatment sequence (97.3% vs 81.6%). At this point, it had been speculated that dual therapy followed by triple therapy was able to eradicate the

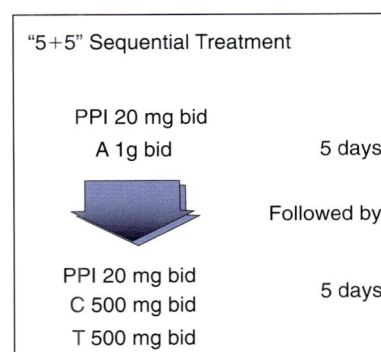

"5+5" Sequential Treatment

PPI 20 mg bid
A 1g bid   5 days

Followed by

PPI 20 mg bid
C 500 mg bid   5 days
T 500 mg bid

6.6 The sequential regimen. A = amoxicillin; C = clar thromycin; T = tinidazole.

Table 6.5 Global eradication rates of *Helicobacter pylori*

Year of study	Country	No. of patients	Eradication (%)
2000	Italy	80	57
2000	Italy	36	69
2000	France	64	64
2000	Ireland	308	73
2000	Japan	55	55
2002	Korea	216	65
2003	Turkey	53	25
2003	Canada	379	74
2004	Italy	115	71
2004	Greece	52	71
2004	Turkey	139	45
2004	Brazil	130	61
2004	USA	77	62
2005	Israel	61	67
2005	Japan	17	41

infection in a very large number of patients. To apply this observation in clinical practice, there was a need to simplify the therapeutic combination, and, for this reason, it was decided to reduce each treatment schedule to no more than 5 days. Indeed, it was known that dual therapy (PPI plus amoxicillin) administered for less than 7 days was able to achieve a cure rate of up to 50%, and that the efficacy of triple therapy (PPI, clarithromycin and tinidazole) was inversely related to the bacterial load, higher eradication rates being achieved in those with a low bacterial density in the stomach.

Therefore, a pioneering 10-day sequential regimen was carried out consisting of a short, initial dual therapy with amoxicillin, aiming to lower the bacterial load in the stomach to favour efficacy of the subsequent short course of triple therapy that immediately followed. Moreover, initial use of amoxicillin may offer another essential

advantage for *Helicobacter pylori* eradication. It has been found that regimens containing amoxicillin prevent selection of secondary clarithromycin resistance. Indeed, it is known that bacteria can develop efflux channels for clarithromycin, which rapidly transfer the drug out of the bacterial cell, preventing binding of the antibiotic to its target. It has been speculated that disruption of the cell wall caused by amoxicillin prevents development of efflux channels. In subsequent years, several therapeutic trials compared this sequential regimen with the standard 7–10-day triple therapies, supporting efficacy of the new treatment even against clarithromycin-resistant strains. To definitively understand whether such a novel therapy is ready to be used as first-line treatment in clinical practice, published studies on the sequential regimen were reviewed by performing a pooled-data analysis of the available results. In the first pilot study, a very high eradication rate (98%) was achieved with the sequential regimen, and such an unexpectedly remarkable result was virtually duplicated in a further two centres, plus a pilot study. These findings suggested that the basic theory of the sequential combination of antibiotics was successful when applied to clinical practice, eliciting a number of trials on the use of such a therapy regimen, which have been published over the course of the last nine years. A descriptive analysis of the 22 available studies on sequential therapy is provided in *Table 6.6*. Of these, two are pilot studies and 20 randomized trials, including 19 single centre and seven multicentre trials, which have been performed in nine different units covering the whole of Italy, and also includes studies from Korea, Panama, Romania, Spain and Taiwan. Five of the studies were in a paediatric population. All but six of these trials have been published as a full paper.

As shown in *Table 6.6* the sequential regimen achieved an average eradication rate of 92% at intention-to-treat (ITT) analysis in a total study population of 2324 patients.

Primary clarithromycin resistance seems to be the only factor reducing the efficacy of this therapy regimen. However, even in these patients, an acceptable >75% eradication rate can be achieved following the sequential therapy, a success rate significantly higher than that observed with the standard 7–10-day triple therapies (<35%).

Comparison with standard 7–10-day triple therapy

A head-to-head comparison between the sequential regimen and standard 7-day triple therapy has been performed in eight randomized trials. At ITT analysis, the infection was cured in 1073 of 1145 patients (93.7%) and in 878 of 1156 (75.9%) patients following the sequential regimen and the 7-day triple therapy, respectively. The difference was statistically significant (93.7% vs 75.9%; $P < 0.0001$).

A head-to-head comparison between the sequential regimen and standard 10-day triple therapy has been performed in four randomized trials. At ITT analysis, infection was cured in 354 of 379 (93.4%) patients and in 309 of 388 (79.6%) patients following the sequential regimen and 10-day triple therapy, respectively. The difference was statistically significant (93.4% vs 79.6%; $P < 0.0001$) (*Table 6.7*).

Triple therapy with a PPI, clarithromycin and either amoxicillin or metronidazole is the most popular treatment regimen to cure *Helicobacter pylori* infection among primary care physicians and gastroenterologists in the USA and Europe. The success of eradication therapy is often reported as a modified ITT rate (patients who do not take a single dose of the medication are excluded from the analysis), and this should be borne in mind when comparisons of studies are made. Two recent double-blind, US multicentre studies found disappointingly low eradication rates with triple therapy. In one study, 75.6% of 402 patients and in the other, 77.2% of 307 patients were cured of *Helicobacter pylori* infection by modified ITT analysis following a 10-day triple regimen. Low eradication rates have also been reported with triple therapy in Europe, Australia and Asia. The study recently published confirms these reports on the poor eradication success with conventional triple therapy and suggests that this may be largely due to clarithromycin resistance.

The outcome of *Helicobacter pylori* therapy depends to a substantial degree on compliance with the regimen and presence of antibiotic resistance. Clarithromycin resistance is a major problem in many Western countries; its prevalence is 12.9% (varying from 6.1% to 14.5%) in the USA and may be as high as 24% in some European countries. A systematic review of *Helicobacter pylori* therapy reported a 53% decrease in eradication rates if clarithromycin resistance was present and a clarithromycin-containing regimen was used. In the study mentioned above, the prevalence of primary clarithromycin resistance was 17%, confirming data recently reported in Italy. In this Italian study, nearly 90% of patients infected with clarithromycin-resistant strains were cured following the sequential regimen, an eradication rate that is three times higher than with the standard regimen in this subgroup. The sequential treatment regimen may be preferable when the prevalence of clarithromycin-resistant *Helicobacter pylori* is high, as is the case in many developed countries.

It is known that bacteria can develop efflux channels for clarithromycin, which rapidly transfer the drug out of the bacterial cell, preventing binding of the antibiotic to the ribosome. Since amoxicillin acts on the bacterial cell wall and weakens it, the initial phase of treatment may prevent the development of efflux channels by weakening the cell wall of the bacterium. This may

Table 6.6 Eradication rates using the sequential regimen

Author	PPI	No. Patients	Eradication %
Zullo[1]	Omeprazole	52	98
Zullo[2]	Rabeprazole	522	92
Zullo[3]	Esomeprazole	40	95
De Francesco[4]	Omeprazole	45	95
De Francesco[5]	Rabeprazole	116	95
De Francesco[6]	Esomeprazole	63	94
De Francesco[7]	Rabeprazole	162	94
Hassan[8]	Rabeprazole	152	93
Scaccianoce[9]	Esomeprazole	72	94
Focareta[10]	Omeprazole	94	96
Focareta[11]	Esomeprazole	174	95
Francavilla[12]	Omeprazole	38	95
Lionetti[13]	Omeprazole	40	82
Lerro[14]	–	25	92
Hurduc[15]	–	45	87
Vaira[16]	Pantoprazole	146	93
Francavilla[17]	–	90	85
Sanchez-Delgado[18]	Omeprazole	139	91
Wu[19]	–	66	98
Choi[20]	Omeprazole	77	86
Ruiz-Obaldia[21]	–	76	85
Paoluzi[22]	–	90	89
TOTAL		**2324**	**92[a]**

– = not recorded; [a] = arithmetic average: median 90; mode 95% eradication

Table 6.7 Eradication rates of sequential versus standard regimens

Analysis	Sequential (no.)	Standard (no.)	Difference	P value
ITT	92% (481/522)	74% (389/572)	18	<0.0001
PP	95% (481/506)	77% (389/507)	18	<0.0001
ITT PUD	97% (124/128)	75% (101/135)	22	<0.0001
PP PUD	98% (124/127)	76% (101/133)	22	<0.0001
ITT NUD	91% (357/394)	73% (288/392)	18	<0.0001
PP NUD	94% (357/379)	77% (288/174)	17	<0.0001
C-RES	78% (7/9)	17% (1/6)	61	0.04
F-RES	94% (34/36)	70% (26/37)	24	0.01
C+M-RES	80% (8/10)	40% (2/5)	40	0.2

C = clarithromycin; F = furazolidone; M = metronidazole; NUD = non-ulcer disease; RES = resistant

improve the efficacy of clarithromycin in the second phase of treatment. Another possibility is that the higher efficacy of the sequential regimen is related to the larger number of antibiotics (three) to which the organism is exposed with this regimen, or to the use of tinidazole, which is not contained in the standard triple regimen. A Medline search in November 2011 using the key words 'sequential therapy' and 'Helicobacter pylori' yielded 188 citations. In areas with high levels of antibiotic resistance, sequential therapy or quadruple therapy are advocated as first line treatment, giving the highest eradication rates.

Cost is a major consideration in many countries. In Europe, the cost of the sequential regimen is similar to that of the standard regimen, making it an attractive alternative to current triple therapy. Tinidazole has recently become available in the USA and the cost of sequential therapy based on retail prices is lower than that of triple therapy. Sequential therapy may therefore be a reasonable alternative to standard therapy.

Large, prospective double-blind controlled studies have demonstrated the superiority of a sequential treatment regimen for *Helicobacter pylori* compared with conventional triple therapy. The sequential regimen is cheaper and more effective than conventional therapy in patients with clarithromycin-resistant organisms. Side effects with both regimens were similar and consisted mostly of diarrhoea and abdominal discomfort. The data suggest that sequential therapy may have a role as a first-line treatment for *Helicobacter pylori* infection.

Attention given to the sequential therapy regimen is steadily increasing in the literature. Several authoritative experts have defined such a therapeutic approach as 'appealing', and the Maastricht III Consensus Statement advised that 'sequential therapy deserves further evaluation in different regions'. Indeed, the sequential regimen, equal to the standard 7–14 triple therapies, was also advised as a first-line treatment in updated Italian National Guidelines on *Helicobacter pylori* management. Gastroenterologists should therefore be encouraged to validate the sequential therapy in other geographical areas where data are still lacking. If patients are our first priority—as they always should be—the time for change is overdue!

Eradication rate in peptic ulcer and non-ulcer dyspepsia patients

Some data suggest that following standard triple therapies the eradication rate in non-ulcer dyspepsia tends to be lower than in peptic ulcer patients. A head-to-head comparison between sequential regimen and standard triple therapy (7–10-day) in these two patient subgroups are available in four studies. Overall, *Helicobacter pylori* infection was cured in 199 of 204 (97.5%) peptic ulcer patients and in 496 of 540 (91.8%) non-ulcer dyspepsia patients with the sequential regimen, and in 217 of 293 (74.1%) and 433 of 576 (75.2%) patients, respectively, following triple therapy. The difference between sequential and standard therapy was statistically significant in both peptic ulcer (97.5% vs 74.1%; $P<0.0001$) and in non-ulcer dyspepsia (91.7% vs 75.2%; $P = 0.0000001$) patients. On the contrary, the eradication rate did not differ between peptic ulcer and non-ulcer dyspepsia matched subgroups following either sequential or standard therapy.

Role of different proton pump inhibitors
Different PPIs have been used in the sequential combination. Bacterial eradication was achieved in 271 of 287 (94.4%) patients following the omeprazole-based regimen; in 133 of 146 (91.1%) patients with pantoprazole; in 1011 of 1086 (93.1%) patients with rabeprazole; and in 272 of 286 (95.1%) patients with esomeprazole. The difference in success rates shown between the different PPIs used was not statistically significant. No data with lansoprazole are available.

Eradication rate in children
The eradication rate following standard 7-day triple therapy in children is known to range from 68% to 75%. To date, two small trials performed in the same centre are available on the use of sequential regimen in dyspeptic children (median age 12.3 years, range 3.3–18). In the first randomized study, *Helicobacter pylori* infection was cured in 36 of 38 (94.7%) and in 28 of 37 (75.7%) children following a sequential regimen and 7-day triple therapy, respectively ($P = 0.02$). In the second study, bacterial eradication was achieved in 33 of 40 (82.5%) children receiving the sequential regimen (with or without probiotic supplementation). Therefore, the cumulative analysis found that *Helicobacter pylori* infection was cured in 69 of 78 (88.5%) treated children.

Eradication rate in elderly patients
The results of Italian studies, overall enrolling 387 patients, showed that *Helicobacter pylori* eradication in elderly patients was 79.3% following the standard 7-day triple therapy. To date, only one randomized study involving 179 peptic ulcer geriatric patients (mean age 69.5 y, range 65–83 y) is available on the use of the sequential regimen. At ITT analysis, the infection was cured in 84 of 89 (94.4%) and in 72 of 90 (80%) patients following sequential and 7-day triple therapy, respectively ($P = 0.008$).

Factors affecting eradication rate

Several factors have been found to affect the efficacy of standard triple therapies, such as bacterial resistance to antibiotics, compliance to therapy, bacterial load in the stomach, CagA status, smoking habit and gastroduodenal pathology. However, among these factors, bacterial clarithromycin resistance and patient compliance to therapy both play major roles in predicting therapeutic outcome. In particular, primary clarithromycin resistance is regarded as the main factor affecting the efficacy of treatment, reducing the success rate of standard triple therapies to mean values of 18–44%.

Clarithromycin resistance
Data on primary clarithromycin resistance and *Helicobacter pylori* eradication following the sequential regimen are available in three trials. Overall, infection was cured in 41 of 53 (77.4%) patients and in 18 of 54 (33.3%) patients infected with clarithromycin-resistant strains following sequential and standard triple therapy, respectively (this was irrespective of metronidazole resistance). Therefore, a significantly higher eradication rate was achieved following sequential therapy as compared with the 7–10-day triple therapies (77.4% vs 33.3%; $P = 0.0001$). The sequential regimen was much more effective than triple therapy even in those patients harbouring a clarithromycin-resistant strain due to, for example, the A2143G point mutation (*see* p. 116), which was found to play a major role in reducing the eradication rate of triple therapy. Other studies found that, in contrast to the standard triple therapy, the cure rate achieved by sequential therapy is not significantly affected by gastroduodenal pathology (peptic ulcer vs non-ulcer dyspepsia), bacterial strain (CagA-positive vs CagA-negative), bacterial load in the stomach (low vs high) or smoking habits.

Compliance and side effects

Compliance to therapy is another major factor influencing outcome. Generally, good compliance is defined as consumption of more than 90% of prescribed drugs. Full data on patient compliance and the incidence of side effects are available from eight trials comparing sequential and triple therapies. Overall, no difference emerged between the two treatments; a good compliance to the therapy was observed in 1004 of 1085 (92.6%) patients receiving the sequential regimen and in 1203 of 1280 (94%) patients treated with triple therapy. In the same studies, the incidence of side effects was 9.9% and 9.8%, respectively. Overall, side effects required the interruption of therapy in only 3 of 1085 (0.27%) and in 9 of 1280 (0.70%) patients receiving sequential and triple therapy, respectively. All of these observations suggest that the sequential regimen and standard triple therapy are characterized by a similar patient compliance, incidence of side effects and therapy interruption rate.

Rescue therapy after sequential regimen failure

When a novel therapy for *Helicobacter pylori* eradication is suggested for clinical practice, it is of paramount importance to identify a second-line therapy that may be used in the event of failure. A levofloxacin–amoxicillin-based triple therapy has been proved to be acceptably effective as second- or even third-line therapy. Two recent meta-analyses showed a higher eradication rate of this regimen as compared with standard quadruple therapy as a retreatment. One of the authors (DV) recently performed a pilot study on 35 patients who failed the sequential regimen. Following a 10-day triple therapy (rabeprazole 20 mg, levofloxacin 250 mg and amoxicillin 1 g, all twice daily), *Helicobacter pylori* infection was successfully cured in 30 patients, accounting for a 85.7% eradication rate at ITT analysis (95% confidence interval = 74–97). These data seem to indicate that levofloxacin–amoxicillin triple therapy is a suitable approach for second-line treatment for patients in whom sequential therapy failed. Therefore, the 10-day sequential regimen plus the 10-day levofloxacin-based triple therapy appears to be a convincing 'therapeutic package' for *Helicobacter pylori* management in clinical practice.

To improve the efficacy of triple therapy in those areas with more than 15–20% primary clarithromycin resistance, the use of a 14-day regimen or 10–14-day quadruple therapy has been recently proposed in the updated European guidelines. However, as mentioned above (p. 122), quadruple therapy is not necessarily available in all countries, and the prolonged 14-day triple therapy has an unfavourable cost/efficacy ratio. On the other hand, over the past five years, only a few novel compounds have been identified as having bactericidal activity against *H. pylori* with the potential to be developed in the near future.

Novel approaches to eradication of *Helicobacter pylori*

The increasing prevalence of antibiotic resistance and falling eradication rates presents therapeutic problems that may be addressed using alternative strategies.

Probiotics

The use of live bacteria as an adjunct to anti-infective treatment either for their immunomodulatory activity (proven in some cases), or because they out-compete potential pathogens in a particular ecological niche and re-establish a normal flora, has been advocated for many years. More recently, the role of probiotics in relation to the eradication of *Helicobacter pylori* has become more fashionable because of increasing antibiotic resistance of the organism and the fact that many bacteria have an inhibitory action upon *Helicobacter pylori* (*Table 6.8*). Many organisms inhibit the growth of *Helicobacter pylori*, some of which are traditionally thought to be probiotic bacteria (e.g. *Lactobacillus* spp.) and others not (e.g. *Salmonella* spp.). However, the results are inconsistent between studies and are very much method- and strain-dependent. *Lactobacillus acidophilus* is a commensal bacterium found in the gastrointestinal tract and used in the preparation of yoghurt. It is an acid-resistant organism and is retained in the stomach unharmed. In mixed cultures, the *Helicobacter* is killed by any of the *Lactobacillus* spp. and this is thought to be caused by the production of lactic acid by the *Lactobacillus*. However, recent studies have demonstrated that L-lactic acid is a growth factor for *Helicobacter pylori* and indeed may facilitate colonization. The growth-promoting activity of L-lactic acid for *Helicobacter pylori* has been incorporated into a screening method for anti-*Helicobacter* substances. Some of these probiotic bacteria have immunomodulatory activity.

Table 6.8 Inhibitory activity of bacteria spp. against *Helicobacter pylori*

	Gram-positive cocci	Gram-positive bacilli	Gram-negative bacilli
Inhibitory activity	Enterococcus faecium	Bacillus subtilis	Acinetobecter baumannii
	Staphylococcus aureus	Bifidobacterium dentium	Bacteroides fragilis
	Staph. auricularis	Clostridium difficile	Enterobacter cloacae
	Staph. cohnii	Corynebacterium butyricum	Escherichia coli
	Staph. epidermidis	Lactobacillus acidophilus	Fusobacterium nucleatum
	Staph. hominis	Lactobacillus casei	Klebsiella pneumoniae
	Staph. warneri	Lactobacillus gasseri	Morganella morganii
		Lactobacillus johnsonii	Pseudomonas aeruginosa
		Lactobacillus salivarius	Salmonella spp.
		Weissella confusa	Serratia marcescens
			Stenotrophomonas maltophilia
No inhibitory activity	Enterococcus faecalis	Bacillus cereus	Enterobacter aerogenes
	Lactococcus lactis	Bifidobacterium longum	Klebsiella oxytoca
	Streptococcus acidophilus		
	Strep. agalactiae		
	Strep. anginosus		
	Strep. oralis		
	Strep. pneumoniae		
	Strep. pyogenes		
	Strep. salivarius		

Lactobacillus bulgaricus modulates the expression of TLR4, inhibits TAK-1 and p38MAPK phosphorylation, preventing NFκB activation and subsequent upregulation of IL-8 by *Helicobacter pylori* lipopolysaccharide (*see* Chapter 4). The molecular mechanism of the reduction in inflammation caused by *Helicobacter pylori* with *Lactobacillus acidophilus* is due to the production of conjugated linoleic acids, which dissociate the IKKγ–Hsp90 complex, resulting in inhibition of NFκB signalling and a reduction in IL-8 secretion.

Of the following probiotic bacteria—*Lactobacillus rhamnosus* GG, *L. rhamnosus* LC705, *Proprionibacterium freudenreichii* ssp *shermanii* JS and *Bifidobacterium breve*—all inhibit adhesion of *Helicobacter pylori* to Caco-2 cells and *Helicobacter pylori*-induced cell leakage, although none of them improve epithelial barrier function, but rather cause deterioration. *L. rhamnosus* and *P. freudenreichii* inhibit *Helicobacter pylori*-induced IL-8 release; *L. rhamnosus* and *B.*

breve prevent PGE$_2$ release. However, when used in combination, the *Helicobacter pylori*-induced anti-inflammatory effects are not evident. Similarly, *L. casei* L26 and *B. lactis* B94 in *Helicobacter pylori*-infected mice decrease neutrophil infiltration and IL-1β levels while increasing IL-10 levels.

In clinical trials, the regular consumption of cranberry juice with the probiotic bacterium *L. johnsonii* LA1 results in a 22% eradication rate in asymptomatic children colonized with *Helicobacter pylori*. Clinical studies of fermented milk-based probiotics have demonstrated an improvement in the eradication rate from 5% to 15%. *L. reuteri*, when given to *Helicobacter pylori*-colonized dyspeptic patients, decreases the gastric load of the organism and improves symptoms. In combination with standard triple therapy, yoghurt containing *L. acidophilus* HY2177, *L. casei* HY2743, *B. longum* HY8001 and *Strep. thermophilus* B-1 (Will yoghurt) enhanced eradication of *Helicobacter pylori* (87% vs 78%) but did not alter the side effects of treatment. On the other hand, *L. reuteri* had no effect on the eradication rate.

Phytoceuticals

Infection with *Helicobacter pylori* causes an inflammatory process in which reactive peroxygen and nitryl radicals are produced, which can induce lipid peroxygenation and DNA damage for the host. As eradication of *Helicobacter pylori* is generally only recommended for symptomatic individuals, asymptomatic individuals who are colonized will continue to have gastritis. Moreover, as long-term gastritis may lead to pre-neoplastic and neoplastic changes, agents that are part of a normal diet and that are antimicrobial or anti-inflammatory have been sought. There is increasing interest in the activity of various food sources such as tea, wine, spices and sprouts in enhancing health by reducing cancer and cardiovascular risks. Many of these foods contain compounds that are bactericidal to *Helicobacter pylori* (**6.7**). Plants contain multiple organic components, including phenols, quinones, flavones, tannins, terpenoids and alkaloids, all of which are known to have bactericidal effects. Green tea, for example, is rich in epigallocatechin gallate, honey rich in glucose oxidase and caffeic acid phenethyl ester, broccoli is rich in sulforaphane and wine in flavenoids. The constituents of one potent bactericide, the spice turmeric, are listed in *Box 6.1*.

Plants also contain many water-soluble proteins—lectins and carbohydrates—which may bind specifically to sugar residues, polysaccharides, glycoproteins or glycolipids, such as those that make up adhesins present on the cell surface of *Helicobacter pylori*. In the event of such interactions occurring, the result would be to block the availability of the adhesin to its receptor. Successful inhibition of adhesion has been shown *in vitro* with cranberry juice against *Helicobacter pylori*. In addition, seaweed (*Cladosiphon fucoidan*), acidic high molecular weight galactans from blackcurrant seeds, and fresh juice preparations of the fruit of the okra plant (*Abelmoschus esculentus* L. Moench) all inhibit adhesion of *Helicobacter pylori*. Polysaccharide fractions of *Panax ginseng* and *Artemisia capillaris* were shown to inhibit *Helicobacter pylori* adhesion to a human gastric adenocarcinoma epithelial cell line.

In a study that tested 25 plants for their bactericidal activity against *Helicobacter pylori*, eight did not have any activity after 60 min of incubation: bengal quince, nightshade, garlic, dill, black pepper, coriander, fenugreek and black tea. Spices with activity include turmeric (the most efficient), ginger, cumin, chilli,

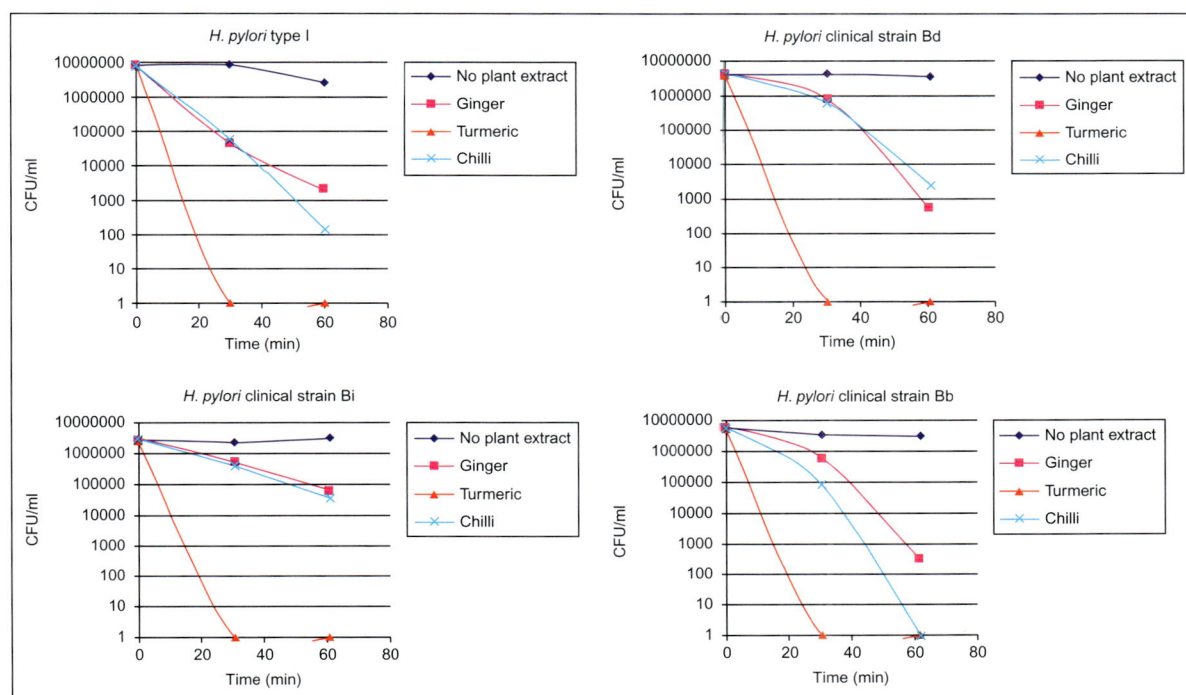

6.7 Kill curves of *Helicobacter pylori* induced by extracts from certain spices.

Box 6.1 Constituents of turmeric

Ascorbic acid	Boron	1,8-cineole; 2-bornanol; 2-hydroxy-methyl-anthraquinone; 4-hydroxy-cinnamoyl-(feruloyl)-methane; α-atlantone; α-pinene; α-terpineol; turmerone; arabinose; azulene; β-carotene; β-pinene; β-sesquiphellandrene; bis(para-hydroxy cinnamoyl)-methane; bis-desmethoxycurcumin; bisabolene; borneol; caffeic acid; caprylic acid; caryophyllene; cineole; cinnamic acid; cuminyl-alcohol; curcumene; curcumenol; curcumin; curdione; curlone; curzerenone; curzerenone-c; cyclo-isoprenemyrcene; D-α-phellandrene; D-camphene; D-camphor; D-sabinene; dehydroturmerone; desmethoxycurcumin; di-p-coumaroyl-methane; dicinnamoylmethane; didesmethoxycurcumin; diferuloyl-methane; dihydrocurcumin; eugenol; feruloyl-p-coumaroyl-methane; γ-atlantone; guaiacol; isoborneol; L-α-curcumene; L-β-curcumene; limonene; monodesmethoxycurcumin; o-coumaric acid; p-coumaric acid; p-cymene; p-methoxycinnamic acid; p-tolymethylcarbinol; protocatechuric acid; syringic acid; terpinene; terpinol; turmerone; ukonan-a; ukonan-b; ukonan-c; ukonan-d; vanillic acid.
Niacin	Calcium	
Riboflavin	Cobalt	
Thiamin	Chromium	
	Copper	
	Manganese	
	Nickel	

liquorice, oregano, black caraway and borage. The bactericidal activity of cinnamon was strain-dependent. Less bactericidal activity was shown by colombo weed, yellow-berried nightshade, long pepper, threadstem carpetweed, sage, tarragon, nutmeg and parsley.

Some of these studies have been validated in animals and confirm the potential benefit of using plants as the source of antimicrobial agents targeting *Helicobacter pylori*, although garlic and cinnamon have been tested in human clinical trials with no significant effect. A recent study has shown that consumption of broccoli sprouts is associated with the eradication of *Helicobacter pylori* in some patients.

Photodynamic therapy

Photodynamic therapy is used widely for superficial malignancies and involves giving a non-toxic photosensitive dye followed by exposure to visible light—usually delivered by a laser—which induces the generation of free radicals in the dye, thus killing the cells that have absorbed the dye. The sensitivity of *Helicobacter pylori* to photodynamic therapy was first demonstrated by one of the authors (JH) (**6.8**). After exposure to laser light, electrons in the photosensitizer dye molecule are excited from a ground singlet state to an excited singlet state, undergoing intersystem crossing (in which the spin of the excited electron is reversed) to produce a longer-lived excited triplet state. Molecular oxygen in tissue has a ground triplet state (represented as $^3O_2$) and when the activated photosensitizer is in

proximity to it, the photosensitizer transfers energy to the O_2 molecule, allowing the dye to fall back to the ground singlet state. This process creates an excited, highly reactive singlet state oxygen molecule ($^1O_2$) that rapidly reacts with adjacent biomolecules, causing cell death.

In the first *in vitro* demonstration of the action of PDT on *Helicobacter pylori*, 100% kill of 50 μl of *Helicobacter pylori* at a concentration of 1.0×10^8 cfu/ml was obtained after incubating the organism with 25 μmol/l of aluminium sulphonated phthalocyanine for 4 hours before exposure to laser light of 675 nm (1.5 J/cm²). Other studies demonstrated a bactericidal activity on *Helicobacter pylori* using coproporphyrin and protoporphyrin IX after exposure to white light (>400 nm) at 30 J/cm² and 405 nm at 20 J/cm². Studies in an animal model of killing *Helicobacter mustelae* on explanted gastric tissue showed 90% reduction in counts using toluidine blue (0.75 mg/kg) and methylene blue (75 mg/kg) and an exposure of 200 J/cm². Phthalocyanine and haematoporphyrin were not effective.

Inhibition of adhesion

The initial step of most infectious diseases is adhesion of the pathogenic organism to the host tissue. Once adherent, the organism is able to avoid removal by the host's clearance mechanisms and establishes an infection. *Helicobacter pylori* causes a chronic mucosal infection when adherent to the mucosal epithelium of the stomach. *Helicobacter*

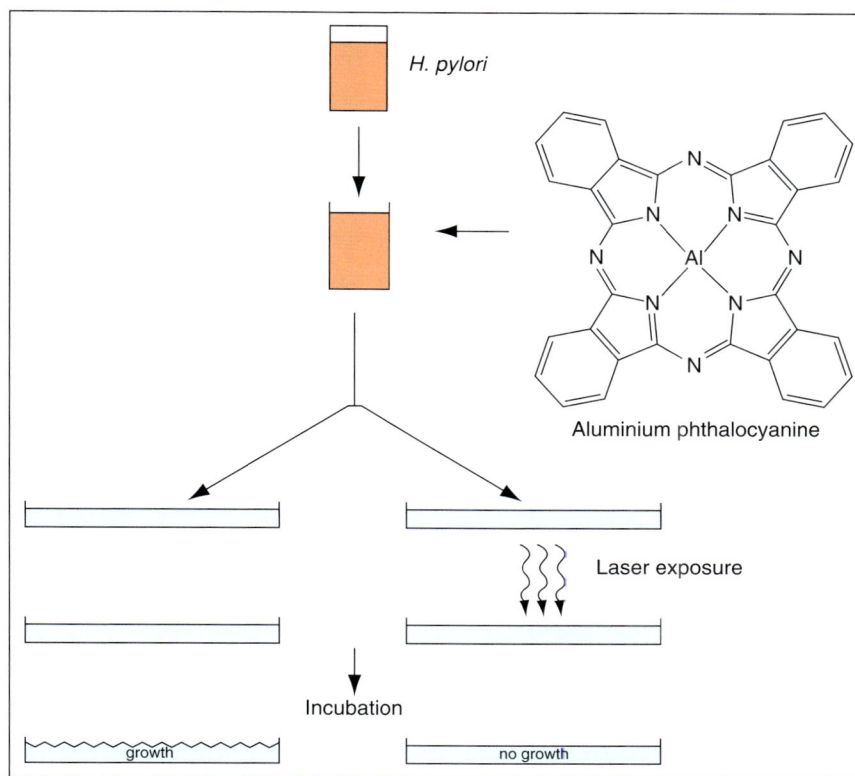

6.8 Photodynamic therapy uses a photosensitizer molecule, such as aluminium phthalocyanine, to induce killing of *Helicobacter* cells after exposure to laser light.

has a number of binding specificities to gangliosides GM1 and GM2, phosphatidyl ethanolamine and, possibly, the trefoil peptide TFF1. However, the most-studied *Helicobacter pylori* adhesin receptor interaction, and the one thought to be the most important, is between the blood group antigen binding adhesin (BabA) and the Lewis[b] (Le[b]) antigen, the blood group antigen expressed by gastric epithelial cells. Patients expressing Le[b] have a higher *Helicobacter pylori* density on the mucosal surface compared with Le[b]-negative patients. However, in Le[b]-negative patients, results suggest that Le[x] and Le[a] may become the alternative major receptors for *Helicobacter pylori* due to the interaction between sialyl-Le[x] and the *H. pylori* protein, SabA.

Inhibiting the binding of *Helicobacter pylori* is a potential therapeutic target (**6.9**). Several naturally occurring products can prevent adhesion of *Helicobacter pylori* to the human stomach as discussed above in the sections on phytoceuticals and probiotics. Additionally, the sodium salt of 3′-sialyllactose (an oligosaccharide found in human and bovine milk) was shown to inhibit adhesion of *Helicobacter pylori in vitro* and in animal models of infection. However, 3′-sialyllactose failed to suppress or cure *Helicobacter pylori* colonization.

A recombinant BabA analogue partially inhibits binding of *Helicobacter pylori* to gastric epithelial cells. Also, an anti-TFF1 monoclonal antibody has been shown to inhibit binding of *Helicobacter pylori* to TFF1-dimer-coated beads and, if TFF1 is an important adhesion molecule for *Helicobacter*, this may be a useful therapeutic. Specific adhesin inhibitors targeted at the BabA ligand have been developed by the authors based upon domain antibodies against BabA or neoglycoconjugates of Le[b] multivalently coupled to poly-D-lysine. Domain antibodies are the smallest functional binding units of antibodies, corresponding to the variable regions of either the heavy (V_H) or light (V_κ) chains of human antibodies.

Poly-D-lysine not only provides a means of oligomerizing Le[b], and hence increasing the avidity of the inhibitor, but also makes use of a protease-resistant backbone to which Le[b] can be coupled. Inhibition of adhesion was demonstrated for both the domain antibodies and the poly-D-lysine glycoconjugate as

Table 6.9

Inhibitor	Adhesin	% Inhibition
dAb9	BabA	56
dAb25	BabA	73
dAb28	BabA	12
dAb26	BabA	23
Le^b-HAS	BabA	57.9
Le^b (tet) PL	BabA	30
Le^b(hex) PL	BabA	92.4
sLe^x	SabA	41
sLe^x + Le^{b}HSA	SabA + BabA	93.4
sLe^x + Le^b(hex)PL	SabA + BabA	95.9
	SabA + BabA	66.3

Inhibitor	Adhesin	% Removal
Le^b-HAS	BabA	68.8
Le^b(hex)PL	BabA	71.5

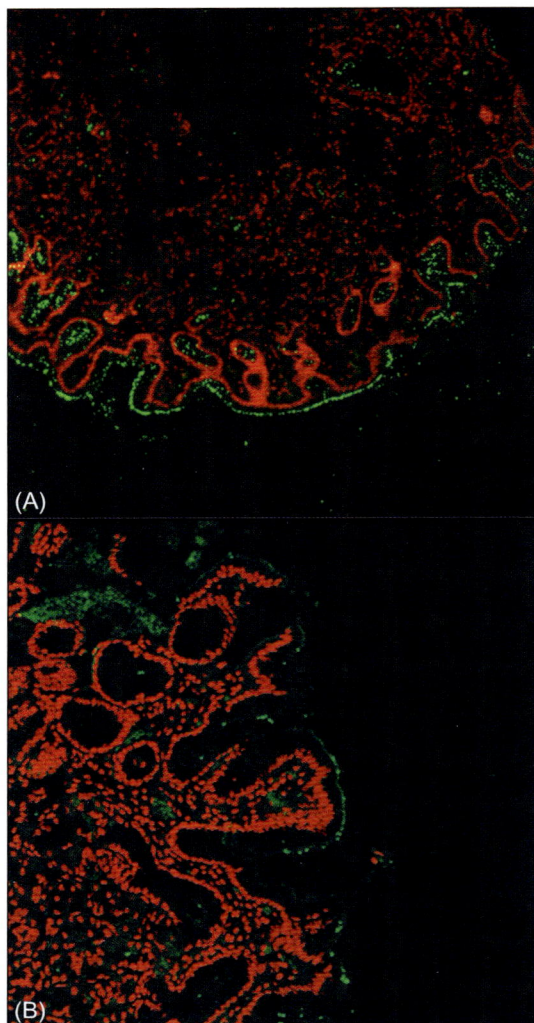

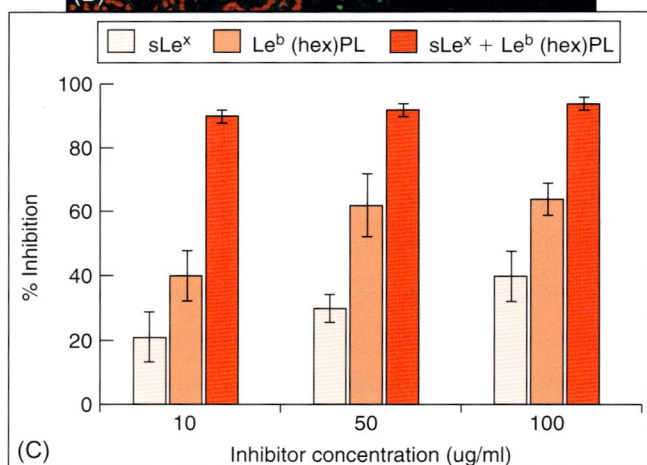

6.9 (A) Photomicrograph of fluorescein isothiocyanate-labelled *Helicobacter pylori* binding to human stomach. (B) Photomicrograph of fluorescein isothiocyanate-labelled *Helicobacter pylori* binding to human stomach in the presence of a domain antibody. (C) Histogram illustrating inhibition of binding of *Helicobacter pylori* in the presence of neoglycoconjugates.

shown in *Table 6.9*. More importantly, removal of bound *Helicobacter* was also demonstrated.

Nanotechnology

Nanoparticles can be used as carriers for antibiotics and/or inhibitors of adhesion and may have the advantage of increasing the local concentration of antibiotic or inhibitor thereby enhancing its effect. To this end, one of the authors (JH) has investigated the use of gold nanoparticles as carriers of amoxicillin (**6.10**).

Gold nanoparticles are prepared from a mixed solution of a gold salt and disulphide-bonded molecules of interest, which form covalent bonds with the gold as the nanoparticles develop. The nanoparticles contain about 120 atoms of gold and are about 5 nm in diameter. Because of their size they enter the total body water and can be cleared in the urine in about 11 min.

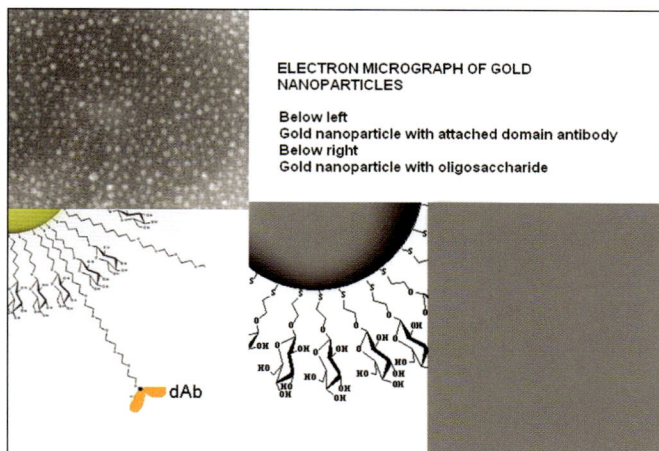

ELECTRON MICROGRAPH OF GOLD NANOPARTICLES

Below left
Gold nanoparticle with attached domain antibody
Below right
Gold nanoparticle with oligosaccharide

dAb

6.10 Gold nanoparticles.

Toxicity profiles demonstrate they have no effect on cellular proliferation nor are they cytotoxic. Gold nanoparticles with attached antibiotic (amoxicillin) do not lose any antimicrobial activity against *Helicobacter pylori* and are slightly more active than the equivalent free antibiotic. Attachment of the domain antibodies or coating with the glycoconjugate of Le[b] to the nanoparticles may increase the activity of the attached antibiotics by ensuring close adherence of the nanoparticle carrier. Additionally, nanoparticles coated with anti-adhesins should act as effective therapeutics, removing bound organisms.

More interestingly, dispensing with any antibiotic and using only gold/iron nanoparticles with attached domain antibodies or Le[b] glycoconjugate, one could, in principle, eradicate even antibiotic-resistant bacteria by induced hysteresis heating. Under these circumstances, hysteresis heating can be generated by exposure to an external radiofrequency-induced oscillating magnetic field (100 kHz–1.2 MHz with a field strength of up to 30 kA/m), which couples with the magnetic dipole moment on the conjugated metallic nanoparticles. This induced rapid heating of the nanoparticles, which are closely adherent to the organism, will kill organisms irrespective of any antibiotic resistance. There is an anticipated minimal effect on adjacent cells, but at this frequency the body water does not heat up. In principle, this technique could be used for any infecting micro-organism irrespective of resistance to antimicrobial agents. The nanoparticles could also be targeted to intracellular sites using specific ligands.

Further reading

Bedwell J, Holton J, Vaira D, MacRobert AJ, Bown SG. *In vitro* killing of *Helicobacter pylori* with photodynamic therapy. *Lancet* 1990; 335: 1287.

Del Giudice G, Covacci A, Telford JL, Montecucco C, Rappuoli R. The design of vaccines against *Helicobacter pylori* and their development. *Annu Rev Immunol* 2001; 19: 523–63.

Isenberg JI. H2 receptor antagonists in the treatment of peptic ulcer. *Ann Intern Med* 1976; 84: 212–14.

Kubas H, Stark H. Medicinal chemistry of H2 receptor antagonists. *Pharm Unserer Zeit* 2007; 36: 24–32.

Laine L, Takeuchi K, Tarnawski A. Gastric mucosa defense and cytoprotection: bench to bedside. *Gastroenterology* 2008; 135: 41–60.

Lü L, Cao HD, Zeng HQ, *et al.* Recombinant *Mycobacterium smegmatis* m(2)155 vaccine expressing outer membrane protein 26kDa antigen affords therapeutic protection against *Helicobacter pylori* infection. *Vaccine* 2009; 27: 972–8.

Millar MR, Pike J. Bactericidal activity of antimicrobial agents against slowly growing *Helicobacter pylori*. *Antimicrob Agents Chemother* 1992; 36: 185–7.

Nagate T, Numata K, Hanada K, Kondo I. The susceptibility of *Campylobacter pylori* to anti-ulcer agents and antibiotics. *J Clin Gastroenterol* 1990; 12(Suppl 1): S135–8.

O'Mahony R, Al-Kitheeri H, Weerasekera D, *et al.* Bactericidal and anti-adhesive properties of culinary and medicinal plants against *Helicobacter pylori*. *World J Gastroenterol* 2005; 47: 7499–507.

Sachdeva A, Nagpal J. Effects of fermented milk-based probiotic preparations on *Helicobacter pylori* eradication: a systematic review and meta analysis of randomized controlled trials. *Eur J Gastroenterol Hepatol* 2009; 21: 45–53.

Selgrad M, Malfertheiner P. Treatment of *Helicobacter pylori*. *Curr Op Gastroenterol* 2011; 27: 565–570

Shin JM, Sachs G. Pharmacology of proton pump inhibitors. *Curr Gastroenterol Rep* 2008; 10: 528–34.

Vorobjova T, Watanabe T, Chiba T. *Helicobacter* immunology and vaccines. *Helicobacter* 2008; 13(Suppl 1): 18–22.

Wallace JL. Prostaglandins, NSAIDs, and gastric mucosal protection: why doesn't the stomach digest itself. *Physiol Rev* 2008; 88: 1547–65.

Wallensten S. Results of the surgical treatment of peptic ulcer by partial gastrectomy according to Billroth I and II methods: a clinical study based on 1256 operated cases. *Acta Chir Scand* 1954; 191(Suppl): 1–161.

Younson J, O'Mahony R, Basset C, *et al.* A human domain antibody and Lewis b glycoconjugate that inhibit binding of *Helicobacter pylori* to Lewis b receptor and adhesion to gastric epithelium. *J Infect Dis* 2009; 200: 1574–82.

Zullo A, Rinaldi V, Winn S, *et al.* A new highly effective short-term therapy schedule for *Helicobacter pylori* eradication. *Aliment Pharmacol Ther* 2000; 14: 715–18.

References for published trial results on sequential therapy, cf. Table 6.6

1 Zullo A, Rinaldi V, Winn S, *et al.* A new highly effective short-term therapy schedule for *Helicobacter pylori* eradication. *Aliment Pharmacol Ther* 2000; 14: 715–18.

2 Zullo A, Vaira D, Vakil N, *et al.* High eradication rates of *Helicobacter pylori* with a new sequential treatment. *Aliment Pharmacol Ther* 2003; 17: 719–26.

3 Zullo A, Hassan C, Campo SMA. Elevata efficacia della terapia sequenziale nel trattamento dell'infezione da *Helicobacter pylori*. *Ospedale e Territorio – Gastroenterologia* 2004; 5: 87–90.

4 De Francesco V, Zullo A, Margiotta M, *et al.* Sequential treatment for *Helicobacter pylori* infection does not share the risk factors of triple therapy failure. *Aliment Pharmacol Ther* 2004; 19: 407–14.

5 De Francesco V, Zullo A, Hassan C, *et al.* The prolongation of triple therapy for *Helicobacter pylori* does not allow reaching therapeutic outcome of sequential scheme: a prospective, randomized study. *Dig Liver Dis* 2004; 36: 322–6.

6 De Francesco V, Zullo A, Hassan C, *et al.* Two new treatment regimens for *Helicobacter pylori* eradication: a randomised study. *Dig Liver Dis* 2001; 33: 67–9.

7 De Francesco V, Della Valle N, Stoppino V, *et al.* Effectiveness and pharmaceutical cost of sequential treatment for *Helicobacter pylori* in patients with non-ulcer dyspepsia. *Aliment Pharmacol Ther* 2004; 19: 993–8.

8 Hassan C, De Francesco V, Zullo A, *et al.* Sequential treatment for *Helicobacter pylori* eradication in duodenal ulcer patients: improving the cost of pharmacotherapy. *Aliment Pharmacol Ther* 2003; 18: 641–6.

9 Scaccianoce G, Hassan C, Panarese A, *et al. Helicobacter pylori* eradication with either 7-day or 10-day triple therapies, and with 10-day sequential regimen. *Can J Gastroenterol* 2006; 20: 113–17.

10 Focareta R, Forte G, Ciarleglio A, *et al. Helicobacter pylori* eradication: one week triple therapy vs. 10-day sequential regimen. *Dig Liver Dis.* 2002; 34(Suppl 1): A17

11 Focareta R, Forte G, Forte F, *et al.* Could the 10-days sequential therapy be considered a first choice treatment for the eradication of *Helicobacter pylori* infection? *Dig Liver Dis.* 2003; 35(Suppl 4): S33

12 Francavilla R, Lionetti E, Castellaneta SP, *et al.* Improved efficacy of 10-day sequential treatment for *Helicobacter pylori* eradication in children: a randomized trial. *Gastroenterology* 2005; 129: 1414–19.

13 Lionetti E, Miniello VL, Castellaneta SP, *et al.* Lactobacillus reuteri therapy to reduce side-effects during anti-*Helicobacter pylori* treatment in children: a randomized placebo controlled trial. *Aliment Pharmacol Ther* 2006; 24: 1461–8.

14 Lerro P, Ruvidi M, Baldi M, Calvo PL, Barbera C. A 10-day sequential therapy: new option for *Helicobacter pylori* eradication in children. *Dig Liver Dis* 2006; 38: A104.

15 Hurduc V, Dragomir D, Leseany G, Sajin M. Comparison of sequential and triple therapies in the eradication of H. pylori infection in symptomatic children. *Gut* 2007; 56(Suppl III): A243.

16 Vaira D, Zullo A, Vakil N, *et al.* Sequential therapy versus standard triple-drug therapy for *Helicobacter pylori* eradication. A randomized trial. *Ann Int Med* 2007; 146: 556–63.

17 Francavilla R, Lionetti E, Cavallo L. Sequential treatment for *Helicobacter pylori* eradication in children. *Gut* 2008; 57: 1178.

18 Sánchez-Delgado J, Calvet X, Bujanda L, Gisbert JP, Tito L, Castro M. Ten-day sequential treatment for *Helicobacter pylori* eradication in clinical practice. *Am J Gastroenterol* 2008; 103: 2220–3.

19 Wu DC, Hsu PI, Wu JY, Opekun AR, Graham DY. Randomized controlled comparison of sequential and quadruple (concomitant) therapies for H. pylori infection. *Gastroenterology* 2008; 134(Suppl 1): A24.

20 Choi WH, Park DI, Oh SJ, *et al*. Effectiveness of 10 day-sequential therapy for *Helicobacter pylori* eradication in Korea. *Korean J Gastroenterol* 2008; 51: 280–4.

21 Ruiz-Obaldia JR, Torrazza EG, Carreno NO. *Helicobacter pylori* eradication with either conventional 10-day triple therapy or 10-day modified sequential regimen. Preliminary report. *Gastroenterology* 2008; 134(Suppl 1): A24.

22 Paoluzi OA, Visconti E, Andrei F, *et al*. Sequential regimens have greater efficacy and better tolerability than standard triple therapy in the eradication of *Helicobacter pylori* infection. *Dig Liver Dis* 2008; 40: S40.

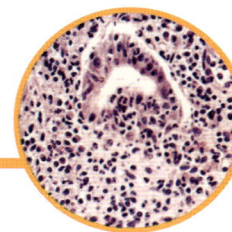

Case studies

Case 1: Indigestion

Edward, a 40-something architect, had suffered from indigestion for several years but noticed in the past few months it was getting worse. He eventually decided to go to his GP, who asked for a faecal sample and gave him antacids, with an appointment the following week. On returning to the GP, he was told that he was positive for *Helicobacter pylori* and was started on a course of tablets for 10 days.

What did his GP give him?

His GP prescribed a proton pump inhibitor with amoxicillin and metronidazole as the standard first-line treatment for *Helicobacter*-related dyspepsia. Most cases of dyspepsia are dealt with in the community and, as the patient was not experiencing alarm symptoms, a 'test and treat' policy was adopted.

Case 2: Reasons to undergo endoscopy

Sandra had just turned 55 years old. For several months she had been experiencing a nagging pain in her upper abdomen that often woke her in the early hours of the morning. She had found that she could gain relief by taking a glass of milk and a digestive biscuit. She eventually decided to go to her GP, who examined her and took a family history. Her weight was 63 kg, which was the same as it had been three years previously, when she had attended because of sprained wrist. Her stool was of normal colour and she did not appear anaemic.

She did not complain of difficulty in swallowing her food. On palpation, her abdomen was normal. Both her parents had died in their eighties, one of pneumonia, the other after a fractured hip.

What course of action did her GP take?

As his patient was aged 55 y, he referred her to a gastroenterologist for an endoscopy, despite the fact she did not have any alarm symptoms of weight loss, anaemia or family history of cancer (*Box 7.1*). Persons aged >45 y (although the minimum age may vary in different geographical regions) should undergo endoscopy as part of the investigation of dyspepsia. On endoscopy, Sandra was found to have a duodenal ulcer and was given sequential *Helicobacter* eradication therapy of amoxicillin for 5 days, followed by clarithromycin for 5 days, along with a proton pump inhibitor for the 10 days of treatment.

Box 7.1: The 'alarm symptoms'

- Anaemia
- Weight loss
- Dysphagia
- Abdominal mass
- Malabsorption
- Family history
- Melaena

Case 3: A pain in the gut

Reginald was at his 35th birthday party and was enjoying himself with friends and colleagues. For several years he had suffered from indigestion and had variously taken different antacids to little avail. More recently, he had started taking low-dose aspirin because of the supposed benefits he had read about in newspapers. He had recently noticed that for several days his faeces had become black and he had been feeling a little tired, which he put down to excessive work. Towards the end of his party, he was suddenly struck with an agonizing pain in his abdomen and he collapsed on to the floor, where he vomited fresh blood. The emergency services were called.

What is to blame for his collapse?

The patient had suffered a perforated duodenal ulcer and was *Helicobacter pylori*-positive. Both *Helicobacter pylori* and non-steroidal anti-inflammatory agents are independent risk factors for the development of a peptic ulcer. It was likely that in this case, the cause of the ulcer was *Helicobacter pylori* as he had only just started taking low-dose aspirin, although this could not be certain (**7.1**, **7.2**).

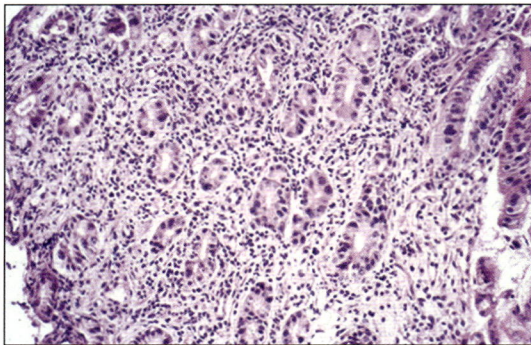

7.1 Histological section illustrating gastritis.

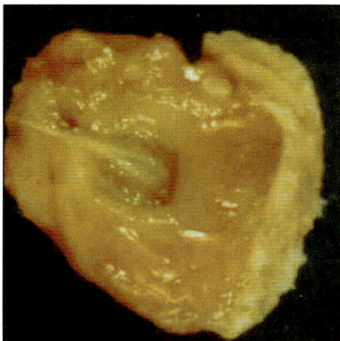

7.2 A peptic ulcer.

Case 4: A worried person

Samantha was concerned: she had read in the newspapers that stomach cancer could be caused by a bug and she wanted to know whether she had it, and if so, how to get rid of it. She made an appointment with her GP, who tried to reassure her, but, as she thought that one of her relatives had died from stomach cancer, her GP decided to perform a urea breath test for *Helicobacter pylori*, which was reported as positive. This increased her anxiety and she then complained of heartburn and stomach pains. Eventually, it was decided to perform an endoscopy, which on examination was macroscopically normal, although both *Helicobacter pylori* and inflammation were seen on histology (**7.3**). Her GP informed her that she had non-ulcer dyspepsia but that there was no sign of any cancer.

Would it be reasonable to give this patient a course of eradication therapy?

The evidence as to whether eradicating *Helicobacter pylori* has any effect on resolution of symptoms generally in non-ulcer dyspepsia is contradictory. The symptoms in this case were likely to have been as a result of anxiety, rather than organic. However, the patient did have a family history of gastric cancer and she was verging on 'cancerophobic'. Consequently, her GP gave a course of a proton pump inhibitor with amoxicillin and clarithromycin for 10 days. The patient had had several courses of metronidazole on previous occasions for gynaecological problems.

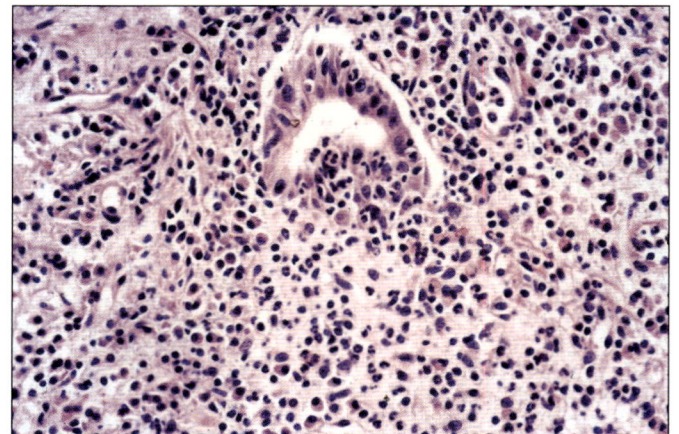

7.3 Photmicrograph showing an example of chronic inflammation.

Case 5: Lost weight

Jeremy was 75 years old and was normally in good health, but he had been feeling unwell for some months with increasing shortness of breath. He made an appointment with his GP, where he complained of cramping upper abdominal pains and that his stools were occasionally black and tarry in consistency. On examination, he appeared a little anaemic and had lost a few kilograms of weight since he had last weighed himself. The GP referred him to the local hospital and an appointment with the gastroenterologist, who performed a gastroscopy. Macroscopically, a mass was seen in the stomach and biopsies showed that an adenocarcinoma of the stomach was present (**7.4A**). He was referred for a surgical opinion.

What type of Helicobacter-related gastritis was likely to be present?

This patient could have pan-gastritis with atrophy and intestinal metaplasia (**7.4B**). Special stains would reveal the presence of sulphomucins (**7.4C**) and, histologically, this would then have been followed by overt carcinomatous changes. In many cases, at this stage, *Helicobacter pylori* may not be detected because of a lack of binding sites.

Case 6: A developing rash

Joan, aged 30 years, noticed a few purplish spots on her legs after playing a game of tennis and thought nothing of it. Over the next few days, further spots appeared and she noticed that she bruised easily. She then had a nosebleed and a heavy period. Worried, she went to her GP. She had not been taking any drugs to account for the symptoms and had not had any recent infection that she could remember. The GP took some blood to test for HIV (negative) and *Helicobacter* (positive), as well as a full blood count (platelets 15000/mm^3; Hb 13g/dL; WBC 9.0/mm^3). A diagnosis of idiopathic thrombocytopenic purpura was made.

Is it worth eradicating Helicobacter pylori?

Antiplatelet antibodies can be found in *Helicobacter*-positive and -negative patients with approximately the same frequency. In those that are positive, about half have anti-CagA antibodies. The evidence suggests that a platelet response can be anticipated in patients who

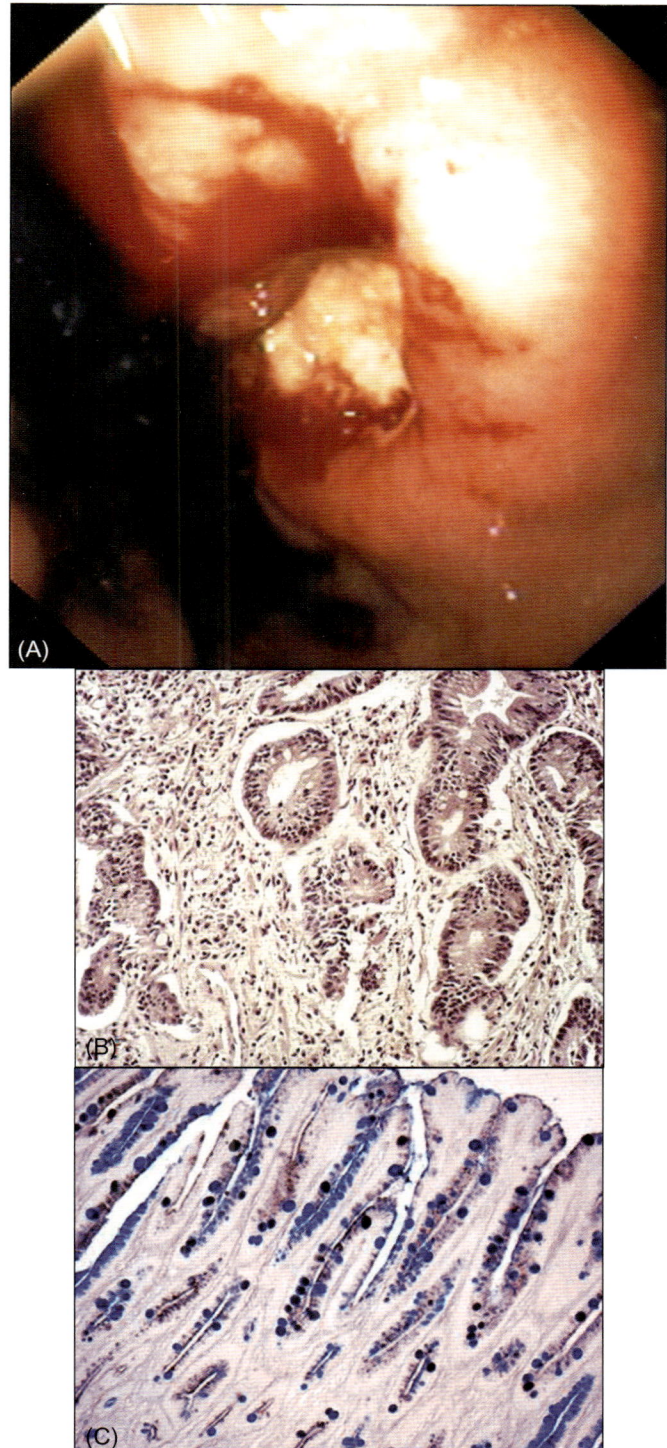

7.4 (A) Endoscopic image of adenocarcinoma. (B) Intestinal metaplasia. (C) Secretion of sialo- and sulphomucins.

have idiopathic thrombocytopenic purpura and are *Helicobacter pylori*-positive in about 50% of patients and it is thus worth giving a course of eradication therapy.

Case 7: The 'slow man'

At his 60th birthday party, Dirk's brother-in-law, who had not seen Dirk for some time, noticed that he appeared to have noticeably slowed up both in speech and in hand movements. The change was marked and could not be put down to excess alcohol. Several possibilities sprang to mind. Over the next few weeks, Dirk's movements did not improve and his speech was a little slow. He was eventually persuaded to visit his GP. A clinical diagnosis of Parkinson's disease was made (7.5).

Is it worth testing for Helicobacter pylori?

As part of the routine examination for Parkinson's disease, probably not. The cause of Parkinson's disease is not known, but the pathological changes are known to be due to the loss of dopaminergic neurons in the substantia nigra. There is a genetic component to some cases—in others, environmental factors (e.g. pesticides) or trauma (e.g. boxing) may be involved. However, some recent, studies have shown that eradication of *Helicobacter pylori* in patients with Parkinson's disease increases their stride length. This interesting finding demonstrates that further work in this area is warranted, particularly in view of the fact that the autoantibodies generated by *Helicobacter pylori* are associated with gastric atrophy and possibly idiopathic thrombocytopenic purpura.

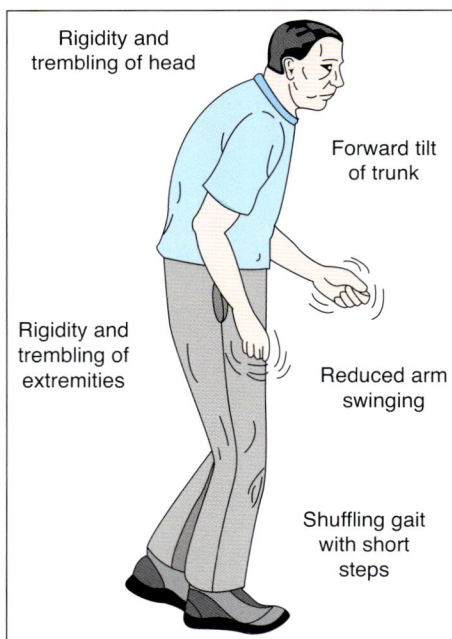

Rigidity and trembling of head

Forward tilt of trunk

Rigidity and trembling of extremities

Reduced arm swinging

Shuffling gait with short steps

7.5 Classic symptoms of Parkinson's disease (the 'slow man').

Case 8: An acid taste

Betty was overweight and was constantly complaining of heartburn and an acid taste in her mouth due to reflux of stomach contents (7.6). She visited her GP who advised her to lose weight and put her on a course of a proton pump inhibitor.

Is it worth eradicating Helicobacter pylori in these circumstances?

It has been suggested that being colonized by *Helicobacter pylori* has its advantages by diminishing the acid load in the stomach and that eradicating the organism can exacerbate reflux disease. Many studies have investigated this and there have been conflicting results. There is no good evidence that eradication of *Helicobacter pylori* will cause reflux disease, nor will it affect the treatment of reflux disease (*see* Chapter 3). However, long-term acid suppression may lead to the development of atrophy and eradicating the organism will reverse atrophy (itself a risk factor for stomach cancer).

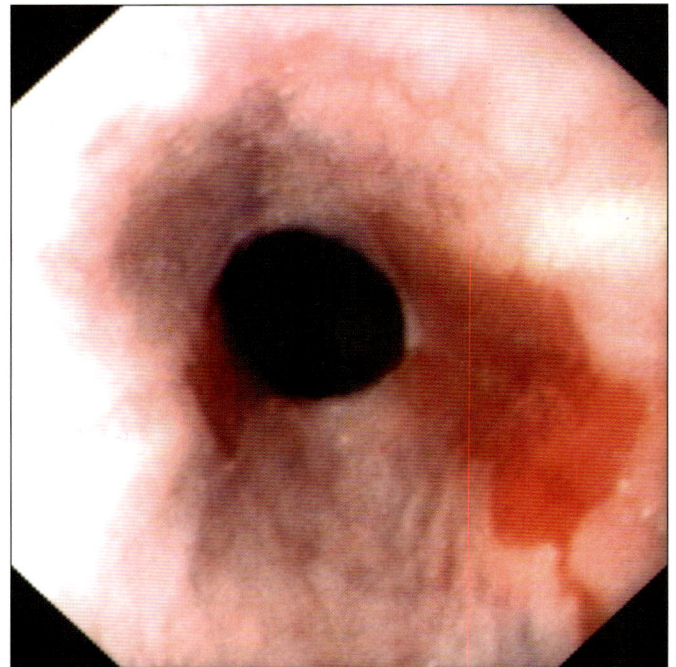

7.6 Endoscopic image of reflux disease.

Index

Note: page numbers in *italics* refer to figures, tables and boxes